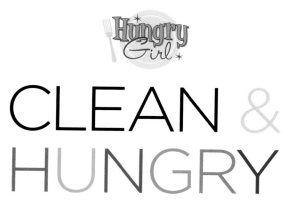

CLEAN &
HUNGRY

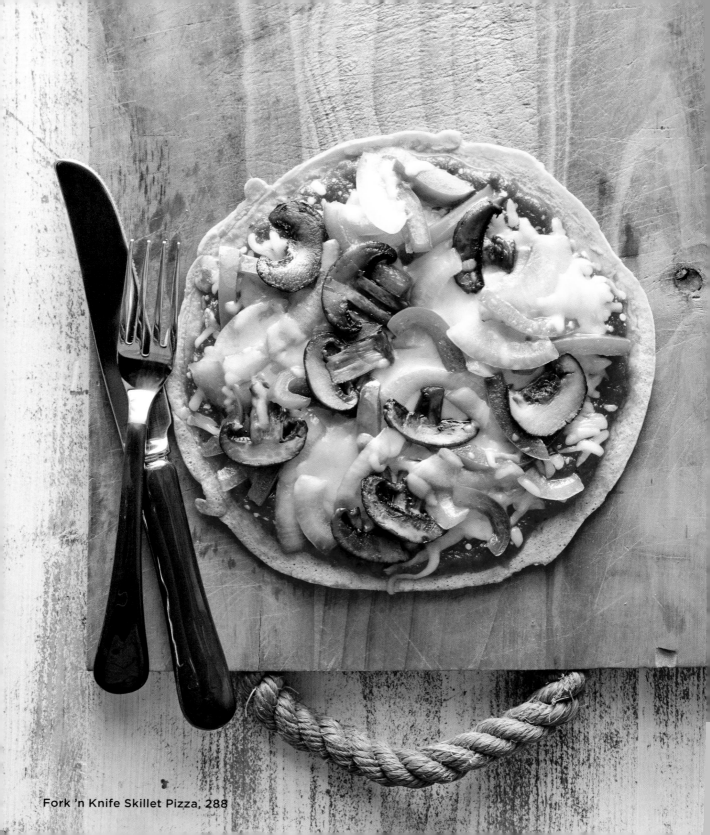

Fork 'n Knife Skillet Pizza, 288

Also by Lisa Lillien

HUNGRY GIRL:
Recipes and Survival Strategies for Guilt-Free
Eating in the Real World

HUNGRY GIRL 200 UNDER 200:
200 Recipes Under 200 Calories

HUNGRY GIRL 1-2-3:
The Easiest, Most Delicious, Guilt-Free
Recipes on the Planet

HUNGRY GIRL HAPPY HOUR:
75 Recipes for Amazingly Fantastic Guilt-Free
Cocktails & Party Foods

HUNGRY GIRL 300 UNDER 300:
300 Breakfast, Lunch & Dinner Dishes Under 300 Calories

HUNGRY GIRL SUPERMARKET SURVIVAL:
Aisle by Aisle, HG-Style!

HUNGRY GIRL TO THE MAX!
The Ultimate Guilt-Free Cookbook

HUNGRY GIRL 200 UNDER 200 JUST DESSERTS:
200 Recipes Under 200 Calories

THE HUNGRY GIRL DIET

THE HUNGRY GIRL DIET COOKBOOK:
Healthy Recipes for Mix-n-Match Meals & Snacks

HUNGRY GIRL: THE OFFICIAL SURVIVAL GUIDES:
Tips & Tricks for Guilt-Free Eating
(audio book)

HUNGRY GIRL CHEW THE RIGHT THING:
Supreme Makeovers for 50 Foods You Crave
(recipe cards)

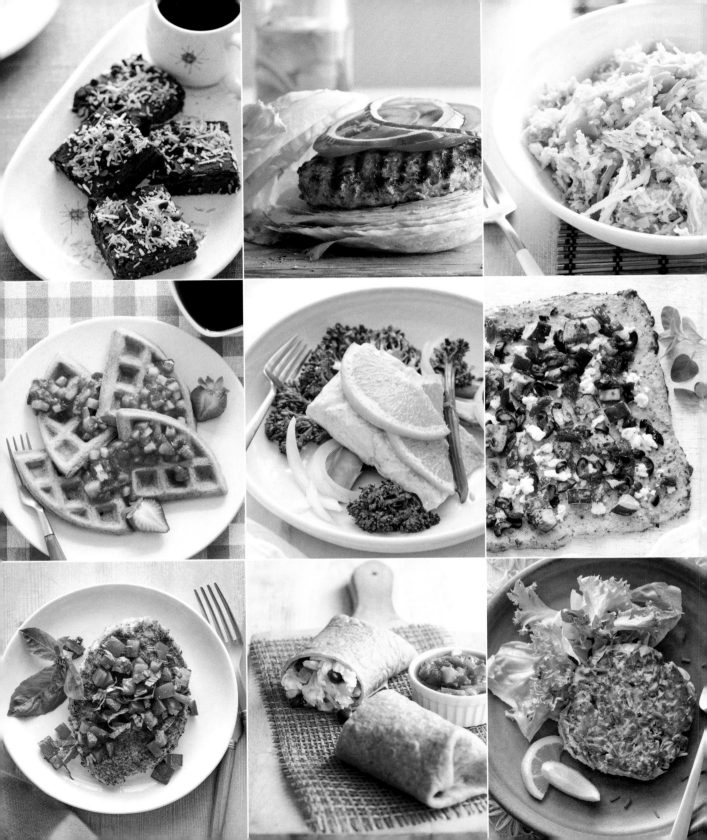

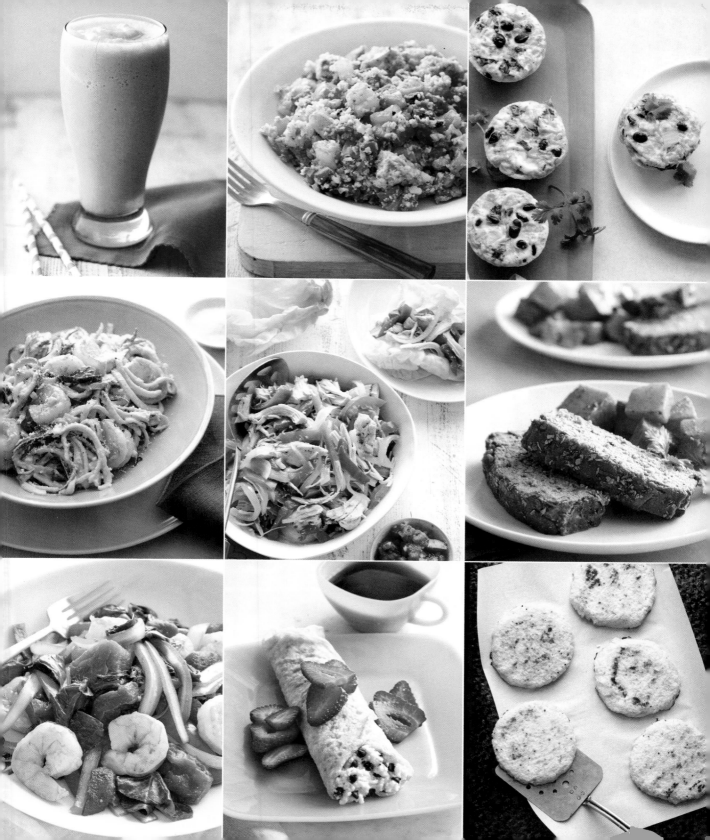

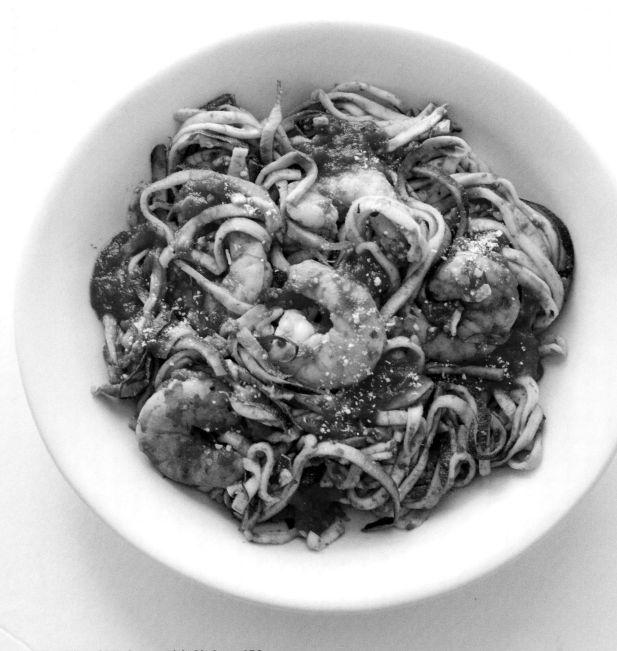

Z'paghetti Marinara with Shrimp, 158

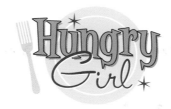

CLEAN &
HUNGRY

EASY ALL-NATURAL RECIPES FOR HEALTHY EATING IN THE REAL WORLD

Lisa Lillien

St. Martin's Griffin ⚜ New York

HUNGRY GIRL CLEAN & HUNGRY: EASY ALL-NATURAL RECIPES FOR HEALTHY EATING IN THE REAL WORLD. Copyright © 2016 by Hungry Girl, Inc. All rights reserved. Printed in the United States of America. For information, address St. Martin's Press, 175 Fifth Avenue, New York, N.Y. 10010.

www.stmartins.com

Cover design by Julie Leonard
Book design by Ralph Fowler
Illustrations by Jack Pullan
Food styling by Adam Pearson
Food photography by Matt Armendariz
Author photography by Jay Lawrence Goldman

The Library of Congress Cataloging-in-Publication Data is available upon request.
ISBN 978-0-312-67677-3 (trade paperback)
ISBN 978-1-250-09194-9 (e-book)

Our books may be purchased in bulk for promotional, educational, or business use. Please contact your local bookseller or the Macmillan Corporate and Premium Sales Department at 1-800-221-7945, extension 5442, or by e-mail at MacmillanSpecialMarkets@macmillan.com.

First Edition: April 2016

10 9 8 7 6 5 4 3 2 1

Contents

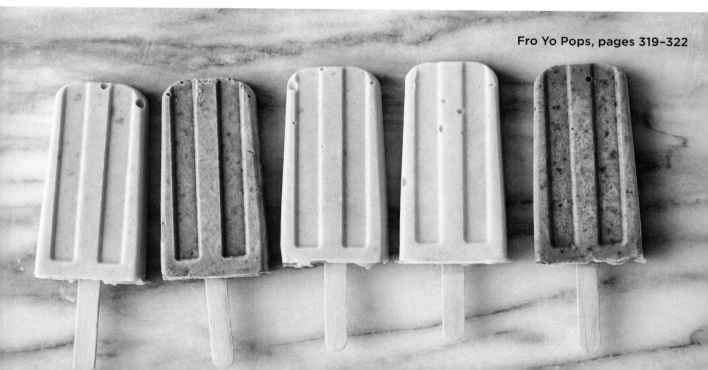

Fro Yo Pops, pages 319–322

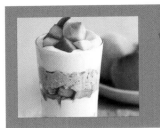

1 Growing Oatmeal, Overnight Oats, Yogurt Bowls & More

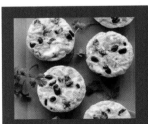

2 Egg Mugs, Skillet Scrambles, Burritos & Bakes

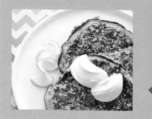

3 Pancakes & Waffles

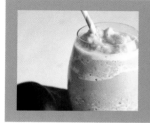

4 Smoothies & Shakes

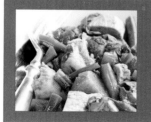

5 Slow-Cooker Soups, Stews & More

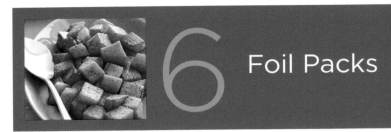

6 Foil Packs

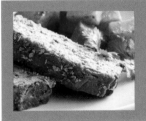

7 Meatloaf & Casseroles

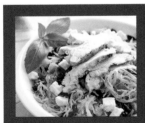

8 Z'paghetti, Spaghetti Squash & More Veggie-Noodle Dishes

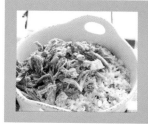

9 Cauliflower Rice & More Cauliflower Creations

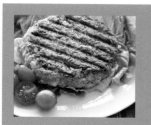

10 Carb-Slashed Sandwiches, Burgers & More

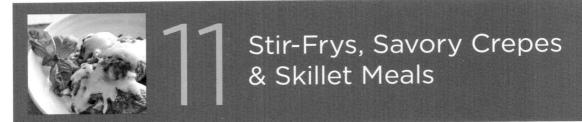

11 Stir-Frys, Savory Crepes & Skillet Meals

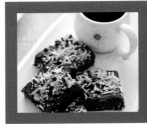

12 Baked Goodies, Frozen Treats & Other Sweets

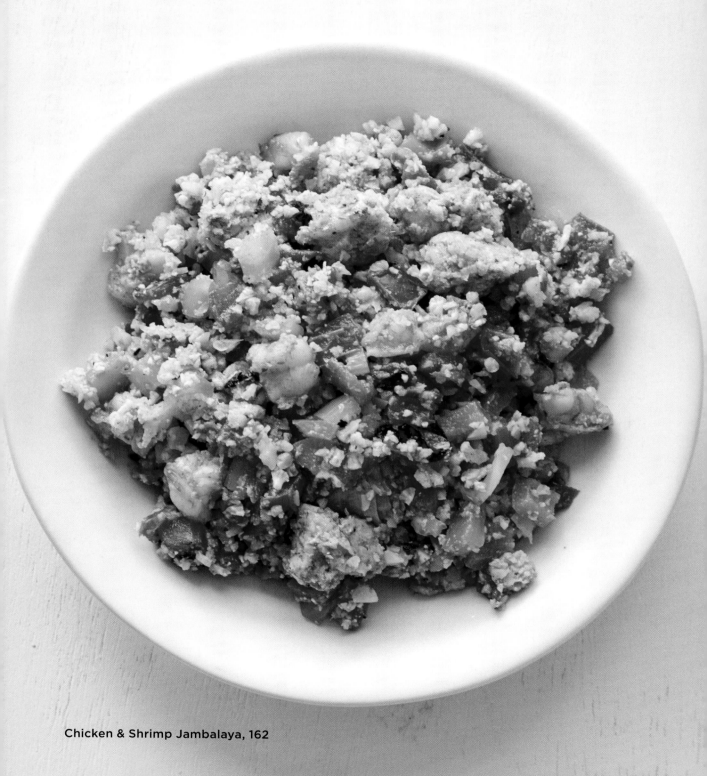

Chicken & Shrimp Jambalaya, 162

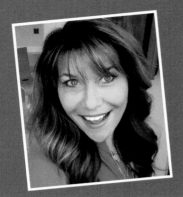

THANK-YOUS!

I couldn't do what I do without the incredibly talented and dedicated HG staff. Please enjoy their faces... and reading about them in 10 words or less! :)

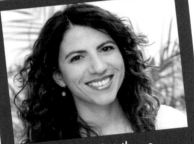

Jamie Goldberg
My left hand & true partner in (fighting food) crime!

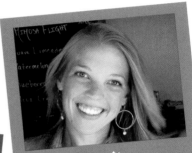

Dana Olsen
Eagle-eyed editor extraordinaire

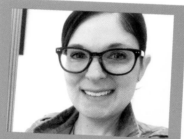

Erin Norcross
Creative & quirky kitchen queen

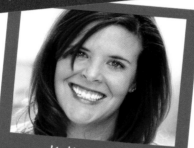

Katie Killeavy
Can-do Katie (She can do anything!)

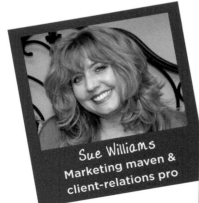

Sue Williams
Marketing maven & client-relations pro

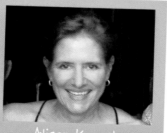

Alison Kreuch
Indispensable advertising whiz

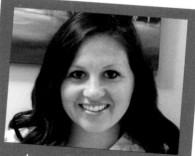

Lynn Bettencourt
Genuine jill-of-all-trades

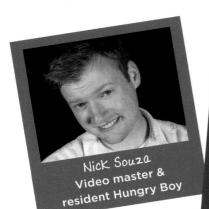

Nick Souza
Video master &
resident Hungry Boy

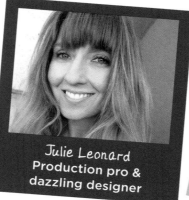

Julie Leonard
Production pro &
dazzling designer

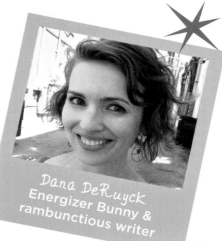

Dana DeRuyck
Energizer Bunny &
rambunctious writer

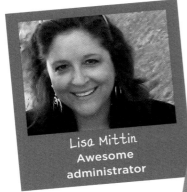

Lisa Mittin
Awesome
administrator

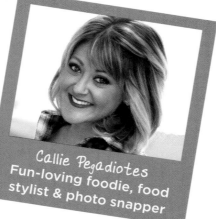

Callie Pegadiotes
Fun-loving foodie, food
stylist & photo snapper

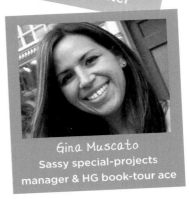

Gina Muscato
Sassy special-projects
manager & HG book-tour ace

Special thanks to these fantastic humans who also help make it happen…

John Vaccaro
Neeti Madan
Jennifer Enderlin
John Karle
Anne Marie Tallberg
Brant Janeway
Angelique Giammarino
Elizabeth Catalano
Caitlin Dareff
James Sinclair
Cheryl Mamaril
Tracey Guest
Bill Stankey

Tom Fineman
Jeff Becker
Cindy Sloop
Olga Gatica
Jackie Mgido
Jennifer Fleming
Emily Warren
Adam Pearson
Matt Armendariz
Jack Pullan
Ralph Fowler
Elizabeth Hodson
Alyssa Bernstein

AND I CAN'T FORGET MY FABULOUS FAMILY…

Daniel Schneider

Florence & Maurice Lillien

Meri Lillien

Jay Lillien

Lolly & Jackson

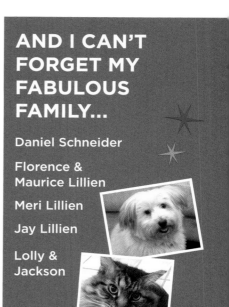

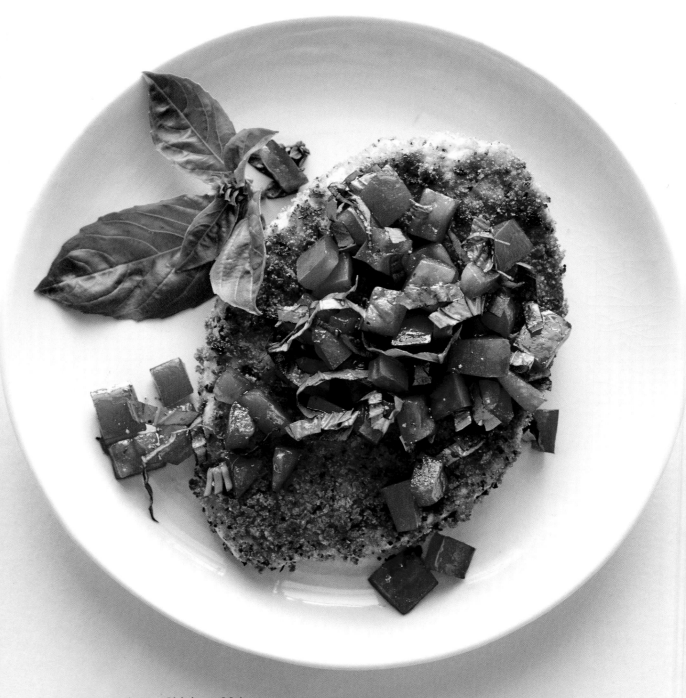

Crispy Bruschetta Chicken, 284

All About Clean & Hungry Recipes

Welcome to Hungry Girl Clean & Hungry, the first-ever all-natural cookbook from Hungry Girl! Here's what you can expect from the 141 recipes on the following pages . . .

- Only all-natural ingredients (like fruits and veggies) and ingredients that are available in all-natural varieties (like cheese and butter)

- Little to no added sugar

- Low in calories and starchy carbs

- High in protein and fiber

They're also GREAT for weight loss and weight maintenance. And you won't believe how easy they are to shop for . . . and simple to make!

Hope you're hungry . . . Enjoy!

Lisa :)

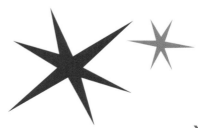

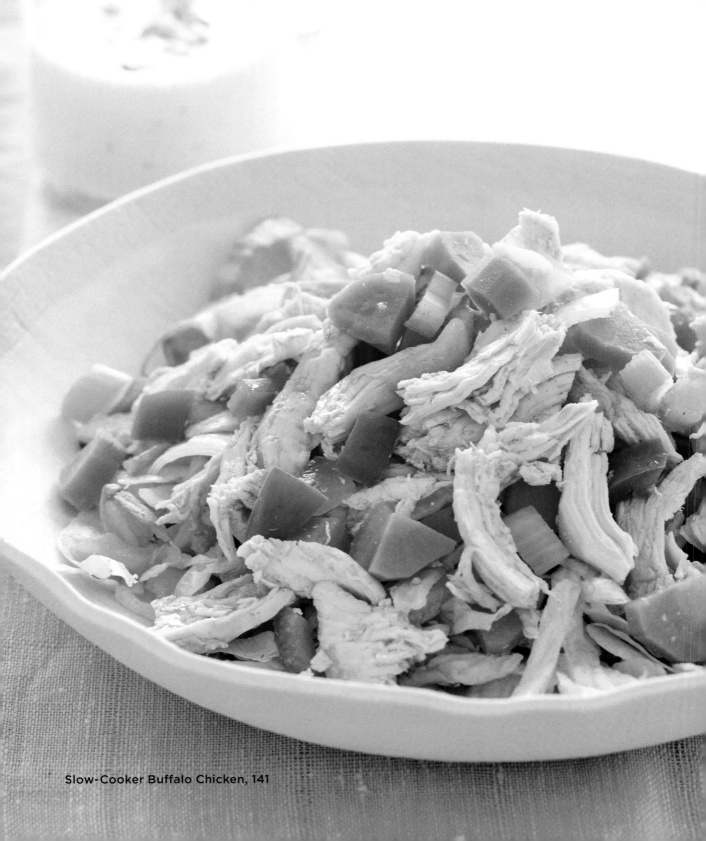

Slow-Cooker Buffalo Chicken, 141

FAQs

Who and what is Hungry Girl?

I'm Lisa Lillien, a.k.a. Hungry Girl! And I'm not a nutritionist . . . I'm just hungry. I don't have any health-related or medical degrees, but I consider myself a "foodologist," because I'm obsessed with food—how incredible it is, and how much of it I can eat and still fit into my pants. And since I've always wanted to share my guilt-free food knowledge with the world, I created Hungry Girl.

Back in 2004, I launched Hungry Girl as a free daily email subscription service. Today, millions of Hungry Girl fans access HG content—as subscribers to the emails (sign up at hungry-girl.com), on social media, in magazines, on television, and more. No matter where it lives, Hungry Girl content consistently delivers guilt-free recipes, food finds, and tips & tricks . . . All of it geared toward helping people eat better, lose weight, and maintain their weight in a fun, real-world way. To date, I have authored ten Hungry Girl books, all *New York Times* Best Sellers. And I could not be more proud of the fact that I've helped millions of people lose hundreds of thousands of pounds. It truly is the best and most satisfying feeling ever.

What is clean eating?

While there's no official definition, clean eating generally focuses on a diet of whole, natural, or "real" foods: fresh fruits and vegetables, whole grains, natural protein, etc. What won't you find in the clean approach to eating? Refined sugar, heavily processed food, and anything artificial. There are most certainly different degrees of "clean eating" . . . and to be honest, some approaches are intimidating. Mine is not—it's more relatable, more realistic, and more real world.

Is clean eating good for weight loss/management?

Not necessarily. (But it certainly *can* be!) It's a misconception that simply eating clean can keep you at a healthy body weight—no matter how many calories you're actually consuming. At the end of the day, CALORIES COUNT. And it's easy to take in too many calories on a diet of all-natural and/or "clean" foods. That's why people who want to make smarter food choices need to look at the whole story and see the big picture. While we're better off choosing healthier ingredients, in order to lose or maintain weight, we need to be mindful of the number of calories we consume. (That's where my calorie-slashed recipes come in . . .)

What does "Clean & Hungry" mean?

Clean & Hungry combines the best of Hungry Girl with the best of clean eating. Like all Hungry Girl creations, Clean & Hungry recipes are guilt-free with huge portions . . . but now I'm highlighting CLEAN ingredients and eliminating artificial and heavily processed foods. It's a delicious, satisfying, real-world approach to eating clean and loving it. I say "real world" because my approach to healthier eating has always been realistic, achievable, and enjoyable, as opposed to restrictive, extreme, or intimidating. The HG philosophy is all about balance. It's okay to have a brownie every now and then—just try to make (or even find!) a better-for-you version. I even feel that it's okay to eat so-called junk foods—I just try to stick with ones made from smarter ingredients. This book is perfect for anyone who wants to incorporate more all-natural recipes into their life—delicious recipes that satisfy cravings without packing on the pounds.

How is this book different from earlier Hungry Girl books?

When I launched Hungry Girl a dozen years ago, the idea of low-calorie food that tasted decadent was a revelation. Diet food didn't really taste good, and no one believed you could lose weight and keep it off eating pizza and chocolate cake. But I knew it was possible, because I had been doing it myself for years. Early Hungry Girl content gave people what they wanted at the time—a lot of low-fat and fat-free ingredients, low-calorie packaged foods, and reduced-calorie finds that were often heavily processed. But as the diet environment shifted and I personally started eating cleaner, the brand evolved and moved in a healthier direction. That doesn't mean I never eat those foods or that I don't enjoy my recipes from years past; I just do so in moderation, and less and less as time goes on. Hungry Girl was always meant to be a bridge between the average fast-food-filled, junk-food-packed diet and the idealistic way of eating perfectly "healthy" at all times. Recent Hungry Girl cookbooks and online content have mostly featured natural foods. But now is the perfect time to take things a step further. So, for the first time ever, I've developed an entire book of delicious, satisfying, low-calorie recipes that are *completely* natural.

Where can I find the Weight Watchers SmartPoints® values for the recipes in this book?

Here at HG, we're fans of Weight Watchers, and we know many of you are too! So we're providing the Weight Watchers **SmartPoints**® value* for each recipe in this book online. Visit hungry-girl.com/books for all the values!

*The SmartPoints® values for these recipes were calculated by Hungry Girl and are not an endorsement or approval of the recipe or developer by Weight Watchers International, Inc., the owner of the SmartPoints® registered trademark.

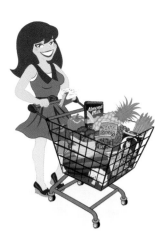

Helpful Shopping Tips

An overall note on shopping for these recipes: Every ingredient in this book is either all-natural (such as apples) or readily available in all-natural varieties (such as cheese). Rather than use the word "natural" over and over again in each recipe's ingredients, I'm telling you now: Look for natural varieties of each ingredient. Unsure if it's natural or not? Flip over the package, and check the ingredient list for anything questionable. Or just shop at natural-food markets.

Unsweetened almond milk

This creamy beverage is a fantastic alternative to regular dairy milk. With around 35 calories per cup, it has less than half the calories of even fat-free dairy milk. Plus, it's virtually sugar-free, while a cup of dairy milk has around 12 grams of sugar. You can find almond milk in refrigerated cartons as well as shelf-stable containers. Favorite brands: Blue Diamond Almond Breeze (refrigerated or shelf stable) and Silk (refrigerated).

When scanning the ingredients on cartons of almond milk, you might come across something called carrageenan. Carrageenan is an FDA-approved natural additive derived from plants. It has been linked to stomach inflammation and related concerns, though, so some people prefer to avoid it. Brands without carrageenan: Silk (refrigerated) and Whole Foods Market 365 (refrigerated or shelf stable).

Cheese

Cheese that comes pre-crumbled, pre-shredded, pre-sliced, or pre-grated—even natural types—sometimes contains anti-caking agents and mold inhibitors, such as cellulose, silica, and calcium sorbate. If you prefer cheese that's completely free of preservatives, check the ingredient lists, or stick with block-style cheese: Then crumble, shred, slice, or grate it yourself. Favorite brands of natural cheese: Sargento and Cabot.

Eggs & poultry

Considering paying more for eggs and poultry marked "no added hormones"? Know the facts: Federal regulations prohibit the use of hormones in *any* poultry. So if it's on store shelves, it's likely free of added hormones.

Ground meat

There's a big difference between lean and extra-lean ground meat. Extra-lean has considerably fewer calories and fat grams. In the case of beef, extra-lean is the way to go—the meat is juicy and flavorful, and the stats are fantastic. Extra-lean ground turkey, on the other hand, is typically dry and lacks flavor—it's worth the additional calories and fat grams to go with lean ground turkey.

Look for extra-lean ground beef, which has about 145 calories and 5g fat per 4-ounce serving. It's often labeled as 4% fat or less, or as being at least 96% fat-free.

Buy lean ground turkey with around 160 calories and 7.5g fat per 4-ounce serving. The packages typically say 7% fat or less, or at least 93% fat-free.

Seafood

Don't hesitate to buy seafood from the freezer aisle. A lot of the fish at the counter was previously frozen anyway, and frozen seafood is just as nutritious. For the best taste and texture, thaw it in the fridge the night before you cook it.

Curious about the difference between wild and farmed seafood? Wild fish are caught in their natural habitats, while farm-raised fish live in commercial aquatic farms. Wild fish tend to be healthier, with less chance of contact with pesticides and contaminated materials.

Canned goods

"BPA"—a.k.a. Bisphenol A—is a major buzzword in the canned-goods aisle. It's a carbon-based synthetic compound found in the lining of some cans. While it's safe as long as the levels are low (which they tend to be in food products), many companies are choosing to eliminate it from their cans as a precaution. Look for products labeled BPA-free.

Frozen fruit

Fruit found in the freezer aisle is just as nutritious and tasty as fresh fruit—sometimes tastier, since it's typically flash frozen at its peak ripeness. Watch out for added sugar, though. Flip over those bags, and check the ingredient lists. Sugar sometimes disguises itself as syrup, fructose, or cane juice . . . all of which can double the calorie count.

Nonstick cooking spray

If you prefer to avoid aerosol containers, Pompeian makes a *great* line of aerosol-free sprays. Another option? DIY! Buy a food-safe mist sprayer bottle, and fill it with your favorite oil. We're big fans of grapeseed oil here at the HG HQ.

Powdered PB and defatted peanut flour

These are made from defatted peanuts, which means that the excess oil has been squeezed out of the peanuts. A 2-tablespoon serving has about 50 calories and 2g fat. The same amount of regular peanut butter, on the other hand, has about 200 calories and 16g fat. Sometimes, Hungry Girl recipes combine the powder/flour with traditional peanut butter to keep the stats low and the texture spot on. Favorite brands: Just Great Stuff Powdered Organic Peanut Butter (made by Betty Lou's), Jif Peanut Powder, and Old Virginia Byrd Mill Light Roast Peanut Flour.

Plain protein powder

The three most popular types of protein powder are whey, casein, and soy. Whey and casein are both derived from milk, while soy comes from plants. Whey is the Hungry Girl top choice because it dissolves really well and tastes the best. Egg white protein powder is also great. Favorite brands: Tera's Whey, Jay Robb, and Quest (All-Purpose Baking Blend).

Semi-sweet chocolate chips

Semi-sweet chocolate has a higher percentage of pure chocolate than milk chocolate, which means less sugar. If you prefer cane sugar to regular, check out the semi-sweet chips by Enjoy Life and Sunspire. And Lily's makes stevia-sweetened dark chocolate chips.

Natural no-calorie sweetener packets

Stevia blends are very common and easy to find. They're made with an extract of the stevia plant, and they typically include another natural calorie-free ingredient for texture and taste. Some favorite brands? Truvia (made with erythritol, a naturally occurring sugar alcohol) and SweetLeaf (made with inulin, a naturally occurring dietary fiber). If you prefer pure stevia, look for liquid varieties or multi-serving jars of stevia powder.

Spoonable natural no-calorie sweetener

While sweetener packets are great in many recipes, sometimes you need larger portions, which is where the spoonable sweeteners come in. Both Truvia and Stevia in the Raw make excellent spoonable versions . . . but Truvia is the hands-down Hungry Girl favorite! Heads up: Truvia is about twice as sweet as the bakers-bag variety of Stevia in the Raw, so you'll only need half as much. To make things easy, the exact amounts of each product are spelled out for each recipe.

Arrowroot powder

Arrowroot powder (sometimes called arrowroot starch) is an alternative to cornstarch, which some people prefer to avoid since it's often made with genetically modified corn. If you're not concerned with GMOs, feel free to use cornstarch instead.

Baking powder

Baking powder often contains cornstarch, which means it may not be GMO-free. However, there are baking powders on shelves made only from non-GMO ingredients, such as Rumford brand. If it's very important to you to avoid all GMOs, seek out baking powder specifically marked as GMO-free.

For the latest shopping tips, brand picks, and more, visit Hungry-Girl.com/CleanAndHungry!

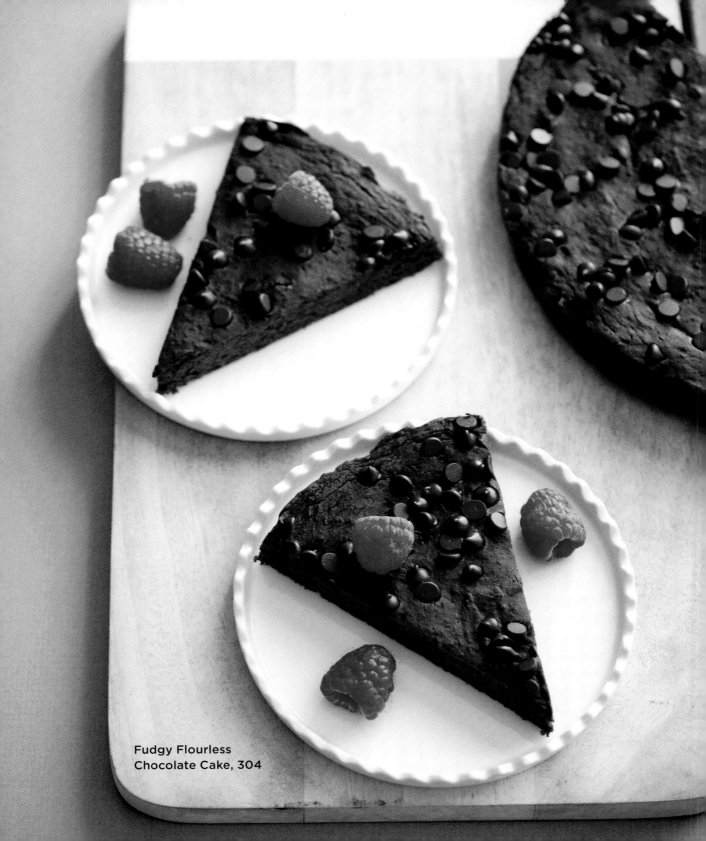

Fudgy Flourless
Chocolate Cake, 304

Recipe Guide

Recipes with five ingredients or less, vegetarian recipes, gluten-free recipes . . . This book is full of all these and so much more! Look for the following symbols throughout the book to find the recipes that suit your needs. And to make things even easier, we've rounded up the recipe names and page numbers on the following pages . . .

5i   5 Ingredients or Less

NC   No-Cook

15m   15 Minutes or Less

30m   30 Minutes or Less

V   Vegetarian

GF   Gluten-Free

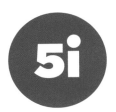

Recipes with 5 Ingredients or Less

The recipes listed here have no more than FIVE main ingredients. FYI: Salt, pepper, no-calorie sweeteners, and basic dried seasonings are not factored into the ingredient totals. It doesn't get much easier than this . . .

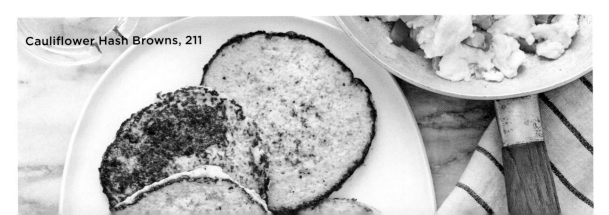

Cauliflower Hash Browns, 211

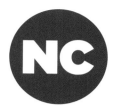

No-Cook Recipes

No baking, no stir-frying, no boiling . . . You won't even need to operate a microwave for these recipes.

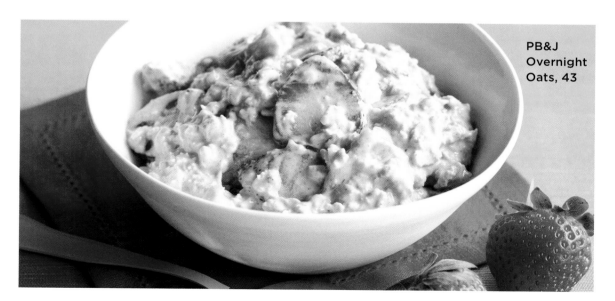

PB&J Overnight Oats, 43

Recipes in 15 Minutes or Less

Each recipe listed here will take you 15 minutes max . . . and that includes both the prep and the cook times!

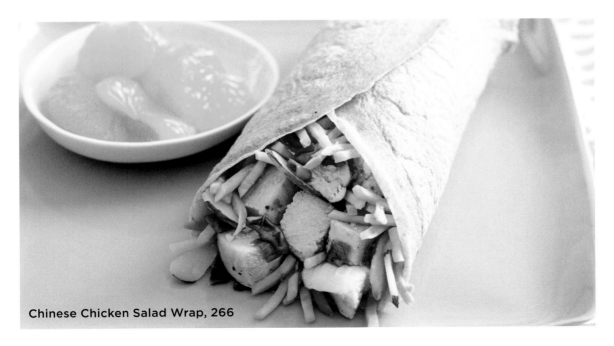

Chinese Chicken Salad Wrap, 266

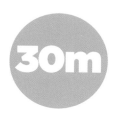

Recipes in 30 Minutes or Less

Each of these recipes can be made in half an hour or less!

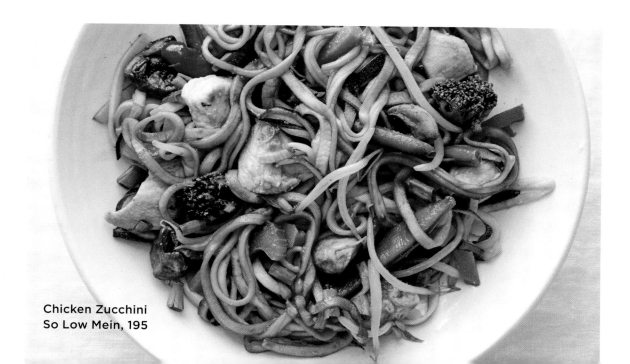

Chicken Zucchini So Low Mein, 195

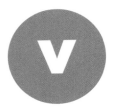

Vegetarian Recipes

These recipes fall under the "lacto-ovo vegetarian" description of vegetarianism, which means they don't include red meat, poultry, seafood, or any ingredients made with those foods (like chicken broth). Keep in mind, these recipes aren't necessarily vegan: They may include dairy and/or egg products.

Heads Up

Although the food itself may be vegetarian friendly, some brands add ingredients derived from animals. For example, some Greek yogurt contains gelatin, and certain cheeses can contain animal rennet. If you're a strict vegetarian, always read labels carefully. When it comes to yogurt, Chobani and Fage are safe vegetarian bets. And in terms of cheese, look for plant-based rennet or rennet-free brands.

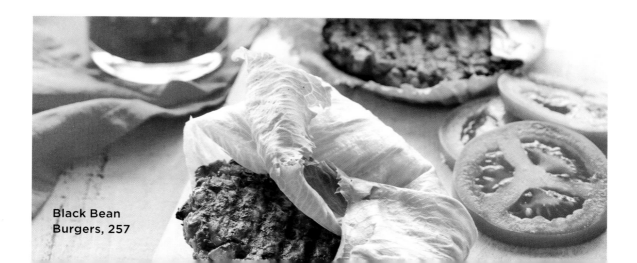

Black Bean Burgers, 257

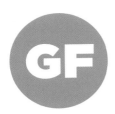

Gluten-Free Recipes

The recipes listed here call for ingredients that are naturally gluten-free. There are some great (and unexpected!) finds here—noodle dishes, pizza, flatbreads, rice dishes . . . even CAKE.

Heads Up

Even foods that are naturally gluten-free might contain a hint of gluten in certain packaged brands. For example, oats are gluten-free, but some companies warn they may contain gluten due to sharing equipment with gluten-containing grains. And about half of the soy sauces found on supermarket shelves have gluten added to them. You know the drill . . . Read labels carefully!

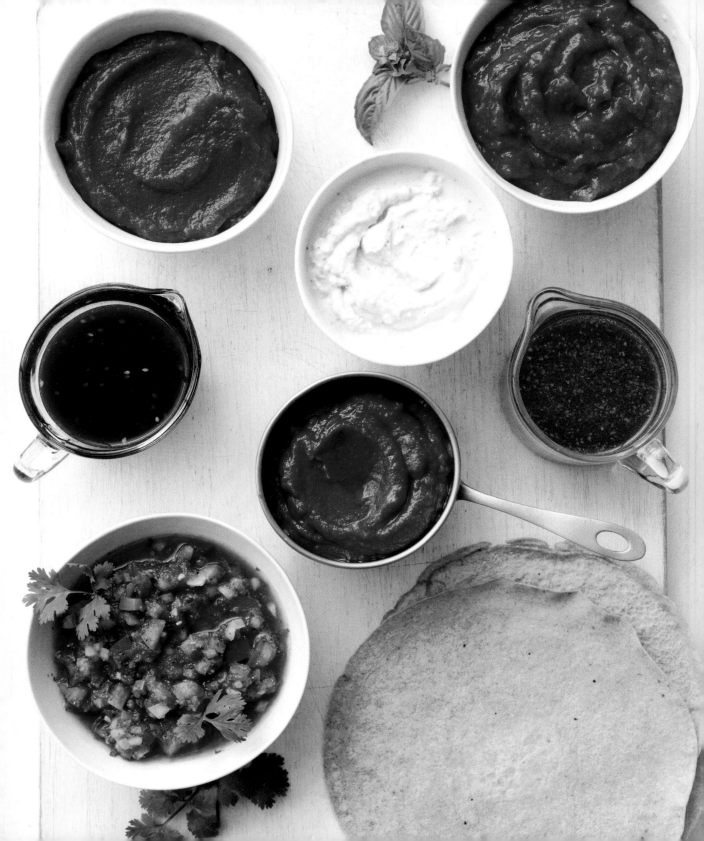

Clean & Hungry Staple Recipes

As you may or may not know, some of the most popular condiments contain a lot of sugar and/or artificial ingredients. Rather than *never* call for favorites like BBQ sauce and teriyaki sauce in this book, I decided to create Clean & Hungry versions. But don't worry: You can still go the premade route. There are helpful tips in this chapter for finding the cleanest condiments on shelves . . .

When a recipe in this book calls for one of these staple recipes or a store-bought alternative, that recipe's nutritional stats were calculated with the staple recipe (not the store-bought product). If you use an alternative from the store, the stats may vary, so look for products with stats that are similar to these staple recipes (or just adjust the recipe's stats accordingly).

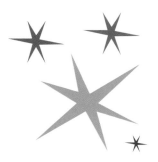

Clean & Hungry Salsa

⅟₁₈ᵗʰ of recipe (about 2 tablespoons): 7 calories, 0g total fat (0g sat fat), 66mg sodium, 1.5g carbs, 0.5g fiber, 1g sugars, <0.5g protein

The natural sweetness from the tomatoes is perfect, and it's got just a hint of jalapeño heat. This salsa is so good, you'll want to put it on EVERYTHING . . .

You'll Need: medium-large sealable container, blender or food processor

Prep: 20 minutes

2 cups chopped tomatoes

½ cup finely chopped onion

½ cup finely chopped green bell pepper

2 tablespoons chopped fresh cilantro

2 tablespoons seeded and finely chopped jalapeño pepper

1½ tablespoons lime juice

½ teaspoon each salt and black pepper

½ teaspoon chopped garlic

¼ teaspoon ground cumin

1. In a medium-large sealable container, combine all ingredients. Mix until uniform.

2. Transfer half of the mixture to a blender or food processor. Pulse until just pureed.

3. Return pureed mixture to the container. Mix well.

4. Seal, and refrigerate until ready to use.

MAKES 18 SERVINGS

HG Alternatives

Enjoy a smoother salsa? Puree the entire mixture instead of just half. Prefer a chunky one? Skip the blending process altogether!

Clean & Hungry BBQ Sauce

¹⁄₁₀ᵗʰ of recipe (about 2 tablespoons): 28 calories, 0g total fat (0g sat fat), 151mg sodium, 6g carbs, 0.5g fiber, 4.5g sugars, 0.5g protein

BBQ sauce is delicious, but it's often full of refined sugar and excess calories. This DIY sauce is made with just the right amount of honey, and the stats are terrific . . .

You'll Need: medium-large bowl, whisk, medium-large sealable container

Prep: 10 minutes

¾ cup canned crushed tomatoes

¼ cup tomato paste

2 tablespoons apple cider vinegar

1 tablespoon molasses

1 tablespoon honey

1 tablespoon Dijon mustard

1 teaspoon reduced-sodium/lite soy sauce

1 teaspoon garlic powder

1 teaspoon onion powder

¼ teaspoon salt

¼ teaspoon paprika

1. In a medium-large bowl, combine all ingredients. Whisk until uniform.

2. Transfer sauce to a medium-large sealable container. Seal, and refrigerate until ready to use.

MAKES 10 SERVINGS

Now Use It!

➤ Flip to "BBQ sauce" in the index (page 336) for a list of recipes that call for this delicious sauce.

Store-Bought Alternatives

➤ Your best bet is a natural BBQ sauce made with clean (not refined) sweetener, like cane sugar or agave nectar. OrganicVille has some fantastic options.

Gluten FYI

Certain brands add gluten to their soy sauce. If you avoid gluten, read labels carefully. Or grab a specially marked product like Kikkoman Gluten-Free Soy Sauce.

Clean & Hungry Marinara Sauce

⅙th of recipe (about ½ cup): 52 calories, 0g total fat (0g sat fat), 354mg sodium, 10.5g carbs, 3g fiber, 5.5g sugars, 2.5g protein

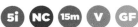

This sauce is loaded with flavor, and it's so easy to make. Try it once, and you might never go back to store-bought sauce . . .

You'll Need: large sealable container

Prep: 5 minutes

3 cups canned crushed tomatoes

¼ cup tomato paste

1 tablespoon white wine vinegar

2 teaspoons Italian seasoning

½ teaspoon garlic powder

½ teaspoon onion powder

¼ teaspoon salt

⅛ teaspoon black pepper

1. Combine ingredients in a large sealable container. Mix until uniform.

2. Seal, and refrigerate until ready to use.

MAKES 6 SERVINGS

Now Use It!

➤ Flip to "marinara sauce" in the index (page 342) for a list of recipes that call for this sauce.

Store-Bought Alternatives

➤ Check out nutritional panels and ingredient lists. Look for a sauce with stats similar to this recipe, made with natural ingredients and no sugar, like the kinds by The Silver Palate and Monte Bene.

Clean & Hungry Sesame Ginger Dressing

⅛ᵗʰ of recipe (about 2 tablespoons): 32 calories, 2.5g total fat (0.5g sat fat), 204mg sodium, 2g carbs, 0g fiber, 1g sugars, 0.5g protein

This sweet stuff is more than just a salad dressing ... Use it as a marinade or sauce too.

You'll Need: medium bowl, whisk, medium sealable container

Prep: 5 minutes

½ **cup plain rice vinegar**

¼ **cup orange juice**

3 tablespoons reduced-sodium/ lite soy sauce

1½ tablespoons sesame oil

2 teaspoons crushed ginger

2 teaspoons crushed garlic

1 packet natural no-calorie sweetener

1. In a medium bowl, combine all ingredients. Whisk until uniform.

2. Transfer to a medium sealable container. Seal, and refrigerate until ready to use.

MAKES 8 SERVINGS

Now Use It!

➤ Flip to page 266 for the Chinese Chicken Salad Wrap.

Store-Bought Alternatives

➤ Look for a natural dressing with similar calorie and fat counts; the less sugar, the better. Newman's Own makes a great one!

Gluten FYI

Certain brands add gluten to their soy sauce. If you avoid gluten, read labels carefully. Or grab a specially marked product like Kikkoman Gluten-Free Soy Sauce.

Clean & Hungry Chunky Blue Cheese Dressing

⅛th of recipe (about 2 tablespoons): 46 calories, 2.5g total fat (1.5g sat fat), 216mg sodium, 1g carbs, 0g fiber, 0.5g sugars, 4g protein

This is more like a dip than a dressing, and it tastes incredible—so creamy! Add a little water for a pourable salad dressing.

You'll Need: medium sealable container

Prep: 5 minutes

½ cup fat-free plain Greek yogurt

2 tablespoons grated Parmesan cheese

¼ teaspoon each salt and black pepper

½ cup crumbled blue cheese

1. In a medium sealable container, combine all ingredients *except* blue cheese. Mix well.

2. Mash and stir blue cheese into the mixture. Seal, and refrigerate until ready to use.

MAKES 8 SERVINGS

Now Use It!

➤ This stuff is a must on the Buffalo Chicken Stuffed Portabellas on page 153. Also try it on the Slow-Cooker Buffalo Chicken (page 141), Buffalo Turkey Meatloaf (page 175), and Big Buffalo Cauliflower Bites (page 247).

Store-Bought Alternatives

➤ Go for a natural salad dressing that's low in fat with 50 or fewer calories per 2-tablespoon serving. Bolthouse Farms is a Hungry Girl favorite.

Clean & Hungry Teriyaki Sauce

1/12th of recipe (about 2 tablespoons): 7 calories, <0.5g total fat (0g sat fat), 184mg sodium, 1g carbs, <0.5g fiber, 0.5g sugars, 0.5g protein

Teriyaki adds major flavor to so many dishes, but your average store-bought sauce is crammed with sugar. Not this sauce ... It's super low in calories and practically sugar-free.

You'll Need: blender or food processor, medium-large sealable container

Prep: 5 minutes

¼ **cup reduced-sodium/lite soy sauce**

3 **tablespoons apple cider vinegar**

2 **packets natural no-calorie sweetener**

1½ **teaspoons chopped garlic**

1½ **teaspoons crushed ginger**

½ **teaspoon xanthan gum**

1 **teaspoon sesame seeds**

1. In a blender or food processor, combine all ingredients *except* sesame seeds.

2. Add 1 cup water. Blend until uniform and slightly thickened, about 20 seconds.

3. Transfer to a medium-large sealable container, and stir in sesame seeds. (It will be a little frothy at first.)

4. Seal, and refrigerate until ready to use.

MAKES 12 SERVINGS

Gluten FYI

Certain brands add gluten to their soy sauce. If you avoid gluten, read labels carefully. Or grab a specially marked product like Kikkoman Gluten-Free Soy Sauce.

Ingredient FYI

Xanthan gum is a natural, plant-based thickener. It gives this sauce a perfect texture. Natural-food stores carry it, as do some mainstream markets. When in doubt, order it online.

Now Use It!

➤ This sauce is essential in the Hawaiian Chicken with Cauliflower Rice (page 138), Shrimp Teriyaki (page 157), Cauliflower Power Fried Rice (page 229), and Hawaiian Shrimp Fried Rice with Pineapple (page 230).

Store-Bought Alternatives

➤ Pick a teriyaki sauce that's made with natural ingredients and not too much sugar. Most are higher in calories and sodium than this recipe, so keep that in mind. A brand called OrganicVille makes really tasty teriyaki sauces that are sweetened with agave nectar.

Clean & Hungry Ketchup

¹⁄₁₆ᵗʰ of recipe (about 1 tablespoon): 14 calories, 0g total fat (0g sat fat), 88mg sodium, 3.5g carbs, 0.5g fiber, 2.5g sugars, 0.5g protein

Creating tasty low-calorie ketchup wasn't easy, but here it is . . . and it ROCKS.

You'll Need: medium bowl, whisk, medium sealable container

Prep: 5 minutes

½ **cup tomato paste**

¼ **cup canned crushed tomatoes**

¼ **cup apple cider vinegar**

1 tablespoon plus 1 teaspoon honey

½ **teaspoon garlic powder**

½ **teaspoon onion powder**

½ **teaspoon salt**

1. Combine ingredients in a medium bowl.

2. Add 2 tablespoons water, and whisk until smooth and uniform.

3. Transfer to a medium sealable container. Seal, and refrigerate until ready to use.

MAKES 16 SERVINGS

Now Use It!

➤ Use this ketchup in the Buffalo Turkey Meatloaf (page 175), drizzle it over the Cheeseburger Crepes (page 279), or spoon some over the Cheeseburger Skillet (page 241). It's also great on Chapter 10's burger patties (pages 257 through 261)!

Store-Bought Alternatives

➤ Look for agave-sweetened ketchup. OrganicVille makes a great one.

Clean & Hungry Whole-Wheat Tortillas

¼th of recipe (1 tortilla): 78 calories, 0.5g total fat (0g sat fat), 280mg sodium, 12g carbs, 2g fiber, 0.5g sugars, 7g protein

These DIY tortillas are SHOCKINGLY easy to make . . . only five ingredients in total!

You'll Need: blender or food processor, large skillet, nonstick spray, offset spatula or flexible rubber spatula

Prep: 10 minutes • **Cook:** 15 minutes

¾ cup (about 6 large) egg whites

½ cup whole-wheat flour

½ teaspoon baking powder

¼ teaspoon each salt and black pepper

1. Place all ingredients in a blender or food processor. Add ½ cup water, and blend until uniform.

2. Bring a large skillet sprayed with nonstick spray to medium heat. Pour ¼th of the batter (about ⅓ cup) into the skillet, quickly tilting the skillet in all directions to evenly distribute.

3. Cook until edges are firm and bottom is lightly browned, about 2 minutes.

4. Carefully flip with an offset spatula or flexible rubber spatula.

5. Cook until lightly browned on the other side, about 1 minute.

6. Repeat three times to make three more tortillas. If needed, remove skillet from heat and re-spray after making each tortilla.

7. Let cool. Cover and refrigerate until ready to use.

MAKES 4 SERVINGS

Now Use 'Em!

➤ Don't miss the California Breakfast Burrito (page 83), Mexican Breakfast Burrito (page 84), Chinese Chicken Salad Wrap (page 266), and BBQ Chicken Wrap (page 269).

Store-Bought Alternatives

➤ Truth be told, it's hard to find clean tortillas that are low in calories. Our pick? La Tortilla Factory Whole Wheat Organic Tortillas, with 100 calories each.

Tortilla Storage Tips & Tricks

To freeze tortillas . . . Stack them with a layer of wax paper in between each tortilla. Place them in a freezer bag, seal, and lay flat in the freezer.

To thaw tortillas . . . Place one tortilla between 2 damp paper towels on a microwave-safe plate. Microwave for 30 seconds, or until thawed.

1

Growing Oatmeal, Overnight Oats, Yogurt Bowls & More

From big portions of hot oatmeal to refreshing fruit and yogurt bowls, this chapter has breakfast lovers covered. Whatever you do, don't bypass the oatmeal bakes—they're AMAZING.

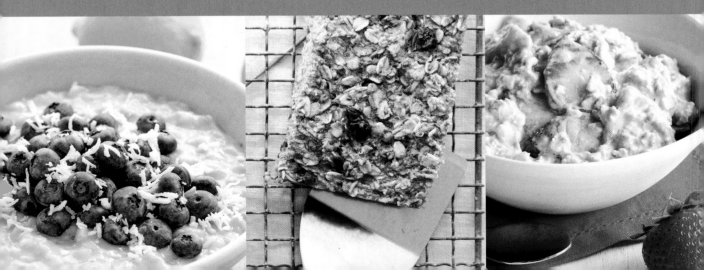

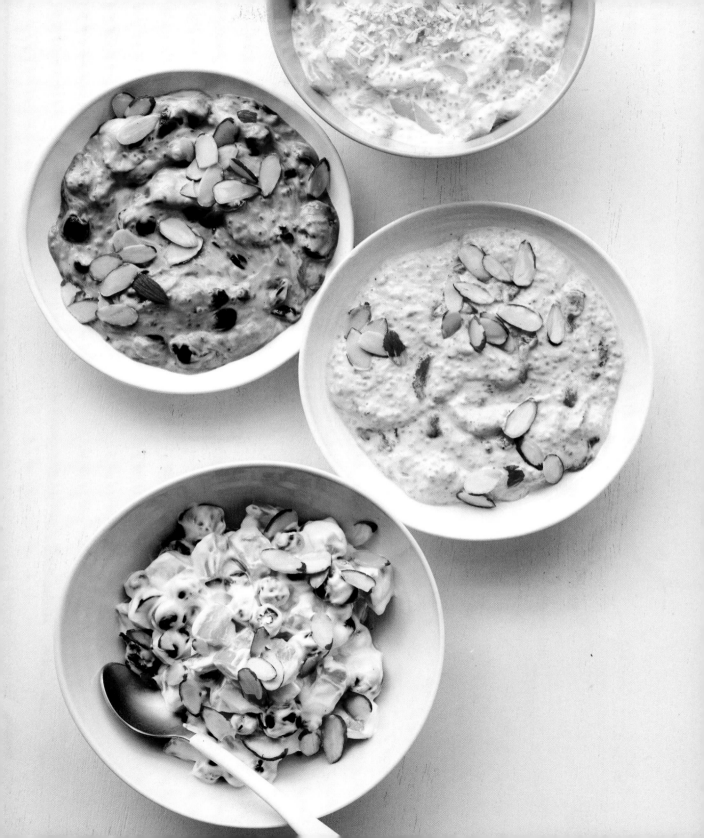

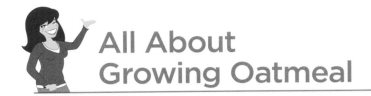

All About Growing Oatmeal

If you're new to the world of Hungry Girl growing oatmeal, prepare to be wowed . . .

Growing oatmeal recipes call for twice the amount of liquid and twice the cook time of ordinary old-fashioned oatmeal. The result? An enormous portion with the same number of calories as traditional oatmeal. So satisfying!

FYI: Old-fashioned oats are a must. Steel-cut oats and instant oats won't easily soak up all the extra liquid or take on an ideal texture, so they're not recommended for these recipes.

Don't be alarmed by the amount of liquid. That's what gives growing oatmeal its super-sizing capability. Although it looks like a lot and hasn't been completely absorbed when the oatmeal's done cooking, your oatmeal will thicken once you've transferred it to a bowl and let it cool for 5 to 10 minutes.

Here's a hot Hungry Girl tip . . . Some natural no-calorie sweeteners can clump when added to hot liquid. To prevent this from happening, sprinkle them in (as opposed to emptying the packets all at once), quickly stirring as you add them.

Hope you're hungry . . . You'll likely *never* go back to ordinary hot oatmeal!

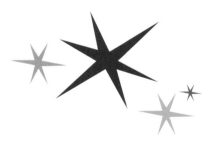

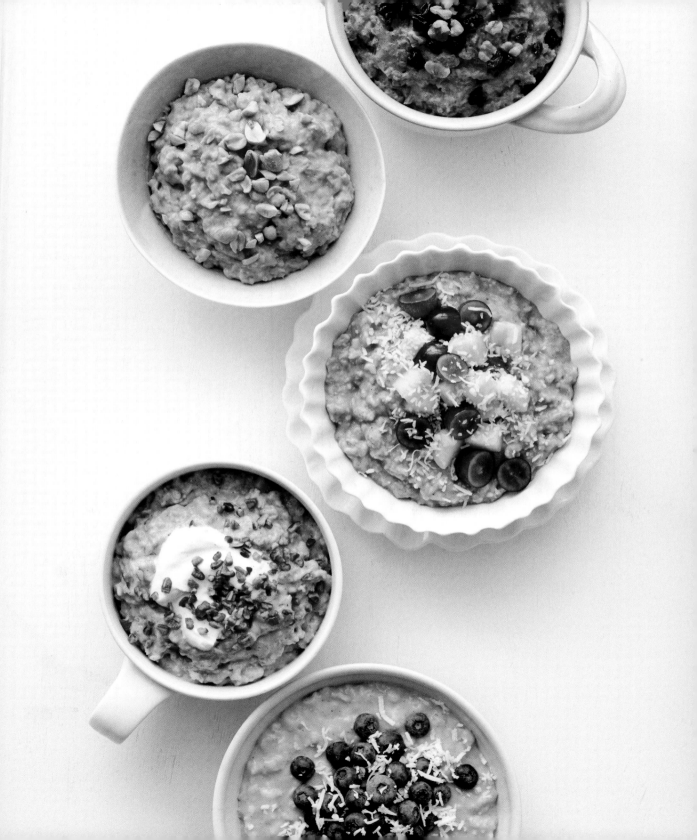

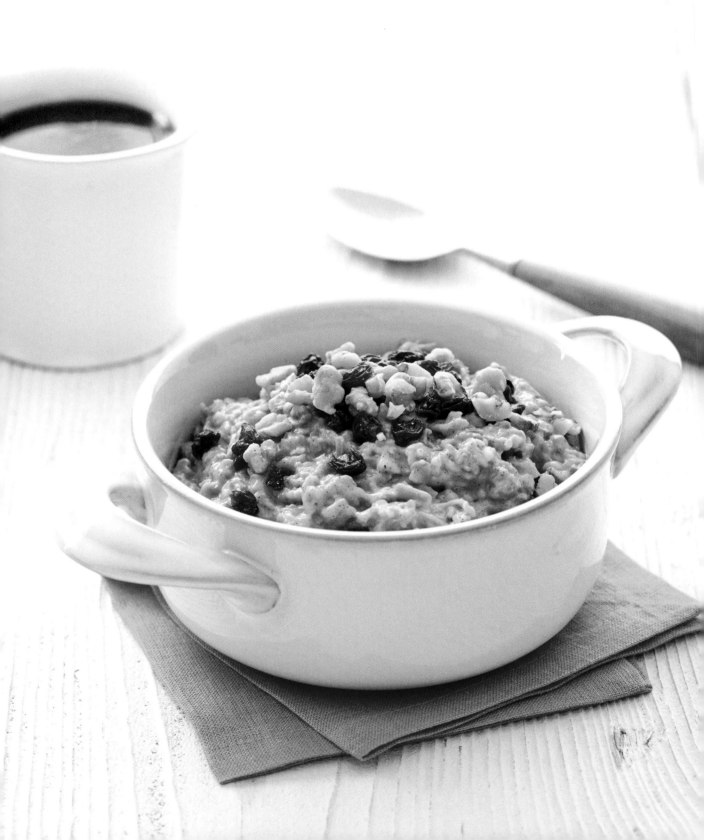

Carrot Cake Growing Oatmeal

Entire recipe: 303 calories, 10.5g total fat (1g sat fat), 373mg sodium, 46g carbs, 8.5g fiber, 11.5g sugars, 8g protein

You'll Need: nonstick pot, medium bowl

Prep: 5 minutes • **Cook:** 20 minutes • **Cool:** 10 minutes

½ **cup old-fashioned oats**

½ **teaspoon vanilla extract**

½ **teaspoon cinnamon**

¼ **teaspoon nutmeg**

Dash salt

1 cup unsweetened vanilla almond milk

½ **cup shredded carrots, finely chopped**

2 packets natural no-calorie sweetener

¼ **ounce (about 1 tablespoon) chopped walnuts**

1 tablespoon raisins, chopped

1. In a nonstick pot, combine oats, vanilla extract, cinnamon, nutmeg, and salt.

2. Add almond milk and 1 cup water. Bring to a boil, and then reduce to a simmer.

3. Stir in carrots. Cook and stir until oats are thick and creamy, 12 to 15 minutes.

4. Transfer to a medium bowl, and stir in sweetener. Let cool until thickened, 5 to 10 minutes.

5. Top with walnuts and chopped raisins.

MAKES 1 SERVING

Peanut Butter Crunch Growing Oatmeal

Entire recipe: 309 calories, 12g total fat (1g sat fat), 385mg sodium, 37g carbs, 8.5g fiber, 3g sugars, 17g protein

You'll Need: nonstick pot, medium bowl

Prep: 5 minutes • **Cook:** 20 minutes • **Cool:** 10 minutes

½ **cup old-fashioned oats**

¼ **teaspoon vanilla extract**

⅛ **teaspoon cinnamon**

Dash salt

1 cup unsweetened vanilla almond milk

3 tablespoons powdered peanut butter or defatted peanut flour

1 packet natural no-calorie sweetener

¼ **ounce (about 1 tablespoon) chopped peanuts**

1. In a nonstick pot, combine oats, vanilla extract, cinnamon, and salt.

2. Add almond milk and 1¼ cups water. Bring to a boil, and then reduce to a simmer.

3. Cook and stir until thick and creamy, 12 to 15 minutes.

4. Transfer to a medium bowl, and stir in powdered peanut butter/peanut flour and sweetener. Let cool until thickened, 5 to 10 minutes.

5. Top with peanuts.

MAKES 1 SERVING

Ingredient FYI

Powdered peanut butter and defatted peanut flour are miracle workers in the kitchen—delicious ones! Flip to page 4 for more info on these ingredients . . .

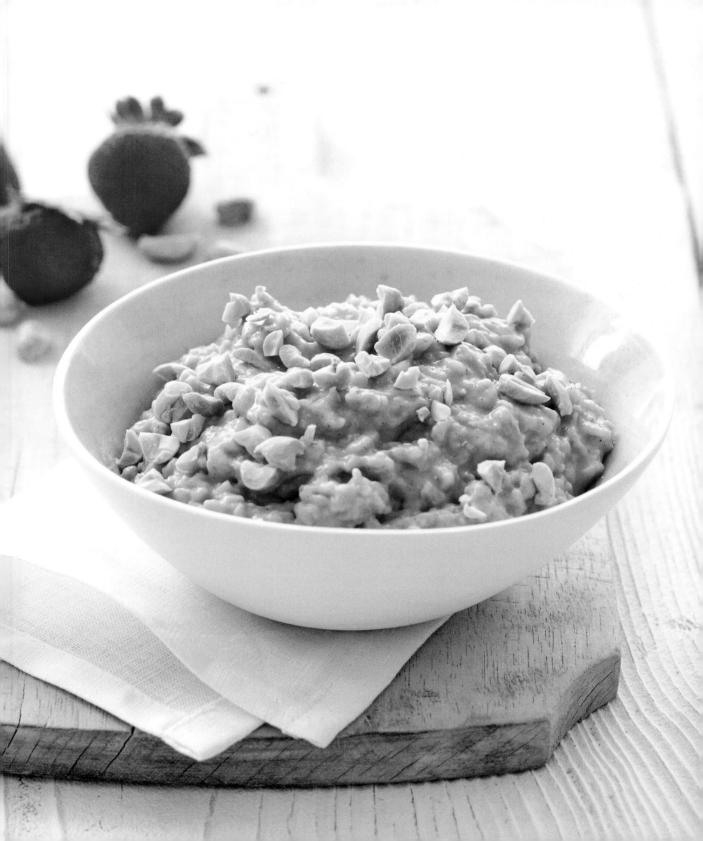

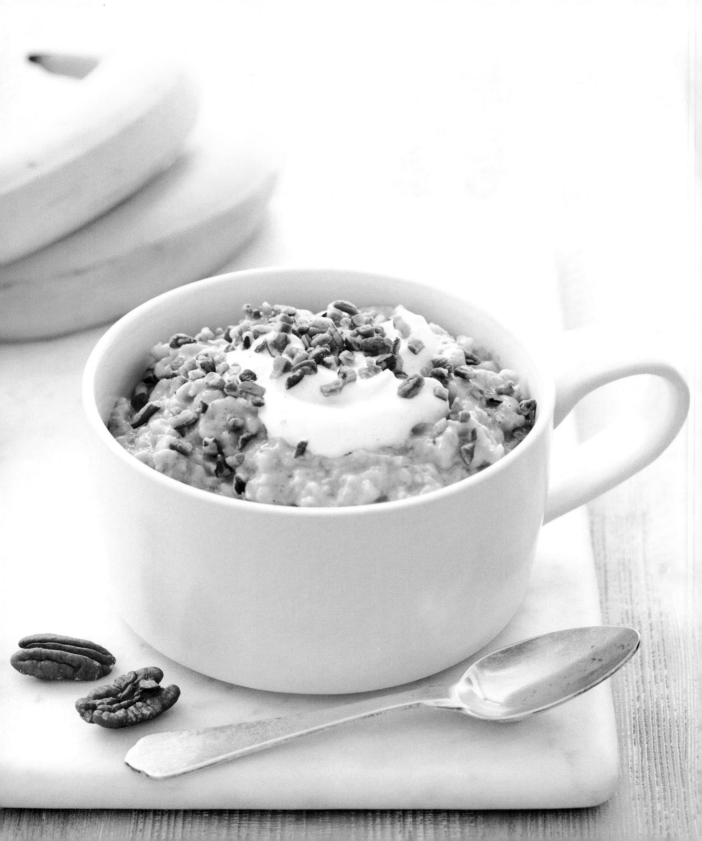

Banana Bread Growing Oatmeal

Entire recipe: 318 calories, 10.5g total fat (1g sat fat), 351mg sodium, 46.5g carbs, 8g fiber, 10g sugars, 12g protein

You'll Need: nonstick pot, medium bowl, small bowl

Prep: 5 minutes • **Cook:** 20 minutes • **Cool:** 10 minutes

½ cup old-fashioned oats

Dash salt

½ teaspoon plus 1 dash cinnamon

⅛ teaspoon plus 1 drop vanilla extract

1 cup unsweetened vanilla almond milk

¼ cup mashed banana

2 packets natural no-calorie sweetener

3 tablespoons fat-free plain Greek yogurt

¼ ounce (about 1 tablespoon) chopped pecans

1. In a nonstick pot, combine oats, salt, ½ teaspoon cinnamon, and ⅛ teaspoon vanilla extract.

2. Add almond milk and 1 cup water. Bring to a boil, and then reduce to a simmer.

3. Stir in banana. Cook and stir until thick and creamy, 12 to 15 minutes.

4. Transfer to a medium bowl, and stir in 1½ sweetener packets. Let cool until thickened, 5 to 10 minutes.

5. Meanwhile, in a small bowl, combine Greek yogurt with remaining dash of cinnamon, drop of vanilla extract, and half of sweetener packet. Mix well.

6. Top oatmeal with yogurt mixture and pecans.

MAKES 1 SERVING

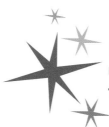

For more healthy recipes, plus the latest food news, tips & tricks, and more, **sign up for free daily emails at Hungry-Girl.com!**

Fruity Coconut Growing Oatmeal

Entire recipe: 271 calories, 8.5g total fat (3g sat fat), 335mg sodium, 44g carbs, 6.5g fiber, 11.5g sugars, 7g protein

You'll Need: nonstick pot, medium bowl

Prep: 5 minutes • **Cook:** 20 minutes • **Cool:** 10 minutes

½ cup old-fashioned oats

¼ teaspoon cinnamon

⅛ teaspoon vanilla extract

⅛ teaspoon coconut extract

Dash salt

1 cup unsweetened vanilla almond milk

1 packet natural no-calorie sweetener

¼ cup chopped pineapple

¼ cup halved grapes

1 tablespoon unsweetened shredded coconut

1. In a nonstick pot, combine oats, cinnamon, vanilla extract, coconut extract, and salt.

2. Add almond milk and 1 cup water. Bring to a boil, and then reduce to a simmer.

3. Cook and stir until thick and creamy, 12 to 15 minutes.

4. Transfer to a medium bowl, and stir in sweetener. Let cool until thickened, 5 to 10 minutes.

5. Top with fruit and coconut.

MAKES 1 SERVING

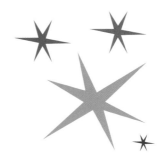

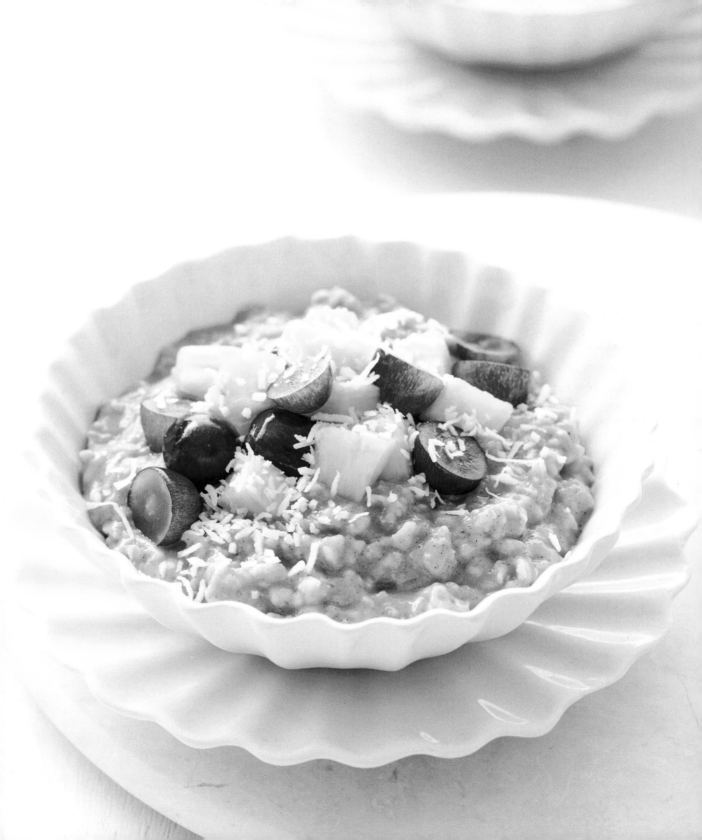

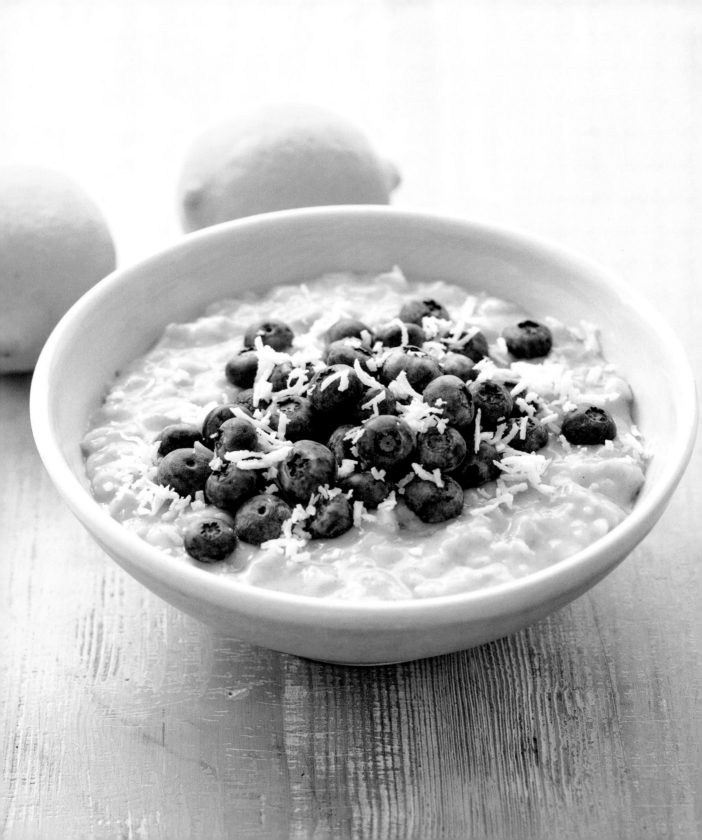

Lemon Blueberry Growing Oatmeal

Entire recipe: 238 calories, 7g total fat (2g sat fat), 469mg sodium, 38.5g carbs, 7g fiber, 6.5g sugars, 7g protein

You'll Need: nonstick pot, medium bowl

Prep: 10 minutes • **Cook:** 20 minutes • **Cool:** 10 minutes

½ **cup old-fashioned oats**

1½ **teaspoons lemon juice**

½ **teaspoon lemon zest**

¼ **teaspoon coconut extract**

⅛ **teaspoon cinnamon**

⅛ **teaspoon salt**

1 **cup unsweetened vanilla almond milk**

1 **packet natural no-calorie sweetener**

⅓ **cup blueberries (fresh or thawed from frozen and drained)**

1½ **teaspoons unsweetened shredded coconut**

1. In a nonstick pot, combine oats, lemon juice, lemon zest, coconut extract, cinnamon, and salt.

2. Add almond milk and 1 cup water. Bring to a boil, and then reduce to a simmer.

3. Cook and stir until thick and creamy, 12 to 15 minutes.

4. Transfer to a medium bowl, and stir in sweetener. Let cool until thickened, 5 to 10 minutes.

5. Top with blueberries and shredded coconut.

MAKES 1 SERVING

Ingredient FYI

If using frozen blueberries rather than fresh, check the ingredient list to make sure no sugar has been added; the only ingredient should be the fruit itself.

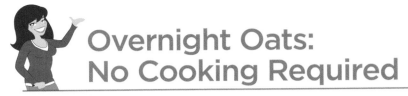

Overnight Oats:
No Cooking Required

Prefer not to cook in the morning? These recipes will be your new BFFs. As the name implies, time does all the work for you. Just combine a few ingredients in the evening, and refrigerate overnight. In the a.m., a delicious breakfast will be waiting.

Skeptical about chilled oatmeal? Don't knock it 'til you've tried it . . . Overnight oats are creamy, sweet, and delicious! But if you discover you'd rather enjoy them heated, you can always pop 'em in the microwave the next morning. Just prepare your recipe in a microwave-safe bowl the night before.

Want to take it to go? Prepare it in a jar with a lid. So convenient!

Have a few extra minutes to spare? Whip up one of the overnight oatmeal parfaits. Those are layered with fruit and yogurt, and they're fantastic.

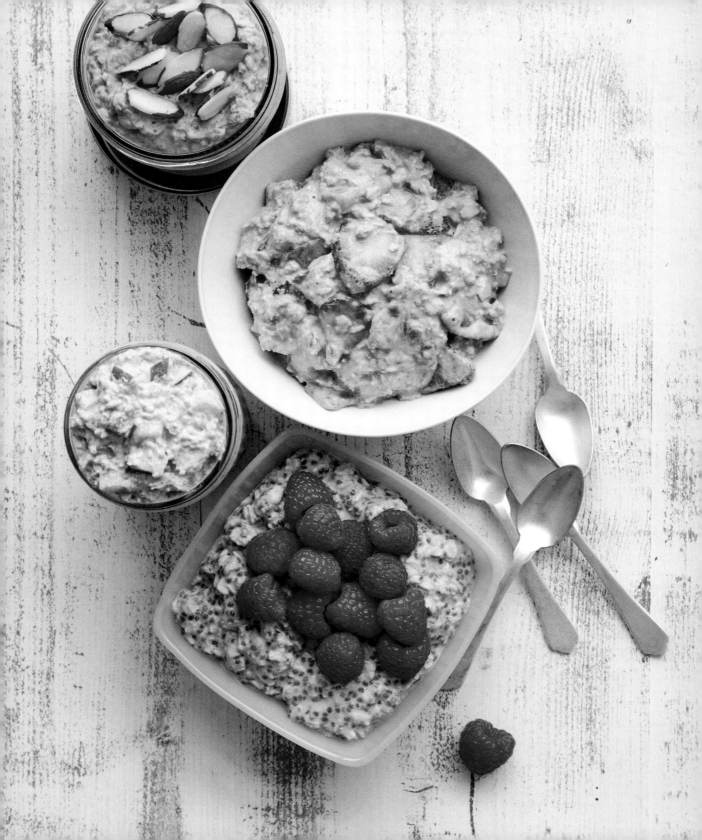

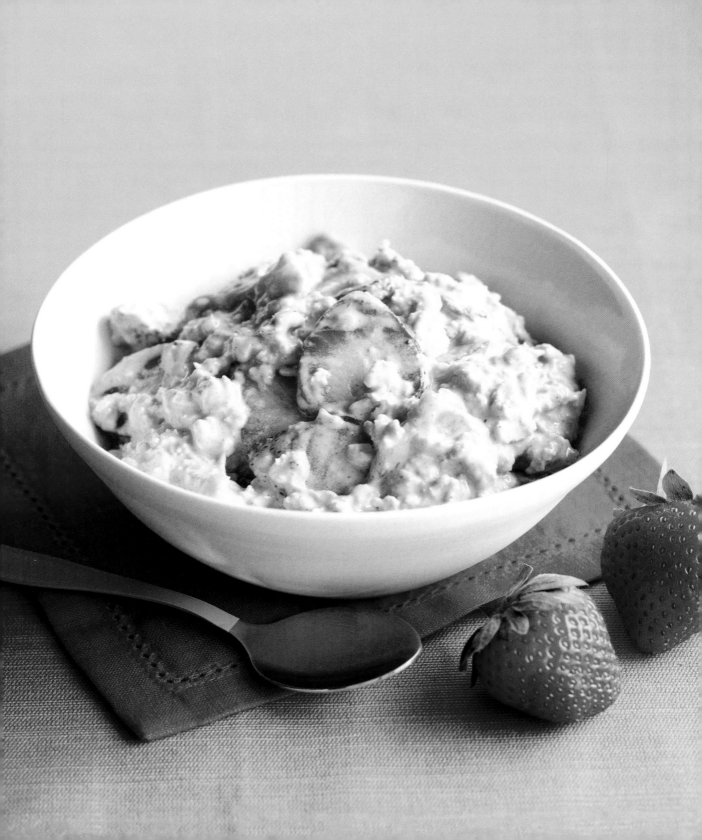

PB&J Overnight Oats

Entire recipe: 293 calories, 10.5g total fat (1g sat fat), 291mg sodium, 38.5g carbs, 8.5g fiber, 5g sugars, 14g protein

You'll Need: medium bowl or jar

Prep: 5 minutes • **Chill:** 6 hours

2 tablespoons powdered peanut butter or defatted peanut flour

½ tablespoon creamy peanut butter (no sugar added)

½ cup old-fashioned oats

½ cup unsweetened vanilla almond milk

⅓ cup sliced strawberries

1 packet natural no-calorie sweetener

⅛ teaspoon cinnamon

⅛ teaspoon vanilla extract

Dash salt

1. In a medium bowl or jar, combine powdered peanut butter/peanut flour, creamy peanut butter, and 2 tablespoons warm water. Mix until smooth and uniform.

2. Add all remaining ingredients. Mix well.

3. Cover and refrigerate for at least 6 hours, until oats are soft and have absorbed most of the liquid.

MAKES 1 SERVING

Ingredient FYI

Combining powdered peanut butter (or defatted peanut flour) with just a small amount of regular peanut butter in this recipe saves a lot of fat and calories. Flip to page 4 for more info . . .

Apple Chia Overnight Oats

Entire recipe: 248 calories, 5.5g total fat (0.5g sat fat), 247mg sodium, 35.5g carbs, 9.5g fiber, 15g sugars, 17g protein

You'll Need: medium bowl or jar

Prep: 5 minutes   •   **Chill:** 6 hours

½ cup fat-free plain Greek yogurt

¼ cup unsweetened vanilla almond milk

2 packets natural no-calorie sweetener

¼ teaspoon cinnamon

¼ teaspoon vanilla extract

Dash salt

¾ cup chopped Fuji or Gala apple

3 tablespoons old-fashioned oats

1 tablespoon chia seeds

1. In a medium bowl or jar, combine yogurt, almond milk, sweetener, cinnamon, vanilla extract, and salt. Mix until smooth and uniform.

2. Stir in apple, oats, and chia seeds.

3. Cover and refrigerate for at least 6 hours, until oats are soft and have absorbed most of the liquid.

MAKES 1 SERVING

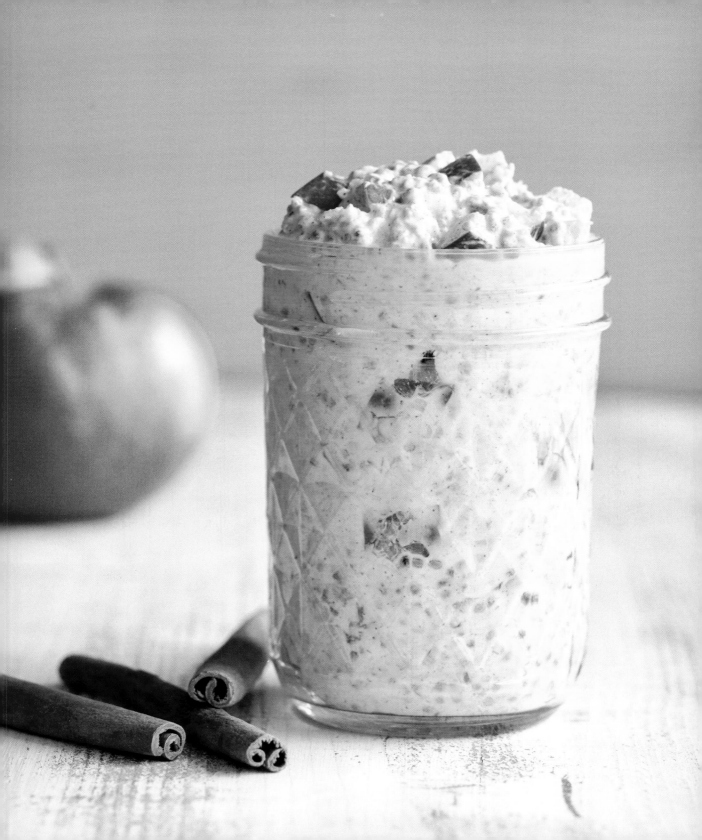

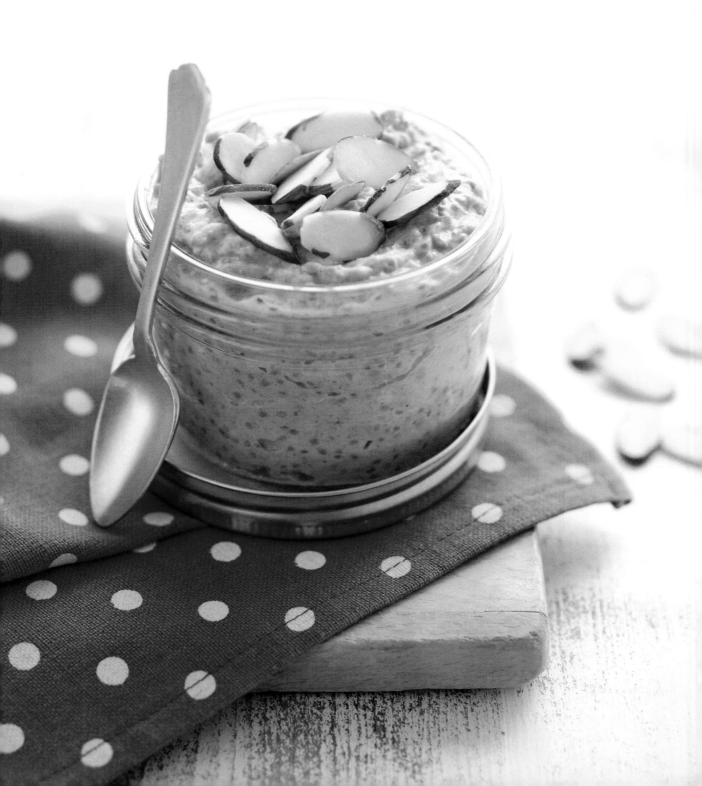

Pumpkin Pie Overnight Oats

Entire recipe: 237 calories, 8.5g total fat (0.5g sat fat), 71mg sodium, 24.5g carbs, 9.5g fiber, 7g sugars, 18g protein

You'll Need: medium bowl or jar

Prep: 5 minutes • **Chill:** 6 hours

½ **cup fat-free plain Greek yogurt**

¼ **cup canned pure pumpkin**

2 **tablespoons unsweetened vanilla almond milk**

2 **tablespoons old-fashioned oats**

1 **tablespoon chia seeds**

2 **packets natural no-calorie sweetener**

¼ **teaspoon pumpkin pie spice**

⅛ **teaspoon vanilla extract**

¼ **ounce (about 1 tablespoon) sliced almonds**

1. In a medium bowl or jar, combine all ingredients *except* almonds. Mix thoroughly.

2. Cover and refrigerate for at least 6 hours, until oats are soft and have absorbed most of the liquid.

3. Top with almonds.

MAKES 1 SERVING

Vanilla Overnight Oats with Raspberries

Entire recipe: 308 calories, 9.5g total fat (1g sat fat), 305mg sodium, 42g carbs, 13.5g fiber, 4.5g sugars, 16g protein

You'll Need: medium bowl or jar

Prep: 5 minutes • **Chill:** 6 hours

¾ **cup unsweetened vanilla almond milk**

½ **cup old-fashioned oats**

2 tablespoons plain protein powder with about 100 calories per serving

1 tablespoon chia seeds

1 packet natural no-calorie sweetener

¼ **teaspoon vanilla extract**

Dash salt

½ **cup raspberries**

1. In a medium bowl or jar, combine all ingredients *except* raspberries. Mix thoroughly.

2. Cover and refrigerate for at least 6 hours, until oats are soft and have absorbed most of the liquid.

3. Top with raspberries.

MAKES 1 SERVING

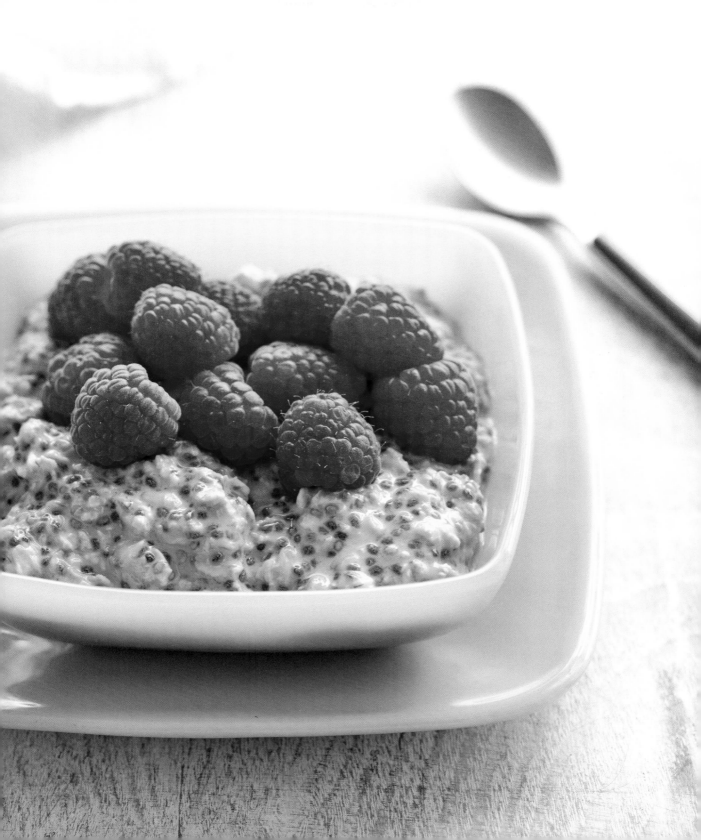

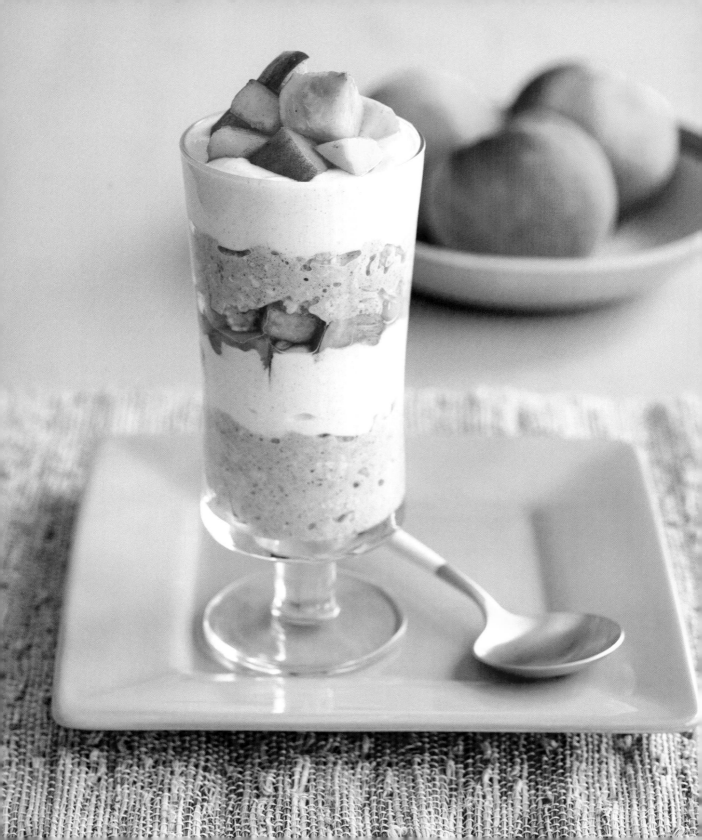

Peach Cobbler Overnight Oatmeal Parfait

Entire recipe: 284 calories, 4.5g total fat (0.5g sat fat), 290mg sodium, 45g carbs, 7g fiber, 14.5g sugars, 18.5g protein

You'll Need: 2 medium bowls, small bowl, tall glass or medium jar

Prep: 5 minutes • **Chill:** 6 hours

½ cup old-fashioned oats

½ cup unsweetened vanilla almond milk

Dash salt

2 packets natural no-calorie sweetener

¼ teaspoon plus ⅛ teaspoon cinnamon

¼ teaspoon vanilla extract

½ cup fat-free plain Greek yogurt

⅔ cup chopped peaches (fresh or thawed from frozen)

1. In a medium bowl, combine oats, almond milk, and salt. Add 1 sweetener packet, ¼ teaspoon cinnamon, and ⅛ teaspoon vanilla extract. Mix well.

2. Cover and refrigerate for at least 6 hours, until oats are soft and have absorbed most of the liquid.

3. In a small bowl, mix yogurt with remaining sweetener packet and ⅛ teaspoon vanilla extract.

4. In another medium bowl, sprinkle peaches with remaining ⅛ teaspoon cinnamon. Stir to coat.

5. Stir oatmeal. In a tall glass or medium jar, layer half of the oatmeal, half of the yogurt, and half of the peaches. Repeat layering with remaining oatmeal, yogurt, and peaches.

MAKES 1 SERVING

Ingredient FYI
If using frozen peaches rather than fresh, check the ingredient list to make sure no sugar has been added.

Dreamsicle Overnight Oatmeal Parfait

Entire recipe: 306 calories, 4g total fat (0.5g sat fat), 301mg sodium, 51.5g carbs, 6g fiber, 20.5g sugars, 18.5g protein

You'll Need: medium bowl, small bowl, tall glass or medium jar

Prep: 5 minutes • **Chill:** 6 hours

½ **cup old-fashioned oats**

½ **cup unsweetened vanilla almond milk**

Dash salt

2 packets natural no-calorie sweetener

½ **teaspoon vanilla extract**

½ **cup fat-free plain Greek yogurt**

⅔ **cup mandarin orange segments packed in juice, drained**

1. In a medium bowl, combine oats, almond milk, and salt. Add 1 sweetener packet and ¼ teaspoon vanilla extract. Mix well.

2. Cover and refrigerate for at least 6 hours, until oats are soft and have absorbed most of the liquid.

3. In a small bowl, mix yogurt with remaining sweetener packet and ¼ teaspoon vanilla extract.

4. Stir oatmeal. In a tall glass or medium jar, layer half of the oatmeal, half of the yogurt, and half of the orange segments. Repeat layering with remaining oatmeal, yogurt, and orange segments.

MAKES 1 SERVING

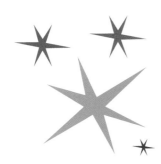

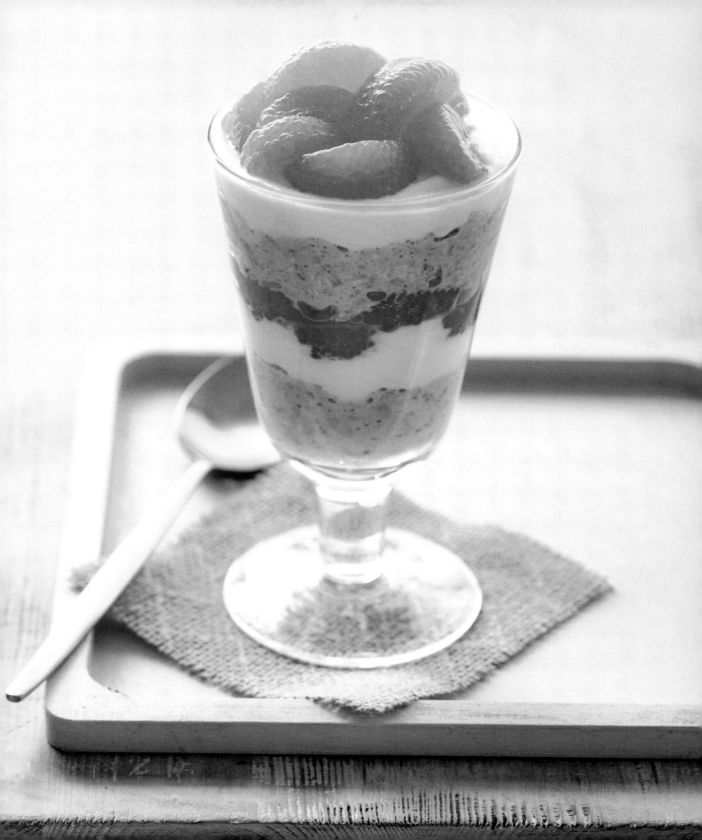

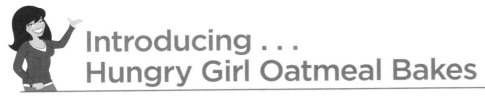

Introducing . . .
Hungry Girl Oatmeal Bakes

I have become completely obsessed with these new Hungry Girl creations. They're satisfying, *comforting,* and perfect when you want to feed the family or whip up a few days' worth of breakfast at once. Here's some more info about them . . .

These bakes taste great hot, warm, or chilled. It's totally your call!

For best results, store leftovers in the fridge. Let them cool completely, and then cover or wrap to keep fresh.

Wanna freeze your oatmeal bake? It's a smart way to always have healthy breakfasts on hand! Here's how to do it . . . Once cool, tightly wrap each serving in plastic wrap. Put individually wrapped pieces in a sealable container or bag, seal, and place in the freezer. To thaw, unwrap one piece, and place on a microwave-safe plate. Microwave for 1½ minutes, or until it reaches your desired temperature.

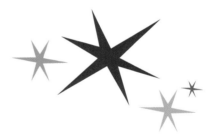

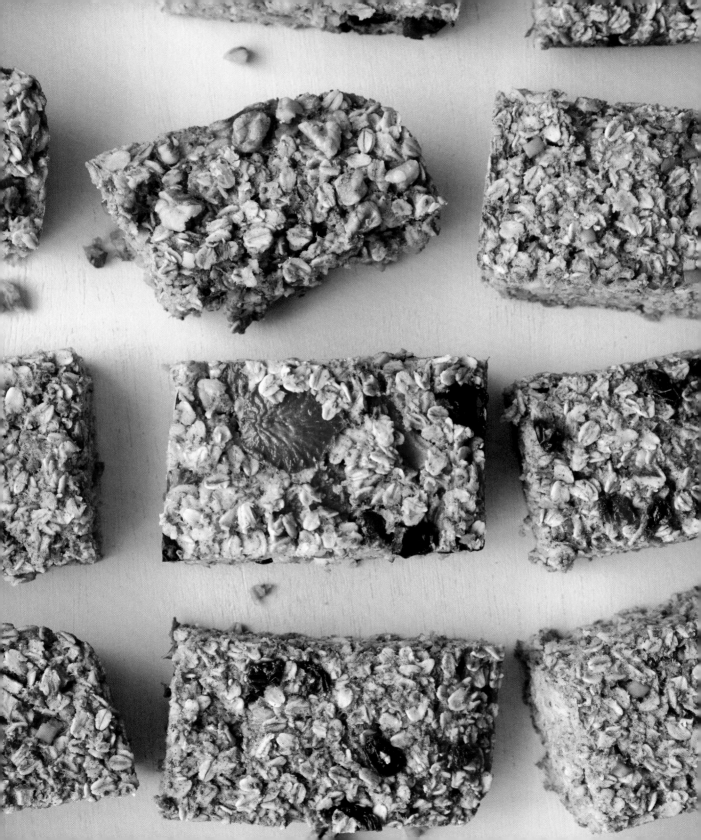

Blueberry Strawberry Oatmeal Bake

⅙ᵗʰ of recipe (about 4 inches by 2½ inches with about ¼ cup topping): 248 calories, 4.5g total fat (0.5g sat fat), 352mg sodium, 39.5g carbs, 7g fiber, 8.5g sugars, 13g protein

You'll Need: 8-inch by 8-inch baking pan, nonstick spray, large bowl, medium-large bowl, medium bowl

Prep: 15 minutes • **Cook:** 35 minutes

3 cups old-fashioned oats

1½ tablespoons chia seeds

2 teaspoons baking powder

¼ teaspoon salt

5 packets natural no-calorie sweetener

1½ teaspoons cinnamon

1½ cups unsweetened vanilla almond milk

½ cup unsweetened applesauce

½ cup (about 4 large) egg whites

2 teaspoons vanilla extract

1 cup blueberries

1 cup sliced strawberries

1 cup fat-free plain Greek yogurt

1. Preheat oven to 350 degrees. Spray an 8-inch by 8-inch baking pan with nonstick spray.

2. In a large bowl, combine oats, chia seeds, baking powder, salt, 4 sweetener packets, and 1 teaspoon cinnamon. Mix well.

3. In a medium-large bowl, combine almond milk, applesauce, egg whites, and 1½ teaspoons vanilla extract. Mix until uniform.

4. Add mixture in the medium-large bowl to the large bowl. Stir until uniform.

5. Gently fold in ½ cup each blueberries and strawberries.

6. Transfer the mixture to the baking pan, and smooth out the surface.

7. Bake until top is light golden brown and entire dish is cooked through, about 35 minutes.

8. Meanwhile, in a medium bowl, combine yogurt with remaining 1 sweetener packet, ½ teaspoon cinnamon, and ½ teaspoon vanilla extract. Mix well. Fold in remaining ½ cup each blueberries and strawberries. Cover and refrigerate.

9. Just before serving, top each piece of the oatmeal bake with ⅙th of the yogurt mixture, about ¼ cup.

MAKES 6 SERVINGS

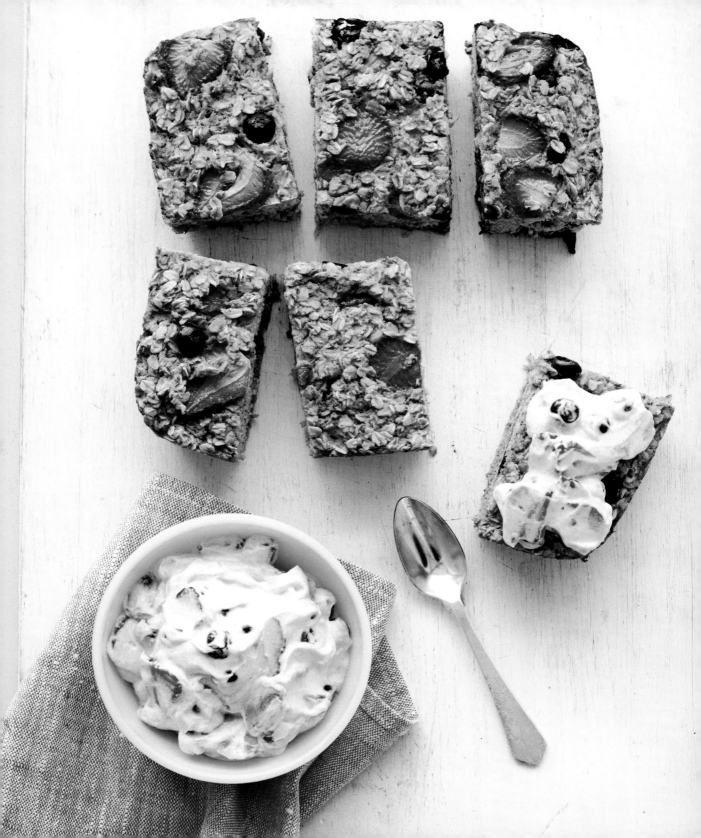

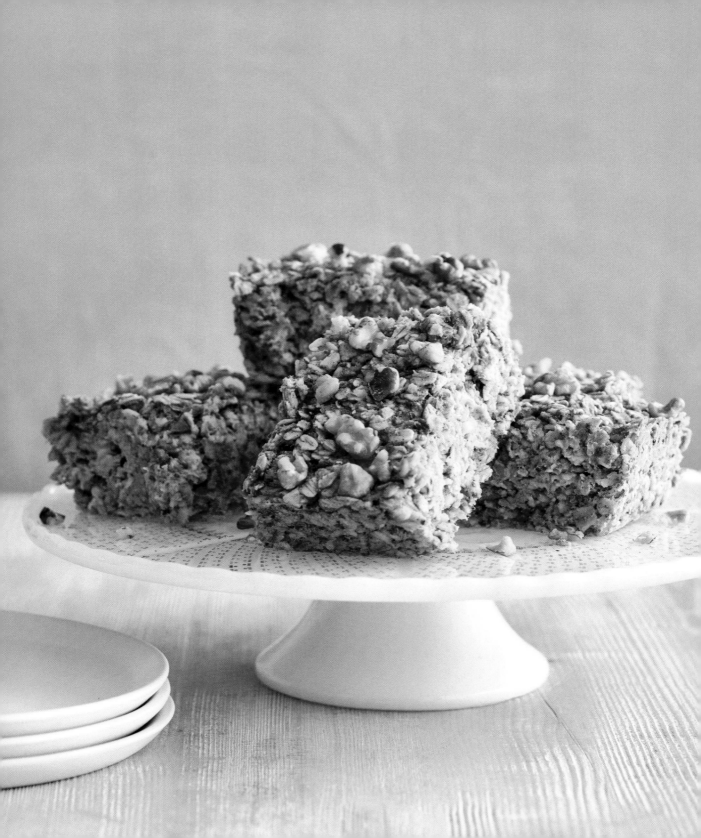

Banana Walnut Oatmeal Bake

⅛ᵗʰ of pan (about 4 inches by 2½ inches): 257 calories, 7.5g total fat (1g sat fat), 336mg sodium, 39.5g carbs, 7g fiber, 6g sugars, 9.5g protein

You'll Need: 8-inch by 8-inch baking pan, nonstick spray, large bowl, medium-large bowl

Prep: 15 minutes • **Cook:** 35 minutes

3 cups old-fashioned oats

1½ tablespoons chia seeds

4 packets natural no-calorie sweetener

2 teaspoons baking powder

1¼ teaspoons cinnamon

¼ teaspoon salt

1½ cups unsweetened vanilla almond milk

1 cup (about 2 medium) mashed extra-ripe bananas

½ cup (about 4 large) egg whites

2 teaspoons vanilla extract

1 ounce (about ¼ cup) chopped walnuts

1. Preheat oven to 350 degrees. Spray an 8-inch by 8-inch baking pan with nonstick spray.

2. In a large bowl, combine oats, chia seeds, sweetener, baking powder, cinnamon, and salt. Mix well.

3. In a medium-large bowl, combine almond milk, bananas, egg whites, and vanilla extract. Mix until uniform.

4. Add mixture in the medium-large bowl to the large bowl. Mix until uniform.

5. Transfer mixture to the baking pan, and smooth out the surface.

6. Top with walnuts, and lightly press them into the mixture.

7. Bake until top is light golden brown and entire dish is cooked through, about 35 minutes.

MAKES 6 SERVINGS

Apple Cinnamon Oatmeal Bake

⅙th of pan (about 4 inches by 2½ inches): 214 calories, 4.5g total fat (0.5g sat fat), 336mg sodium, 36g carbs, 7g fiber, 5.5g sugars, 8.5g protein

You'll Need: 8-inch by 8-inch baking pan, nonstick spray, large bowl, medium-large bowl

Prep: 15 minutes • **Cook:** 35 minutes

3 cups old-fashioned oats

1½ tablespoons chia seeds

4 packets natural no-calorie sweetener

2 teaspoons baking powder

2 teaspoons cinnamon

1 teaspoon pumpkin pie spice

¼ teaspoon salt

1½ cups unsweetened vanilla almond milk

½ cup unsweetened applesauce

½ cup (about 4 large) egg whites

2 teaspoons vanilla extract

1 cup finely chopped Fuji or Gala apple

1. Preheat oven to 350 degrees. Spray an 8-inch by 8-inch baking pan with nonstick spray.

2. In a large bowl, combine oats, chia seeds, sweetener, baking powder, cinnamon, pumpkin pie spice, and salt. Mix well.

3. In a medium-large bowl, combine almond milk, applesauce, egg whites, and vanilla extract. Mix until uniform.

4. Add mixture in the medium-large bowl to the large bowl. Stir until uniform.

5. Fold in apple.

6. Transfer the mixture to the baking pan, and smooth out the surface.

7. Bake until top is light golden brown and entire dish is cooked through, about 35 minutes.

MAKES 6 SERVINGS

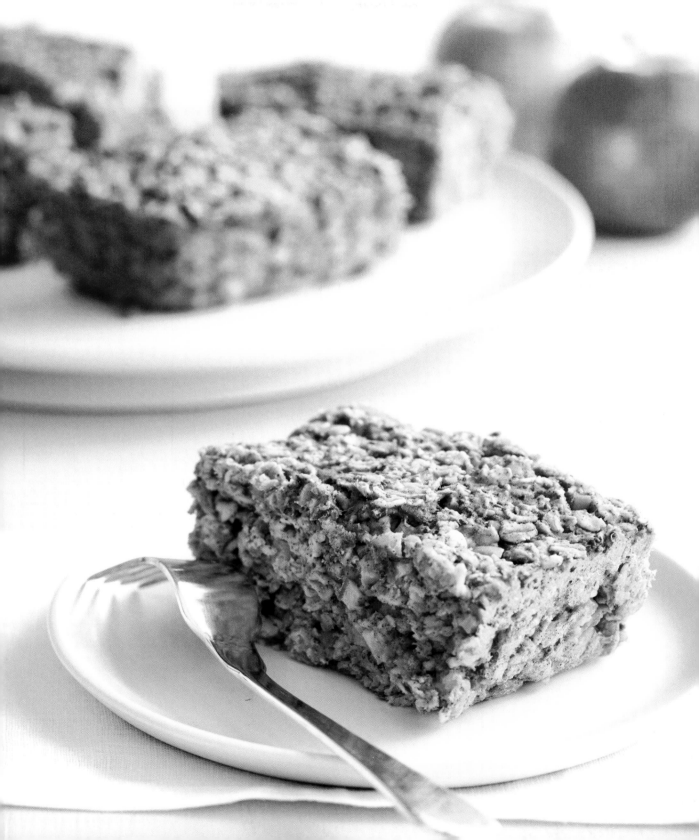

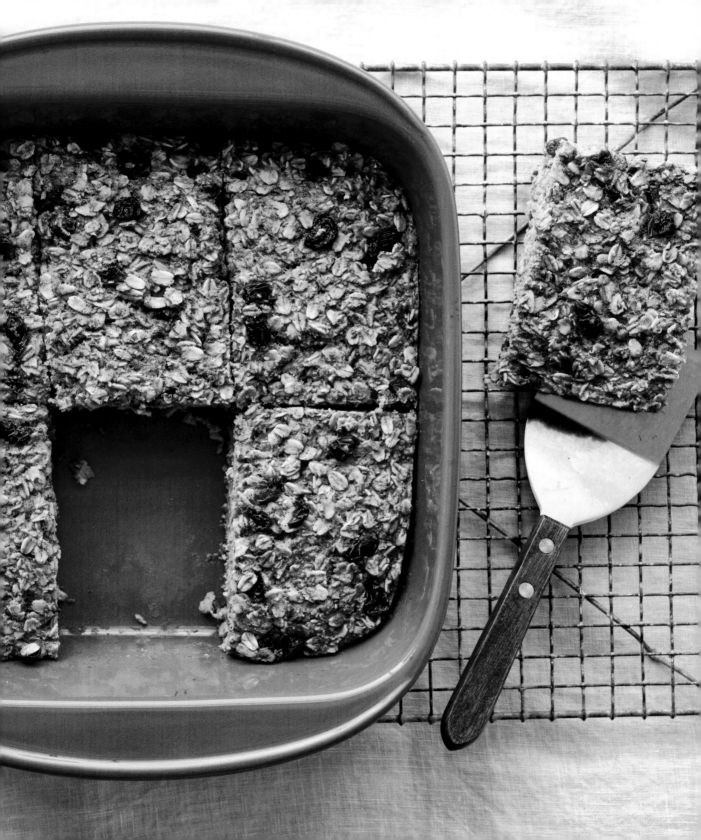

Cinnamon Raisin Oatmeal Bake

⅛th of pan (about 4 inches by 2½ inches): 232 calories, 4.5g total fat (0.5g sat fat), 338mg sodium, 40g carbs, 7g fiber, 9.5g sugars, 8.5g protein

You'll Need: 8-inch by 8-inch baking pan, nonstick spray, large bowl, medium-large bowl

Prep: 15 minutes • **Cook:** 35 minutes

3 cups old-fashioned oats

1½ tablespoons chia seeds

4 packets natural no-calorie sweetener

1 tablespoon cinnamon

2 teaspoons baking powder

¼ teaspoon nutmeg

¼ teaspoon salt

1½ cups unsweetened vanilla almond milk

½ cup unsweetened applesauce

½ cup (about 4 large) egg whites

2 teaspoons vanilla extract

⅓ cup raisins, chopped

1. Preheat oven to 350 degrees. Spray an 8-inch by 8-inch baking pan with nonstick spray.

2. In a large bowl, combine oats, chia seeds, sweetener, cinnamon, baking powder, nutmeg, and salt. Mix well.

3. In a medium-large bowl, combine almond milk, applesauce, egg whites, and vanilla extract. Mix until uniform.

4. Add mixture in the medium-large bowl to the large bowl. Stir until uniform.

5. Fold in chopped raisins.

6. Transfer the mixture to the baking pan, and smooth out the surface.

7. Bake until top is light golden brown and entire dish is cooked through, about 35 minutes.

MAKES 6 SERVINGS

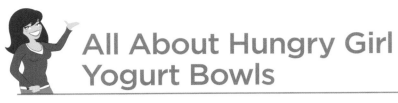

All About Hungry Girl
Yogurt Bowls

It doesn't get much easier than these 5-minute morning meals. (You can chill 'em if you like, but it's definitely not necessary.) Greek yogurt brings so much protein to the table—literally! Combine that with fiber-packed fruit, and you're looking at some seriously satisfying, healthy breakfast options. Plus, Greek yogurt's rich taste and thick, creamy texture are fantastic. And if you're skeptical of its tartness, worry not: The sweetener and extracts in these recipes round out the yogurt's flavor perfectly.

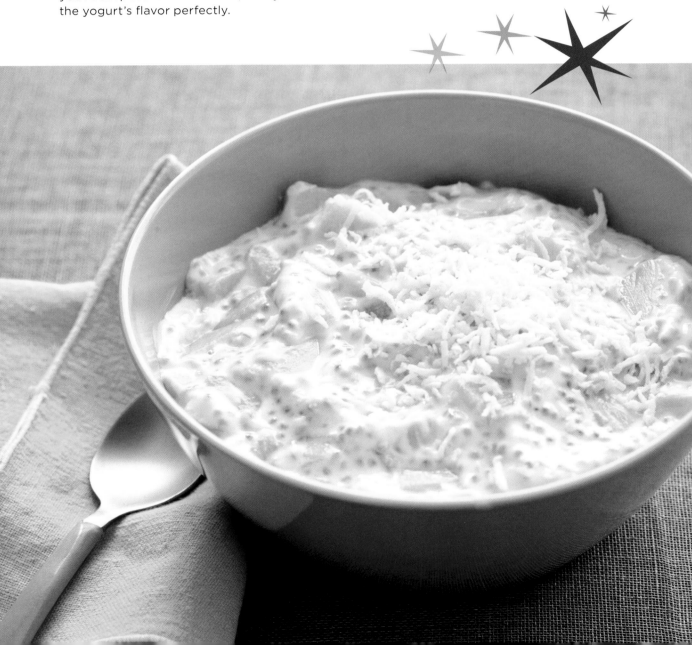

Tropical Chia Yogurt Bowl

Entire recipe: 242 calories, 8g total fat (3g sat fat), 93mg sodium, 32g carbs, 8g fiber, 22g sugars, 16g protein

You'll Need: medium bowl

Prep: 5 minutes • **Chill (optional):** 3 hours

½ **cup fat-free plain Greek yogurt**

¼ **cup unsweetened vanilla almond milk**

2 packets natural no-calorie sweetener

2 drops coconut extract

¾ **cup chopped mango**

1 tablespoon chia seeds

1 tablespoon unsweetened shredded coconut

1. In a medium bowl, combine yogurt, almond milk, sweetener, and coconut extract. Mix until smooth and uniform.

2. Stir in mango and chia seeds.

3. Top with coconut.

4. If you like, refrigerate until yogurt has thickened and chia seeds have expanded, about 3 hours.

MAKES 1 SERVING

Strawberry Chia Yogurt Bowl

Entire recipe: 238 calories, 8g total fat (0.5g sat fat),
64mg sodium, 24g carbs, 8.5g fiber, 12.5g sugars, 20.5g protein

You'll Need: medium bowl

Prep: 5 minutes • **Chill (optional):** 3 hours

¾ **cup sliced strawberries**

⅔ **cup fat-free plain Greek yogurt**

1 tablespoon chia seeds

2 packets natural no-calorie sweetener

½ **teaspoon vanilla extract**

¼ **ounce (about 1 tablespoon) sliced almonds**

1. In a medium bowl, thoroughly mash strawberries with a fork. Add all remaining ingredients *except* almonds. Mix until uniform.

2. Top with almonds.

3. If you like, refrigerate until yogurt has thickened and chia seeds have expanded, about 3 hours.

MAKES 1 SERVING

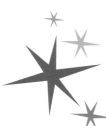

For more healthy recipes, plus the latest food news, tips & tricks, and more, **sign up for free daily emails at Hungry-Girl.com!**

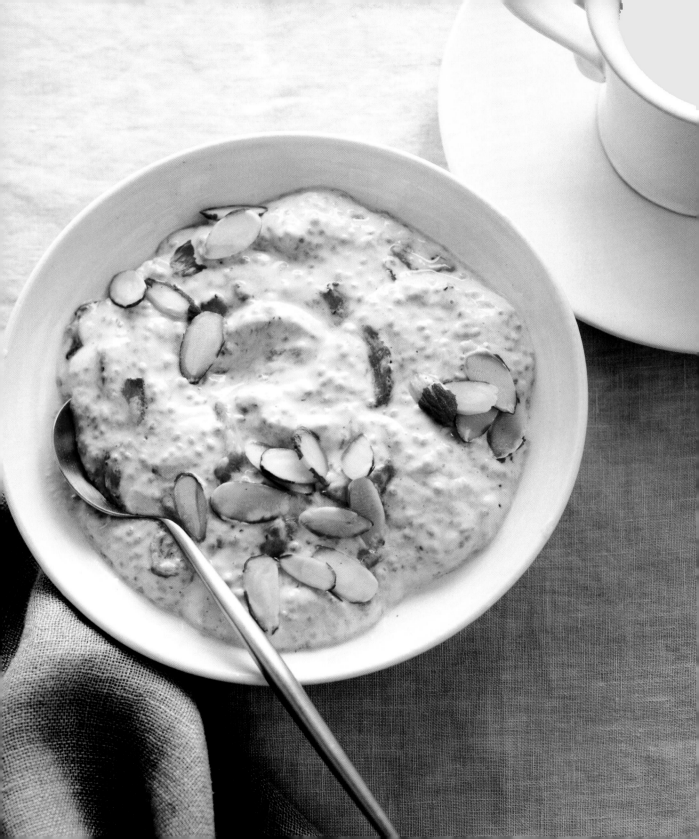

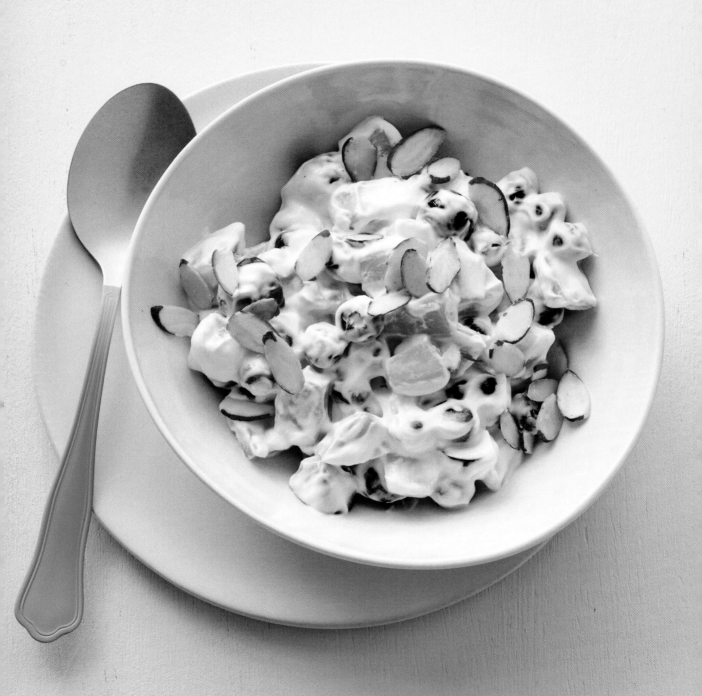

Fruit Salad Yogurt Bowl

Entire recipe: 284 calories, 4g total fat (<0.5g sat fat), 85mg sodium, 46g carbs, 5g fiber, 36.5g sugars, 21g protein

You'll Need: medium bowl

Prep: 5 minutes

¾ **cup fat-free plain Greek yogurt**

1 packet natural no-calorie sweetener

½ **cup chopped cantaloupe**

½ **cup blueberries**

½ **cup halved grapes**

¼ **cup chopped pineapple**

¼ **ounce (about 1 tablespoon) sliced almonds**

1. In a medium bowl, stir sweetener into yogurt. Add all fruit, and mix well.

2. Sprinkle with almonds.

MAKES 1 SERVING

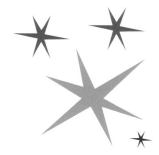

Cherry-Vanilla Super Yogurt

Entire recipe: 251 calories, 6.5g total fat (0.5g sat fat), 85mg sodium, 28.5g carbs, 6g fiber, 20g sugars, 22.5g protein

This one's called Super Yogurt because it's boosted with protein powder and made with chia seeds (a superfood). For tips on choosing the best protein powder, flip to page 5.

You'll Need: medium bowl or jar

Prep: 5 minutes • **Chill (optional):** 3 hours

½ **cup fat-free plain Greek yogurt**

2 **tablespoons plain protein powder with about 100 calories per serving**

2 **tablespoons unsweetened vanilla almond milk**

1 **packet natural no-calorie sweetener**

⅛ **teaspoon vanilla extract**

Dash cinnamon

1½ **teaspoons chia seeds**

¾ **cup pitted dark sweet cherries (fresh or thawed from frozen and drained), chopped**

¼ **ounce (about 1 tablespoon) sliced almonds**

1. In a medium bowl or jar, combine yogurt, protein powder, almond milk, sweetener, vanilla extract, and cinnamon. Mix until smooth and uniform.

2. Stir in chia seeds and chopped cherries.

3. Top with almonds.

4. If you like, refrigerate until yogurt has thickened and chia seeds have expanded, about 3 hours.

MAKES 1 SERVING

Ingredient FYI

If using frozen cherries versus fresh, check the ingredient list to make sure no sugar has been added.

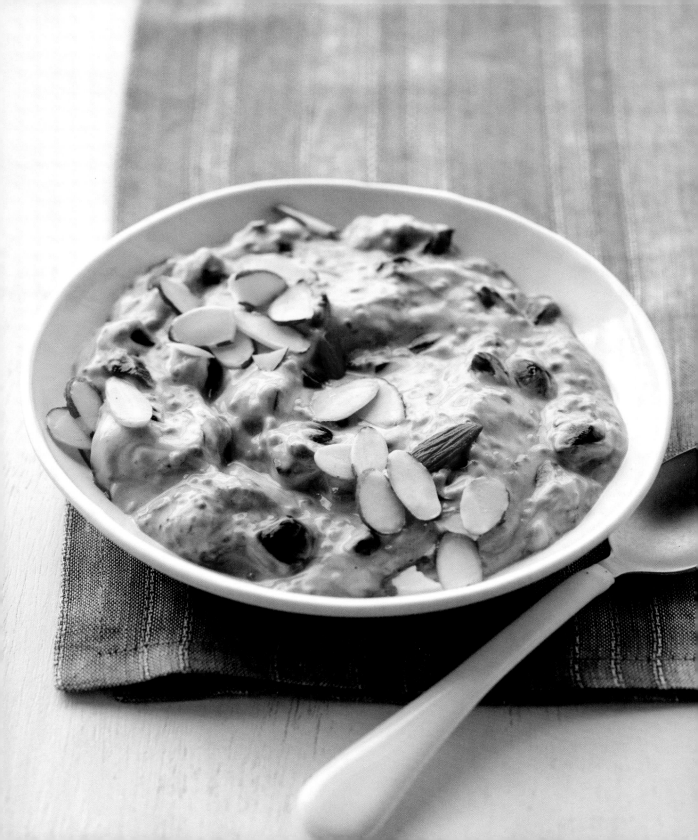

2

Egg Mugs, Skillet Scrambles, Burritos & Bakes

If you like protein-packed, savory, hot meals in the morning, this is the chapter for you . . .

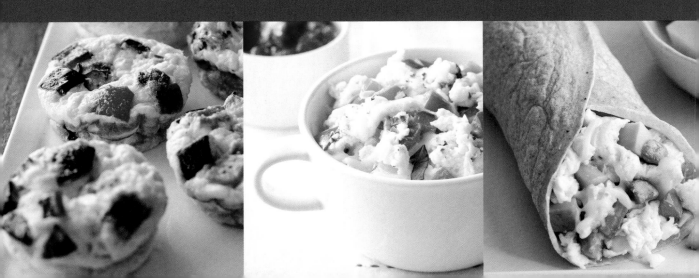

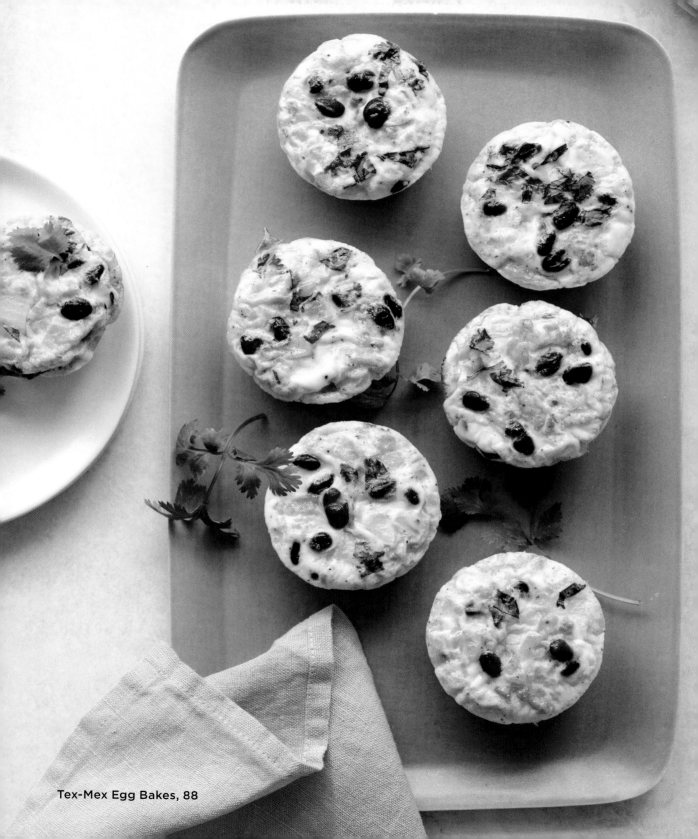

Tex-Mex Egg Bakes, 88

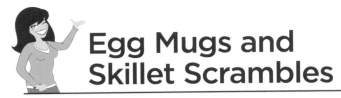

Egg Mugs and Skillet Scrambles

Unfamiliar with the egg mug phenomenon? Hungry Girl egg mugs are scrambles made *in the microwave*. Quick, easy, and you don't even need to turn on the stove or break out a skillet and spatula! If you prefer to go the skillet route, every egg mug recipe in this chapter has alternate stovetop directions. Now about those egg mugs . . .

First things first: Grab a large microwave-safe mug. Why a large one? The egg mixture rises and puffs up while it cooks; a large mug will avoid messy spillover. Your best bet: A tall, wide mug with a 16-ounce capacity. Another option? Any tall or wide microwave-safe bowl will do the trick.

To keep your scramble from sticking to the mug, give the inside of the mug a good spritz with nonstick spray. If you prefer to avoid aerosol containers, go the DIY route: Pour your favorite oil into a food-safe misting bottle. Olive oil works, and grapeseed oil is great too. You can also buy non-aerosol sprays, like the ones from Pompeian.

For easy cleanup, act fast. Right after you're done eating, soak your mug with warm soapy water.

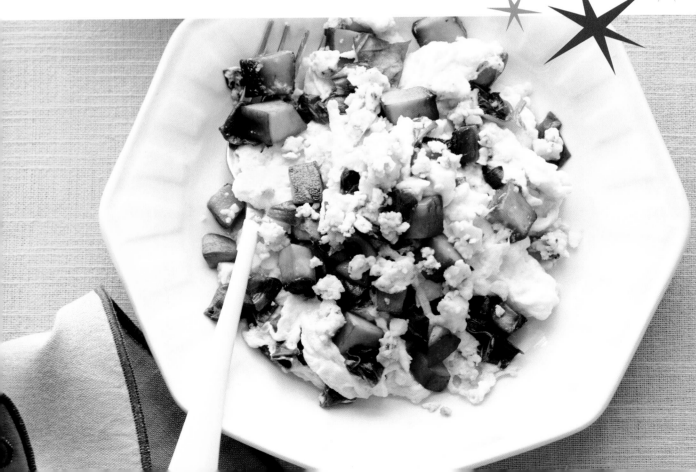

Portabella Blue Egg Mug

Entire recipe: 166 calories, 4.5g total fat (2.5g sat fat), 514mg sodium, 5.5g carbs, 1g fiber, 3g sugars, 24.5g protein

You'll Need: large microwave-safe mug, nonstick spray

Prep: 5 minutes • **Cook:** 5 minutes

½ cup chopped portabella mushrooms

½ cup chopped spinach leaves

¾ cup (about 6 large) egg whites

1 teaspoon dried minced onion

2 tablespoons crumbled blue cheese

1. Spray a large microwave-safe mug with nonstick spray. Microwave mushrooms and spinach for 1 minute, or until mushrooms have slightly softened and spinach has wilted.

2. Blot away excess moisture. Add egg whites and onion, and stir. Microwave for 1 minute.

3. Mix in cheese. Microwave for 1 more minute, or until set.

MAKES 1 SERVING

In a skillet . . .

1. Bring a skillet sprayed with nonstick spray to medium heat. Cook and stir mushrooms until slightly softened and lightly browned, about 2 minutes.

2. Add spinach, and cook and stir until wilted, about 1 minute.

3. Add egg whites and onion. Cook and scramble until mushrooms are soft and egg whites are fully cooked, about 2 minutes.

4. Remove from heat, and stir in cheese.

Swiss Chick Egg Mug

Entire recipe: 218 calories, 4.5g total fat (2g sat fat), 742mg sodium, 7g carbs, 1g fiber, 3.5g sugars, 34.5g protein

You'll Need: large microwave-safe mug, nonstick spray

Prep: 5 minutes • **Cook:** 5 minutes

¼ **cup sliced mushrooms**

¼ **cup chopped onion**

¾ **cup (about 6 large) egg whites**

1 teaspoon Dijon mustard (grainy, if available)

Dash each salt and black pepper, or more to taste

1 ounce cooked and chopped skinless chicken breast

1 slice reduced-fat Swiss cheese, broken into pieces

1. Spray a large microwave-safe mug with nonstick spray. Microwave mushrooms and onion for 1 minute, or until slightly softened.

2. Blot away excess moisture. Add egg whites, mustard, salt, and pepper. Stir well. Microwave for 1 minute.

3. Mix in chicken and cheese. Microwave for 1 more minute, or until set.

MAKES 1 SERVING

In a skillet . . .

1. Bring a skillet sprayed with nonstick spray to medium heat. Add mushrooms and onion. Cook and stir until veggies have slightly softened and lightly browned, about 3 minutes.

2. Add egg whites, chicken, mustard, salt, and pepper. Cook and scramble until veggies are soft, egg whites are fully cooked, and chicken is hot, about 2 minutes.

3. Reduce heat to low. Add cheese, and cook and stir until melted, about 1 minute.

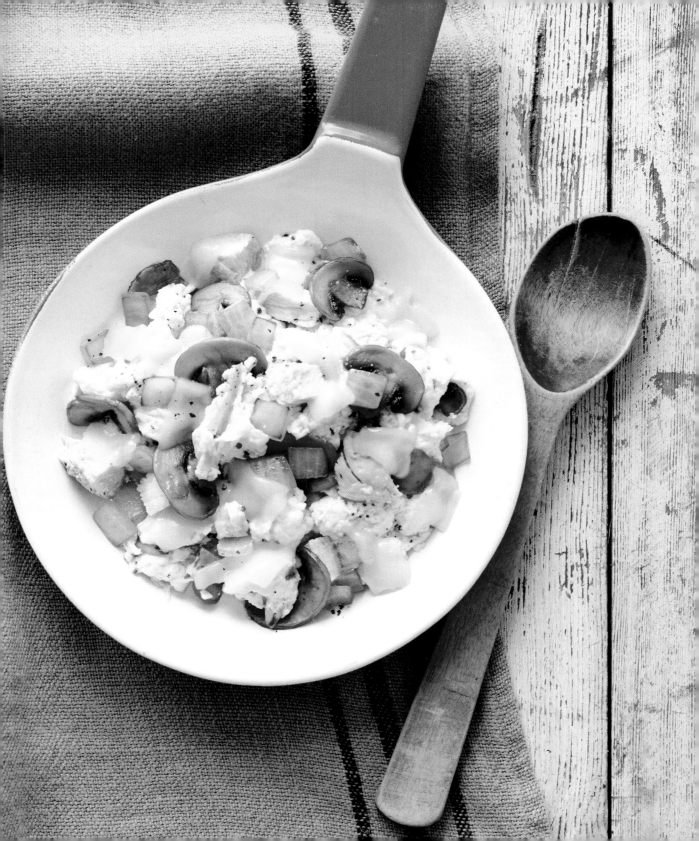

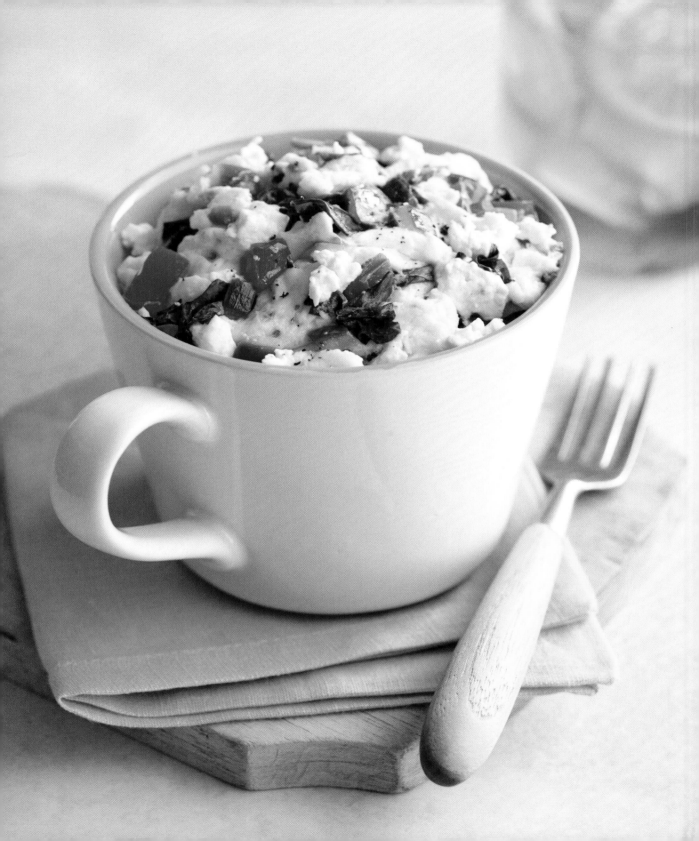

Mediterranean Egg Mug

Entire recipe: 156 calories, 3g total fat (2g sat fat), 500mg sodium, 6.5g carbs, 1.5g fiber, 3.5g sugars, 23.5g protein

You'll Need: large microwave-safe mug, nonstick spray

Prep: 5 minutes • **Cook:** 5 minutes

1 cup chopped spinach leaves

¼ cup seeded and chopped tomato

2 tablespoons chopped red onion

¾ cup (about 6 large) egg whites

⅛ teaspoon oregano

Dash black pepper

2 tablespoons crumbled feta cheese

1. Spray a large microwave-safe mug with nonstick spray. Add spinach, tomato, and onion. Microwave for 1 minute, or until spinach has wilted and tomato and onion have slightly softened.

2. Blot away excess moisture. Add egg whites, oregano, and pepper. Stir, and microwave for 1 minute.

3. Mix in feta cheese. Microwave for 1 more minute, or until set.

MAKES 1 SERVING

In a skillet . . .

1. Bring a skillet sprayed with nonstick spray to medium heat. Cook and stir tomato and onion until slightly softened and lightly browned, about 3 minutes.

2. Add spinach, and cook and stir until wilted, about 1 minute.

3. Add egg whites, oregano, and pepper. Cook and scramble until veggies are soft and egg whites are fully cooked, about 2 minutes.

4. Remove from heat, and stir in cheese.

Cheesy Italian Egg Mug

Entire recipe: 209 calories, 5.5g total fat (3.5g sat fat), 492mg sodium, 10g carbs, 1.5g fiber, 5g sugars, 28.5g protein

You'll Need: large microwave-safe mug, nonstick spray

Prep: 5 minutes • **Cook:** 5 minutes

¼ **cup seeded and chopped tomato**

¼ **cup chopped green bell pepper**

¼ **cup chopped onion**

½ **teaspoon chopped garlic**

⅛ **teaspoon Italian seasoning**

¾ **cup (about 6 large) egg whites**

¼ **cup shredded part-skim mozzarella cheese**

1 **tablespoon chopped fresh basil**

Optional topping: Clean & Hungry Marinara Sauce (recipe and store-bought alternatives on page 20)

1. Spray a large microwave-safe mug with nonstick spray. Add tomato, pepper, onion, garlic, and Italian seasoning. Microwave for 1 minute, or until slightly softened.

2. Blot away excess moisture. Add egg whites, and stir. Microwave for 1 minute.

3. Mix in cheese and basil. Microwave for 1 more minute, or until set.

MAKES 1 SERVING

In a skillet . . .

1. Bring a skillet sprayed with nonstick spray to medium heat. Add tomato, pepper, onion, garlic, and Italian seasoning. Cook and stir until slightly softened and lightly browned, about 4 minutes.

2. Add egg whites. Cook and scramble until veggies are soft and egg whites are fully cooked, about 2 minutes.

3. Remove from heat, and stir in cheese and basil.

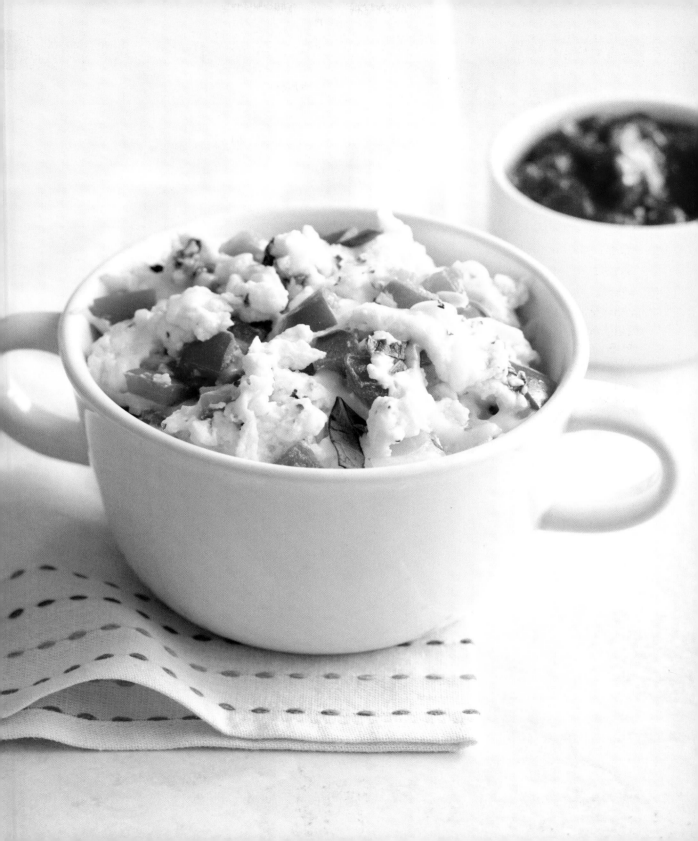

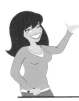

Best-Ever Burritos

All-natural breakfast wraps with no more than 250 calories each? Yup! These recipes call for Clean & Hungry Whole-Wheat Tortillas (page 25). Those are packed with protein and have less than 80 calories each. Keep a batch in the fridge or freezer, and these burritos will be ready in no time. Rather stick with store-bought whole-wheat tortillas? Grab all-natural ones with the lowest calorie count you can find, and adjust the recipe stats accordingly . . .

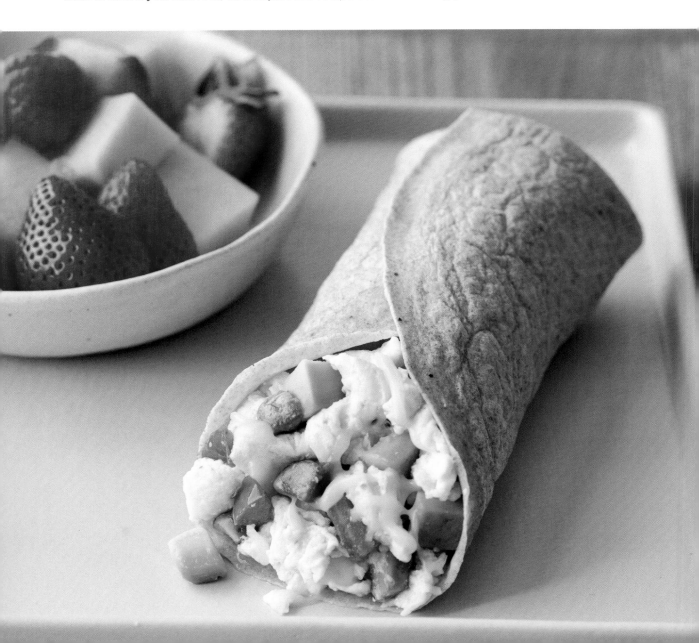

California Breakfast Burrito

Entire recipe: 238 calories, 7.5g total fat (2.5g sat fat), 579mg sodium, 18g carbs, 4.5g fiber, 3g sugars, 25g protein

You'll Need: large microwave-safe mug, nonstick spray, microwave-safe plate

Prep: 5 minutes • **Cook:** 5 minutes

¼ **cup seeded and chopped tomato**

¼ **cup chopped mushrooms**

½ **cup (about 4 large) egg whites**

⅛ **teaspoon garlic powder**

Dash black pepper

2 **tablespoons shredded part-skim mozzarella cheese**

1 **Clean & Hungry Whole-Wheat Tortilla (recipe and store-bought alternatives on page 25)**

1 **ounce (about 2 tablespoons) chopped avocado**

1. Spray a large microwave-safe mug with nonstick spray. Microwave tomato and mushrooms for 1 minute, or until slightly softened.

2. Blot away excess moisture. Add egg whites, garlic powder, and pepper. Stir, and microwave for 1 minute.

3. Mix in cheese. Microwave for 1 more minute, or until set.

4. Microwave tortilla on a microwave-safe plate for 10 seconds, or until warm.

5. Place egg scramble across the middle of the tortilla. Top with avocado.

6. Wrap tortilla up by first folding in one side (to keep filling from escaping) and then tightly rolling it up from the bottom.

MAKES 1 SERVING

To make the egg scramble in a skillet . . .

1. Bring a skillet sprayed with nonstick spray to medium heat. Add tomato and mushrooms. Cook and stir until slightly softened, about 2 minutes.

2. Add egg whites, garlic powder, and pepper. Cook and scramble until veggies are soft and egg whites are fully cooked, about 2 minutes.

3. Remove from heat, and stir in cheese.

Mexican Breakfast Burrito

Entire recipe: 250 calories, 3.5g total fat (1.5g sat fat), 669mg sodium, 28g carbs, 5g fiber, 5.5g sugars, 26.5g protein

You'll Need: large microwave-safe mug, nonstick spray, microwave-safe plate

Prep: 5 minutes • **Cook:** 5 minutes

¼ **cup chopped bell pepper**

¼ **cup chopped onion**

2 tablespoons frozen sweet corn kernels

½ **cup (about 4 large) egg whites**

Dash cayenne pepper

Dash garlic powder

2 tablespoons shredded reduced-fat Mexican-blend cheese

2 tablespoons canned black beans, drained and rinsed

1 Clean & Hungry Whole-Wheat Tortilla (recipe and store-bought alternatives on page 25)

Optional topping: Clean & Hungry Salsa (recipe and store-bought alternatives on page 18)

1. Spray a large microwave-safe mug with nonstick spray. Add bell pepper, onion, and corn. Microwave for 1 minute, or until pepper and onion have slightly softened and corn has thawed.

2. Blot away excess moisture. Add egg whites, cayenne pepper, and garlic powder. Stir, and microwave for 1 minute.

3. Mix in cheese and beans. Microwave for 1 more minute, or until set.

4. Microwave tortilla on a microwave-safe plate for 10 seconds, or until warm.

5. Place egg scramble across the middle of the tortilla.

6. Wrap tortilla up by first folding in one side (to keep filling from escaping) and then tightly rolling it up from the bottom.

MAKES 1 SERVING

To make the egg scramble in a skillet . . .

1. Bring a skillet sprayed with nonstick spray to medium heat. Add bell pepper, onion, and corn. Cook and stir until pepper and onion have slightly softened and corn has thawed, about 3 minutes.

2. Add egg whites, cayenne pepper, and garlic powder. Cook and scramble until veggies are soft and egg whites are fully cooked, about 2 minutes.

3. Add beans, and cook and stir until hot, about 1 minute.

4. Remove from heat, and stir in cheese.

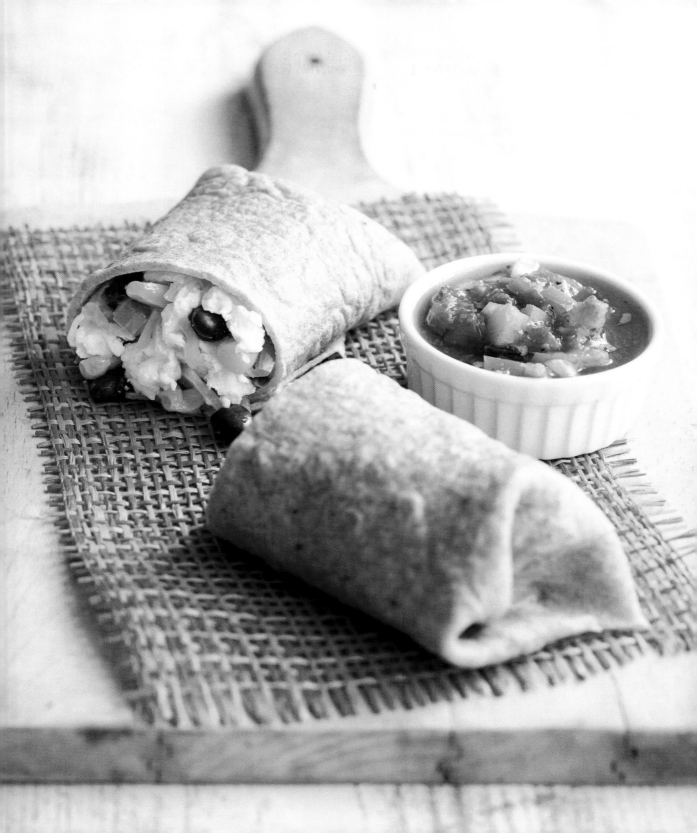

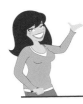

All About Egg Bakes

Looking for great make-ahead morning meals or grab-n-go breakfasts to feed a small crowd? Perfect! Baked in a muffin pan, these egg bakes are convenient, healthy, satisfying, and delicious. They even make *excellent* mid-day snacks . . .

If you're not eating the egg bakes immediately or you have leftovers, let them cool completely. Then cover and refrigerate until you're ready to eat 'em.

For best results, reheat in the microwave. First, wrap an egg bake in a paper towel. Then microwave for 20 seconds, or until hot.

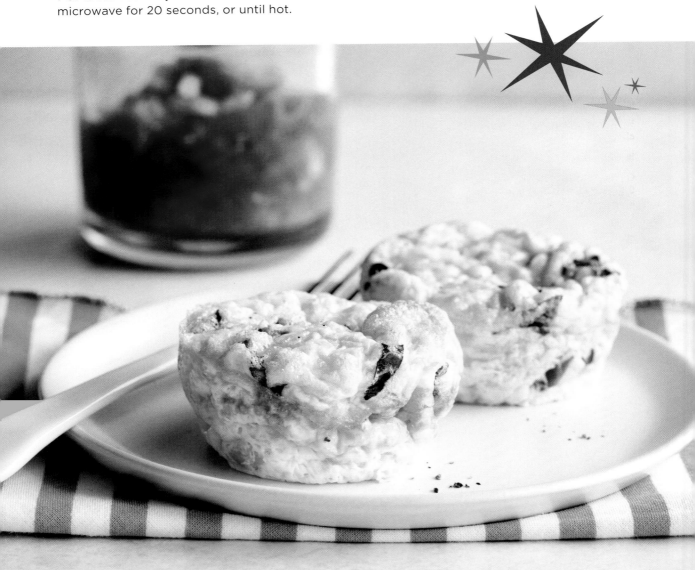

Roasted Veggie Egg Bakes

⅙ᵗʰ of recipe (2 egg bakes): 122 calories, 3g total fat (2g sat fat), 384mg sodium, 7g carbs, 1g fiber, 3g sugars, 15.5g protein

You'll Need: large baking sheet, 12-cup muffin pan, nonstick spray, large bowl, whisk

Prep: 20 minutes • **Cook:** 40 minutes

1 cup chopped bell pepper

1 cup chopped onion

1 cup chopped zucchini

¼ teaspoon each salt and black pepper

2½ cups (about 20) egg whites

2 tablespoons fat-free plain Greek yogurt

¾ cup shredded reduced-fat cheddar cheese

¼ cup chopped fresh basil

Optional topping: Clean & Hungry Salsa (recipe and store-bought alternatives on page 18)

1. Preheat oven to 400 degrees. Spray a large baking sheet and a 12-cup muffin pan with nonstick spray.

2. Lay veggies on the baking sheet, evenly spaced. Season with salt and black pepper.

3. Bake for 10 minutes.

4. Stir/rearrange veggies. Bake until softened and lightly browned, about 10 more minutes.

5. Remove baking sheet from oven, and reduce heat to 350 degrees.

6. In a large bowl, whisk egg whites with Greek yogurt until mostly smooth. Add cheese, basil, and cooked veggies. Stir to mix.

7. Evenly distribute mixture among the cups of the muffin pan. (Cups will be full.)

8. Bake until firm and cooked through, about 20 minutes.

MAKES 6 SERVINGS

Tex-Mex Egg Bakes

⅛th of recipe (2 egg bakes): 177 calories, 5g total fat (2g sat fat), 457mg sodium, 10g carbs, 1.5g fiber, 3g sugars, 22.5g protein

You'll Need: 12-cup muffin pan, nonstick spray, skillet, large bowl, whisk

Prep: 20 minutes • **Cook:** 25 minutes

6 ounces raw lean ground turkey (7% fat or less)

¼ teaspoon garlic powder

¼ teaspoon onion powder

¼ teaspoon each salt and black pepper

1 cup chopped onion

½ cup frozen sweet corn kernels

2½ cups (about 20 large) egg whites

2 tablespoons fat-free plain Greek yogurt

¾ cup shredded reduced-fat Mexican-blend cheese

½ cup canned black beans, drained and rinsed

2 tablespoons chopped fresh cilantro

¼ teaspoon chili powder

¼ teaspoon ground cumin

1. Preheat oven to 350 degrees. Spray a 12-cup muffin pan with nonstick spray.

2. Bring a skillet sprayed with nonstick spray to medium-high heat. Add turkey, and sprinkle with garlic powder, onion powder, and ⅛ teaspoon each salt and pepper. Add onion and corn. Cook, stir, and crumble until turkey is fully cooked, onion has softened and lightly browned, and corn has thawed and slightly blackened, about 4 minutes.

3. In a large bowl, whisk egg whites with Greek yogurt until mostly smooth. Add cheese, beans, cilantro, chili powder, cumin, turkey mixture, and remaining ⅛ teaspoon each salt and pepper. Stir to mix.

4. Evenly distribute mixture among the cups of the muffin pan. (Cups will be full.)

5. Bake until firm and cooked through, about 20 minutes.

MAKES 6 SERVINGS

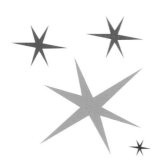

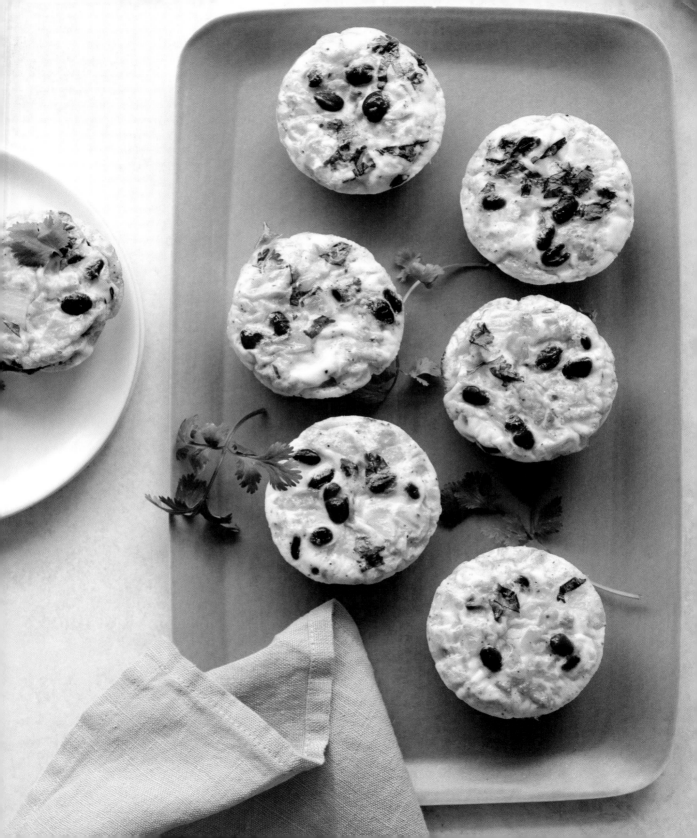

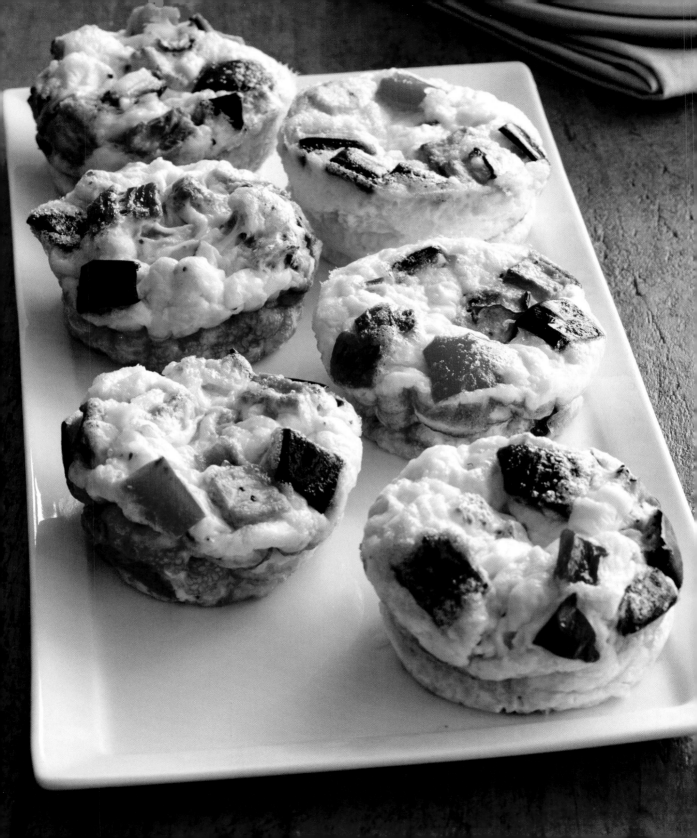

Sun-Dried Tomato & Feta Egg Bakes

⅙th of recipe (2 egg bakes): 124 calories, 3g total fat (2g sat fat), 449mg sodium, 7.5g carbs, 2g fiber, 4.5g sugars, 14.5g protein

You'll Need: baking sheet, 12-cup muffin pan, nonstick spray, large bowl, whisk

Prep: 20 minutes • **Cook:** 45 minutes

1 cup eggplant cut into ½-inch cubes

½ cup chopped red bell pepper

½ cup chopped red onion

¼ teaspoon each salt and black pepper

¼ teaspoon garlic powder

¼ teaspoon onion powder

2½ cups (about 20 large) egg whites

2 tablespoons fat-free plain Greek yogurt

⅓ cup bagged sun-dried tomatoes (not packed in oil), chopped

¾ cup crumbled feta cheese

1. Preheat oven to 400 degrees. Spray a baking sheet and a 12-cup muffin pan with nonstick spray.

2. Lay veggies on the baking sheet, evenly spaced. Sprinkle with salt, black pepper, and ⅛ teaspoon each garlic powder and onion powder.

3. Bake for 10 minutes.

4. Stir/rearrange veggies. Bake until softened and lightly browned, about 10 more minutes.

5. Remove baking sheet from oven, and reduce heat to 350 degrees.

6. In a large bowl, combine egg whites, Greek yogurt, and remaining ⅛ teaspoon each garlic powder and onion powder. Whisk until mostly smooth. Add cooked veggies, sun-dried tomatoes, and feta cheese. Stir to mix.

7. Evenly distribute mixture among the cups of the muffin pan. (Cups will be full.)

8. Bake until firm and cooked through, about 25 minutes.

MAKES 6 SERVINGS

3

Pancakes & Waffles

Pancakes and waffles that are completely guilt-free *and* all-natural are entirely possible. This chapter proves that again, and again, and again . . .

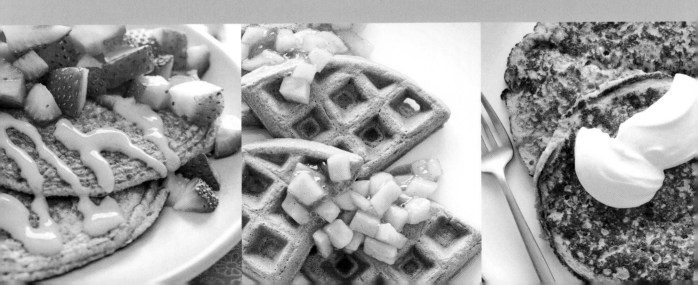

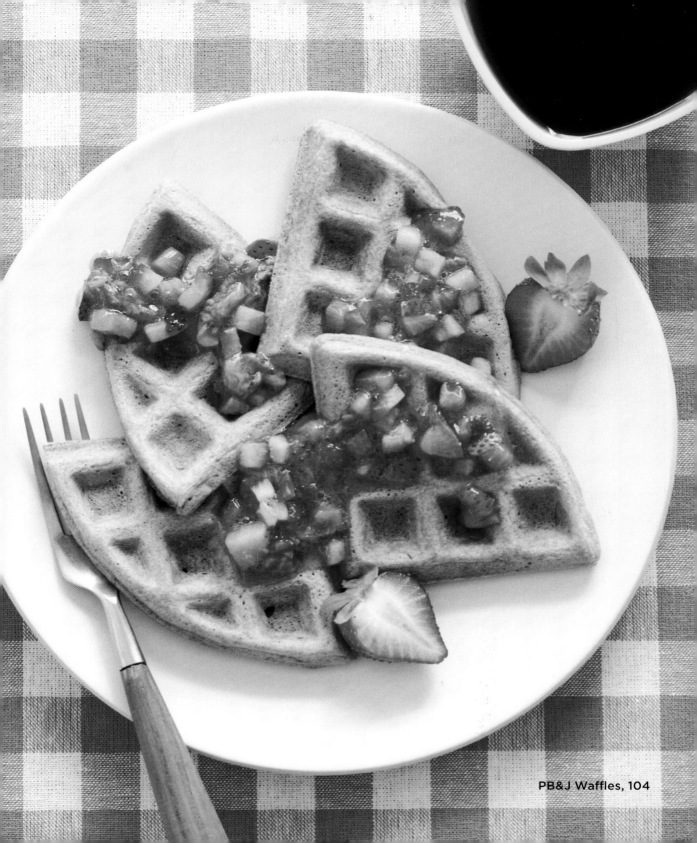

PB&J Waffles, 104

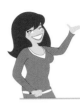

Pancake Perfection

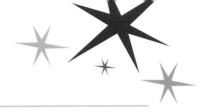

Your average flapjacks are pretty much all carbs. Not these! They're loaded with protein and fiber, thanks to egg whites, oat bran, and whole-wheat flour. They're also light, fluffy, and all-around amazing . . .

Quick tip!

Each of these recipes makes two large pancakes. The first pancake generally takes longer to cook, so keep an eye on that second one; it'll cook faster.

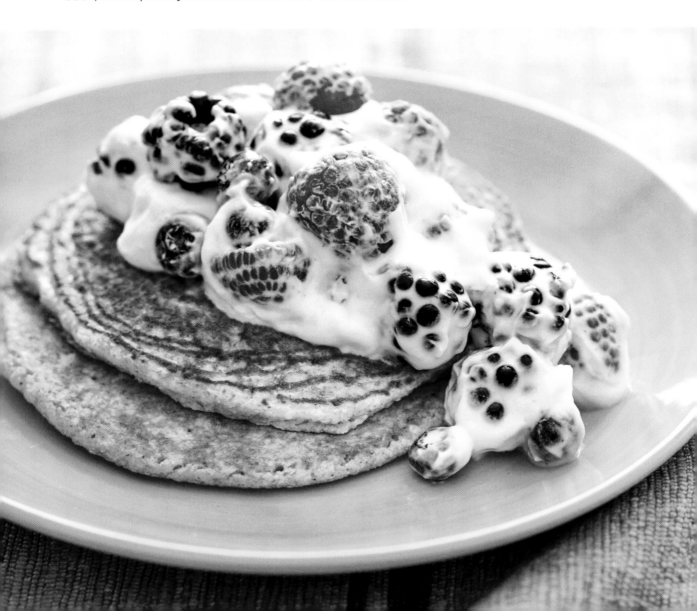

Berries & Cream Pancakes

Entire recipe: 278 calories, 2.5g total fat (<0.5g sat fat),
530mg sodium, 44.5g carbs, 11g fiber, 14g sugars, 21g protein

You'll Need: small bowl, medium bowl, skillet, nonstick spray, plate

Prep: 10 minutes • **Cook:** 10 minutes

Topping

⅓ **cup fat-free plain Greek yogurt**

1 packet natural no-calorie sweetener

⅛ **teaspoon vanilla extract**

¼ **cup blackberries**

¼ **cup raspberries**

2 tablespoons blueberries

Pancakes

¼ **cup (about 2 large) egg whites**

¼ **cup unsweetened applesauce**

¼ **cup oat bran**

1 tablespoon whole-wheat flour

1 packet natural no-calorie sweetener

½ **teaspoon baking powder**

⅛ **teaspoon vanilla extract**

Dash cinnamon

Dash salt

1. To make the topping, place Greek yogurt in a small bowl. Stir in sweetener and vanilla extract. Fold in berries.

2. Combine all pancake ingredients in a medium bowl. Mix until uniform.

3. Bring a skillet sprayed with nonstick spray to medium heat. Add half of the batter to form a large pancake. Cook until it begins to bubble and is solid enough to flip, 1 to 2 minutes.

4. Gently flip, and cook until both sides are lightly browned and inside is cooked through, about 1 minute.

5. Plate your pancake. Remove skillet from heat, re-spray, and return to medium heat. Repeat with remaining batter to make a second pancake.

6. Top pancakes with topping.

MAKES 1 SERVING

Strawberries 'n Peanut Butter Pancakes

Entire recipe: 295 calories, 5g total fat (<0.5g sat fat), 555mg sodium, 47.5g carbs, 10g fiber, 16.5g sugars, 19g protein

You'll Need: small bowl, medium bowl, skillet, nonstick spray, plate

Prep: 10 minutes • **Cook:** 10 minutes

Topping

2 tablespoons unsweetened vanilla almond milk

2 tablespoons powdered peanut butter or defatted peanut flour

1 teaspoon honey

½ cup chopped strawberries

Pancakes

¼ cup (about 2 large) egg whites

¼ cup unsweetened applesauce

¼ cup oat bran

1 tablespoon whole-wheat flour

1 packet natural no-calorie sweetener

½ teaspoon baking powder

¼ teaspoon cinnamon

⅛ teaspoon vanilla extract

Dash salt

1. In a small bowl, combine all topping ingredients *except* strawberries. Mix until uniform.

2. Combine all pancake ingredients in a medium bowl. Mix until uniform.

3. Bring a skillet sprayed with nonstick spray to medium heat. Add half of the batter to form a large pancake. Cook until it begins to bubble and is solid enough to flip, 1 to 2 minutes.

4. Gently flip, and cook until both sides are lightly browned and inside is cooked through, about 1 minute.

5. Plate your pancake. Remove skillet from heat, re-spray, and return to medium heat. Repeat with remaining batter to make a second pancake.

6. Drizzle peanut butter topping over pancakes, and top with strawberries.

MAKES 1 SERVING

Ingredient FYI

Powdered peanut butter and defatted peanut flour have less than *half* the calories of ordinary peanut butter. For more on these magical ingredients, flip to page 4.

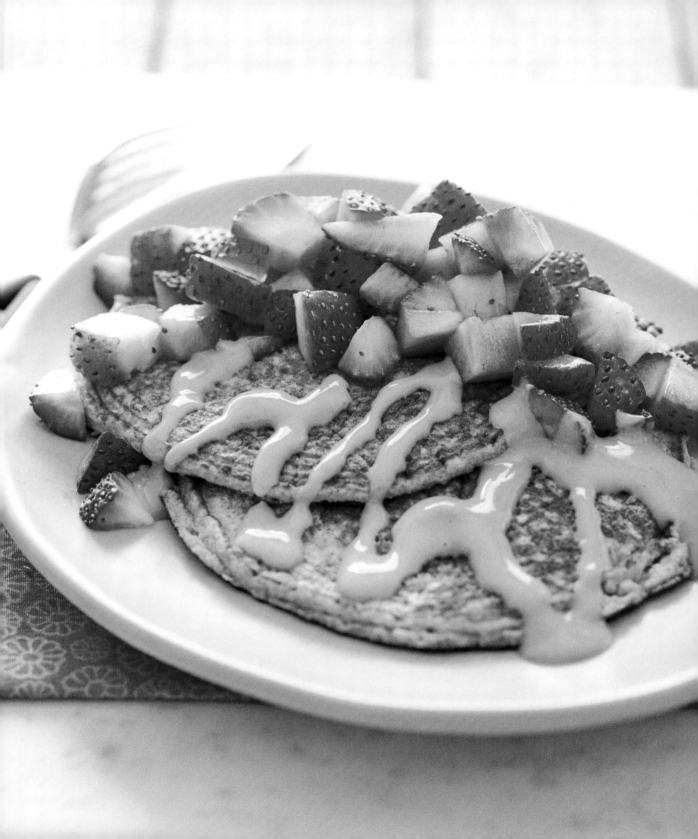

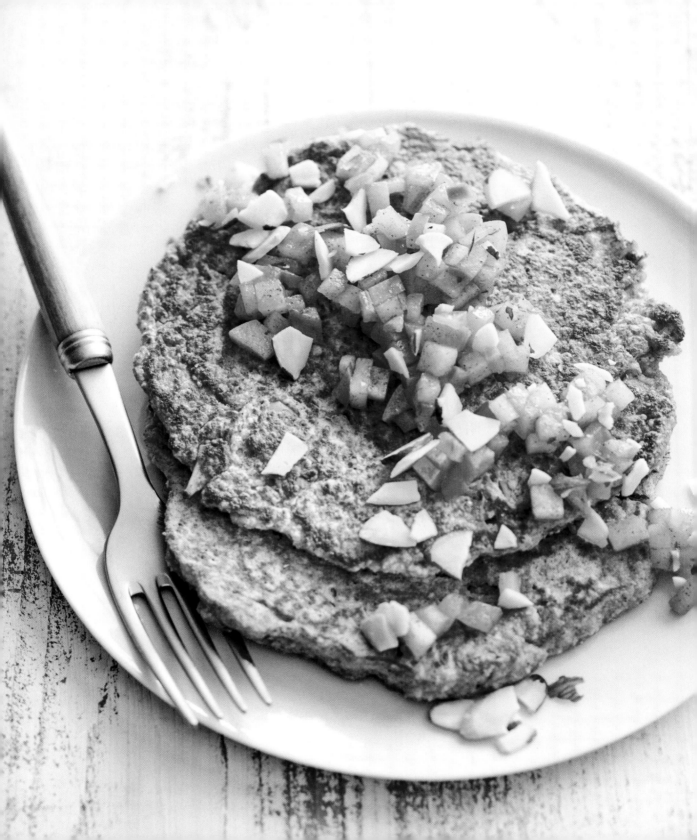

Apple Cinnamon Crunch Pancakes

Entire recipe: 308 calories, 9.5g total fat (1g sat fat), 501mg sodium, 43g carbs, 9.5g fiber, 13g sugars, 16g protein

You'll Need: medium microwave-safe bowl, nonstick spray, medium bowl, skillet, plate

Prep: 10 minutes • **Cook:** 10 minutes

½ **cup finely chopped Fuji or Gala apple**

2 **packets natural no-calorie sweetener**

¼ **teaspoon cinnamon**

¼ **cup (about 2 large) egg whites**

¼ **cup unsweetened applesauce**

¼ **cup oat bran**

1 **tablespoon whole-wheat flour**

½ **teaspoon baking powder**

⅛ **teaspoon vanilla extract**

Dash salt

½ **ounce (about 2 tablespoons) sliced and chopped almonds**

1. Place apple in a medium microwave-safe bowl sprayed with nonstick spray. Sprinkle with 1 sweetener packet and ⅛ teaspoon cinnamon, and stir to coat.

2. Cover and microwave for 1 minute, until apple has softened.

3. To make the pancake batter, in a medium bowl, combine egg whites, applesauce, oat bran, flour, baking powder, vanilla extract, and salt. Add remaining sweetener packet and ⅛ teaspoon cinnamon. Mix until uniform.

4. Add half of the apple mixture (about 2½ tablespoons) and half of the almonds (about 1 tablespoon) to the batter.

5. Bring a skillet sprayed with nonstick spray to medium heat. Add half of the batter to form a large pancake. Cook until it begins to bubble and is solid enough to flip, 1 to 2 minutes.

6. Gently flip, and cook until both sides are lightly browned and inside is cooked through, about 1 minute.

7. Plate your pancake. Remove skillet from heat, re-spray, and return to medium heat. Repeat with remaining batter to make a second pancake.

8. Top pancakes with remaining apple mixture and almonds.

MAKES 1 SERVING

Lemon Ricotta Pancakes

Entire recipe: 262 calories, 5g total fat (2g sat fat), 602mg sodium, 32g carbs, 6g fiber, 6.5g sugars, 24g protein

You'll Need: small bowl, medium bowl, skillet, nonstick spray, plate

Prep: 10 minutes • **Cook:** 10 minutes

¼ **cup fat-free plain Greek yogurt**

2 **packets natural no-calorie sweetener**

¼ **teaspoon vanilla extract**

¼ **cup (about 2 large) egg whites**

¼ **cup light/low-fat ricotta cheese**

¼ **cup oat bran**

1 **tablespoon whole-wheat flour**

2 **teaspoons lemon juice**

1 **teaspoon lemon zest**

½ **teaspoon baking powder**

Dash cinnamon

Dash salt

1. In a small bowl, combine yogurt with 1 sweetener packet and ⅛ teaspoon vanilla extract. Mix until uniform.

2. To make the pancake batter, in a medium bowl, combine all remaining ingredients, including remaining sweetener packet and ⅛ teaspoon vanilla extract. Add 2 tablespoons water, and mix until uniform.

3. Bring a skillet sprayed with nonstick spray to medium heat. Add half of the batter to form a large pancake. Cook until it begins to bubble and is solid enough to flip, 1 to 2 minutes.

4. Gently flip, and cook until both sides are lightly browned and inside is cooked through, about 1 minute.

5. Plate your pancake. Remove skillet from heat, re-spray, and return to medium heat. Repeat with remaining batter to make a second pancake.

6. Top with yogurt mixture.

MAKES 1 SERVING

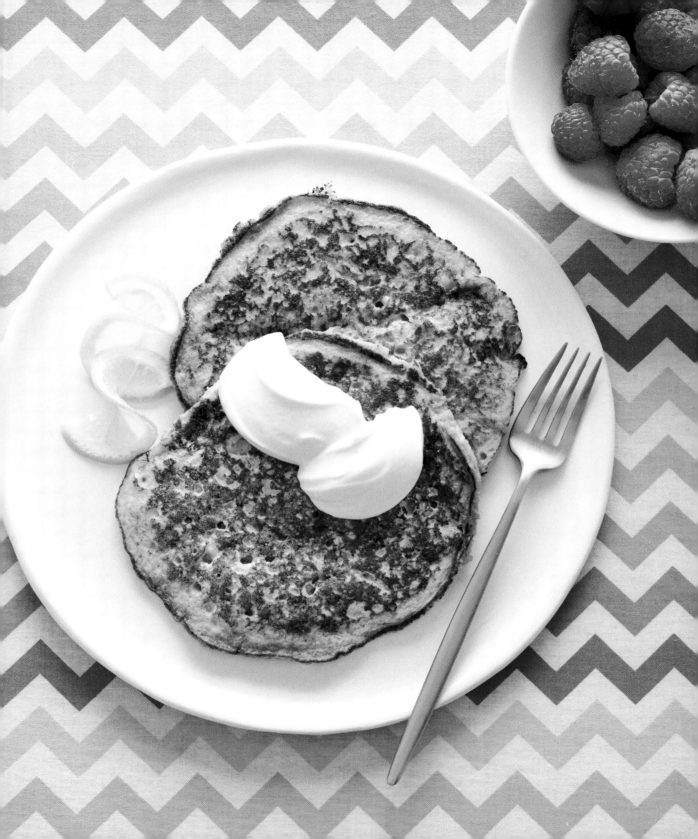

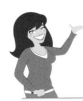
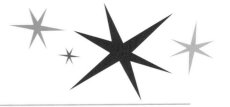

Waffle Tips & Tricks

Never made waffles from scratch before? It's actually pretty easy, and the delicious results are well worth the effort.

When choosing a waffle maker . . . Any standard round waffle maker will do. Look for one that's about 8 inches in diameter.

To store leftovers . . . Let waffles cool completely. Cover and refrigerate until ready to serve. Store (cooled) topping separately, in a covered microwave-safe container in the fridge; before reheating, give it a good stir.

You can even freeze your waffles . . . Just tightly wrap each cooled waffle in plastic wrap. Place individually wrapped waffles in a sealable container or bag, seal, and place in the freezer.

To thaw from frozen . . . For best results, place a single waffle directly on the rack of a toaster oven; toast until hot and crispy, about 5 minutes. Want a quicker method? Microwave on a microwave-safe plate for 1½ minutes, or until hot.

Ingredient FYI: These waffles call for arrowroot powder, a clean cornstarch alternative. Arrowroot powder and cornstarch can be used interchangeably. Check out page 5 for more arrowroot info.

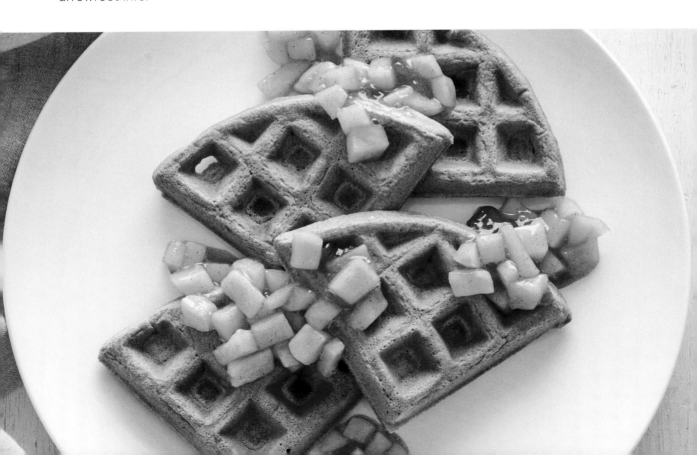

Apple Cinnamon Waffles

¼ᵗʰ of recipe (1 waffle with about ¼ cup topping):
209 calories, 4.5g total fat (2g sat fat), 695mg sodium, 33.5g carbs,
5.5g fiber, 6g sugars, 9g protein

You'll Need: medium-large microwave-safe bowl, medium bowl, electric mixer, large microwave-safe bowl, whisk, standard round waffle maker, nonstick spray, plate

Prep: 20 minutes • **Cook:** 20 minutes

Topping

1 tablespoon arrowroot powder

1½ cups peeled and chopped Fuji or Gala apples

1 packet natural no-calorie sweetener

¼ teaspoon cinnamon

⅛ teaspoon vanilla extract

Dash salt

Waffles

¾ cup (about 6 large) egg whites

2 tablespoons whipped butter

1 cup whole-wheat flour

½ cup unsweetened vanilla almond milk

2 packets natural no-calorie sweetener

2 teaspoons cinnamon

2 teaspoons baking powder

2 teaspoons vanilla extract

½ teaspoon salt

1. To make the topping, in a medium-large microwave-safe bowl, combine arrowroot powder with ¼ cup cold water; stir to dissolve.

2. Add remaining topping ingredients, and mix well. Cover and microwave for 2½ minutes. Mix well, and re-cover to keep warm.

3. Place egg whites in a medium bowl. With an electric mixer set to medium speed, beat until fluffy, 1 to 2 minutes.

4. In a large microwave-safe bowl, microwave butter for 30 seconds, or until melted. Add remaining waffle ingredients (excluding whipped egg whites) and ¾ cup water. Whisk until smooth and uniform.

5. Gently but thoroughly fold egg whites into batter. Stir until just mixed and uniform.

6. Spray a standard round waffle maker with nonstick spray, and set heat to medium. Once hot, pour ¼ᵗʰ of the batter (about ⅔ cup) into the center of the waffle maker. Close and cook for 4 minutes, or until golden brown and crispy.

7. Transfer waffle to a plate. Repeat to make 3 more waffles, re-spraying between waffles if needed.

8. Just before serving, top each waffle with ¼ᵗʰ of the topping (about ¼ cup).

MAKES 4 SERVINGS

PB&J Waffles

¼th of recipe (1 waffle with about ¼ cup topping):
203 calories, 5g total fat (2g sat fat), 673mg sodium, 28g carbs,
5.5g fiber, 4.5g sugars, 11.5g protein

You'll Need: medium-large microwave-safe bowl, medium bowl, electric mixer, large microwave-safe bowl, whisk, standard round waffle maker, nonstick spray, plate

Prep: 20 minutes • **Cook:** 25 minutes

Topping

1 tablespoon arrowroot powder

1½ cups chopped strawberries

1 packet natural no-calorie sweetener

¼ teaspoon vanilla extract

Waffles

¾ cup (about 6 large) egg whites

2 tablespoons whipped butter

¾ cup whole-wheat flour

½ cup unsweetened vanilla almond milk

¼ cup powdered peanut butter or defatted peanut flour

2 packets natural no-calorie sweetener

2 teaspoons vanilla extract

2 teaspoons baking powder

1½ teaspoons cinnamon

½ teaspoon salt

1. To make the topping, in a medium-large microwave-safe bowl, combine arrowroot powder with 2 tablespoons cold water; stir to dissolve.

2. Add remaining topping ingredients, and mix well. Cover and microwave for 2½ minutes. Keep covered so topping remains warm.

3. Place egg whites in a medium bowl. With an electric mixer set to medium speed, beat until fluffy, 1 to 2 minutes.

4. In a large microwave-safe bowl, microwave butter for 30 seconds, or until melted. Add remaining waffle ingredients (excluding whipped egg whites) and ¾ cup water. Whisk until smooth and uniform.

5. Gently but thoroughly fold egg whites into batter. Stir until just mixed and uniform.

6. Spray a standard round waffle maker with nonstick spray, and set heat to medium. Once hot, pour ¼th of the batter (about ⅔ cup) into the center of the waffle maker. Close and cook for 4 minutes, or until golden brown and crispy.

7. Transfer waffle to a plate. Repeat to make 3 more waffles, re-spraying between waffles if needed.

8. Just before serving, top each waffle with ¼th of the topping (about ¼ cup).

MAKES 4 SERVINGS

Ingredient FYI

Unfamiliar with powdered peanut butter, a.k.a. defatted peanut flour? Get the scoop on page 4.

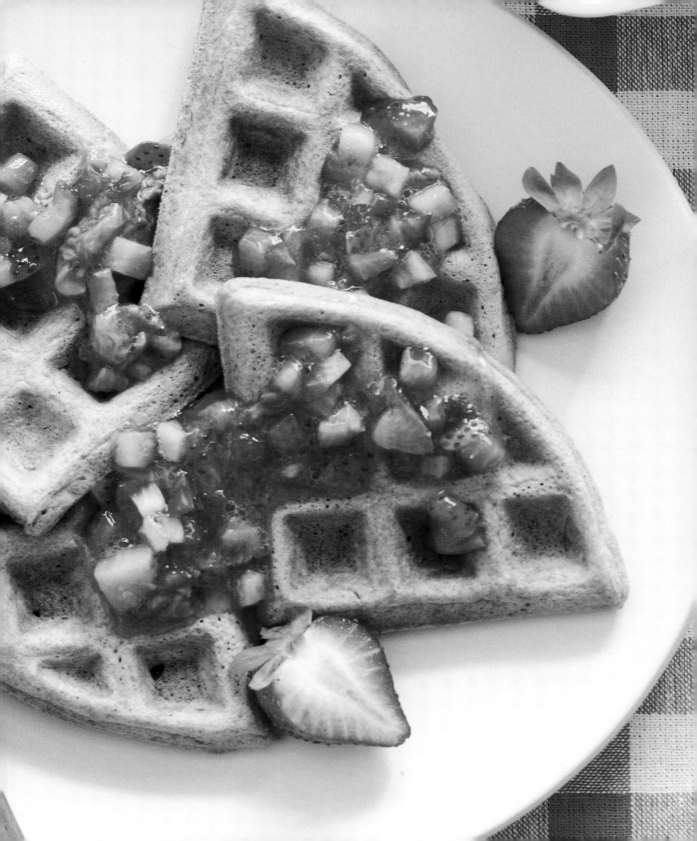

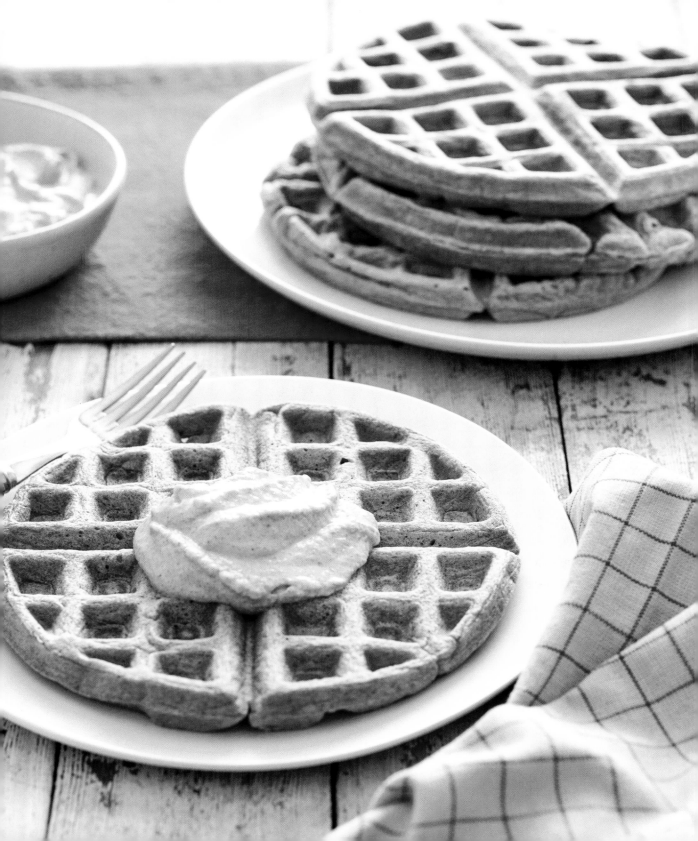

Pumpkin Spice Waffles

¼th of recipe (1 waffle with about ¼ cup topping): 219 calories, 4.5g total fat (2g sat fat), 675mg sodium, 30.5g carbs, 5.5g fiber, 4g sugars, 14g protein

You'll Need: 2 medium bowls, electric mixer, large microwave-safe bowl, whisk, standard round waffle maker, nonstick spray, plate

Prep: 15 minutes • **Cook:** 15 minutes

Topping

¾ cup fat-free plain Greek yogurt

¼ cup canned pure pumpkin

3 packets natural no-calorie sweetener

1 teaspoon cinnamon

½ teaspoon vanilla extract

Waffles

¾ cup (about 6 large) egg whites

2 tablespoons whipped butter

1 cup whole-wheat flour

½ cup unsweetened vanilla almond milk

¼ cup canned pure pumpkin

1 tablespoon pumpkin pie spice

2 packets natural no-calorie sweetener

2 teaspoons baking powder

2 teaspoons vanilla extract

½ teaspoon salt

1. Combine topping ingredients in a medium bowl, and mix until smooth and uniform. Cover and refrigerate.

2. Place egg whites in another medium bowl. With an electric mixer set to medium speed, beat until fluffy, 1 to 2 minutes.

3. In a large microwave-safe bowl, microwave butter for 30 seconds, or until melted. Add remaining waffle ingredients (excluding whipped egg whites) and ¾ cup water. Whisk until smooth and uniform.

4. Gently but thoroughly fold egg whites into batter. Stir until just mixed and uniform.

5. Spray a standard round waffle maker with nonstick spray, and set heat to medium. Once hot, pour ¼th of the batter (about ⅔ cup) into the center of the waffle maker. Close and cook for 4 minutes, or until golden brown and crispy.

6. Transfer waffle to a plate. Repeat to make 3 more waffles, re-spraying between waffles if needed.

7. Just before serving, top each waffle with ¼th of the topping (about ¼ cup).

MAKES 4 SERVINGS

4

Smoothies & Shakes

These healthy, filling, and delicious
smoothies 'n shakes are GREAT snacks
or mini-meals!

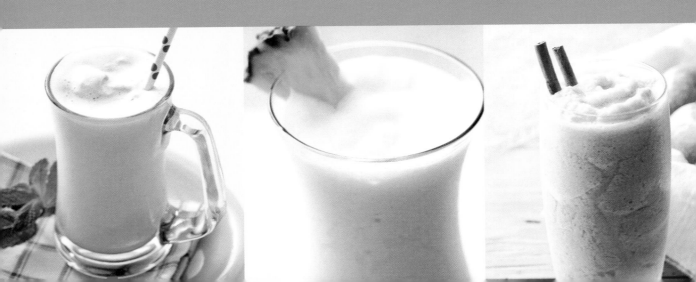

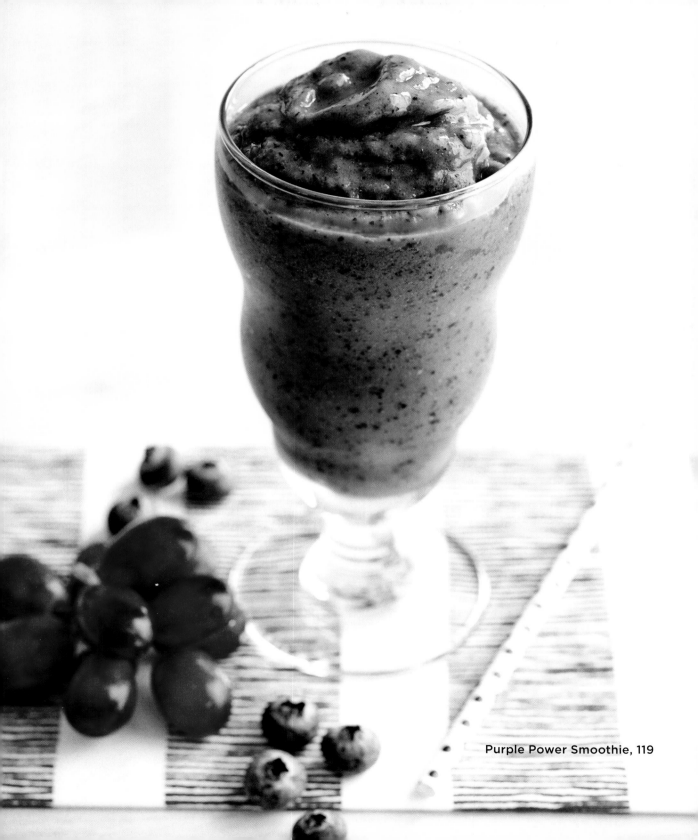

Purple Power Smoothie, 119

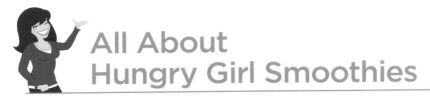

All About
Hungry Girl Smoothies

These drinks are large and in charge! So break out your biggest and best cups or oversized mason jars. Colorful straws optional (but encouraged)!

For best results, use crushed ice. Since ice cubes vary in size—and not every blender can effectively pulverize them—crushed ice will give you the most consistent results. If you don't have crushed ice on hand, DIY. Place ice cubes in a sealable plastic bag, squeeze out the air, and seal. Then crush the cubes through the bag using a (clean) meat mallet, a rolling pin, or another heavy kitchen utensil. Just watch your fingers!

Several of these recipes call for protein powder. Besides the obvious boost of protein, the powder adds creaminess and pumps up the volume of your drink. One other thing about blended drinks made with protein powder: The longer you blend 'em, the bigger and frothier they get! For protein powder shopping tips, flip to page 5.

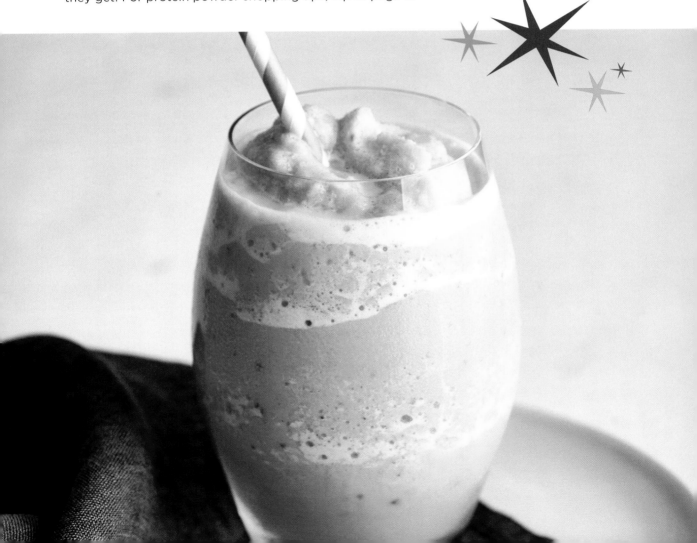

Creamy Peanut Butter Smoothie

Entire recipe (about 16 ounces): 160 calories, 4.5g total fat (<0.5g sat fat), 183mg sodium, 19g carbs, 4g fiber, 8g sugars, 14g protein

This recipe calls for banana, but you'll mostly just taste peanut butter goodness! The banana adds creaminess and texture (plus bonus fiber)...

You'll Need: blender

Prep: 5 minutes

¾ cup unsweetened vanilla almond milk

⅓ cup sliced and frozen banana

2 tablespoons plain protein powder with about 100 calories per serving

2 tablespoons powdered peanut butter or defatted peanut flour

2 packets natural no-calorie sweetener

⅛ teaspoon vanilla extract

1¼ cups crushed ice (about 8 ice cubes)

1. Place all ingredients in a blender. Blend at high speed until smooth, stopping and stirring if needed.

MAKES 1 SERVING

Ingredient FYI
Unfamiliar with powdered peanut butter, a.k.a. defatted peanut flour? Get the scoop on page 4.

HG Tip
Keep some banana slices in your freezer at all times for recipes like this.

Pretty in Green Smoothie

Entire recipe (about 22 ounces): 191 calories, 4g total fat (1.5g sat fat), 184mg sodium, 39.5g carbs, 7.5g fiber, 24g sugars, 4g protein

This drink looks green but tastes PINK! Embrace the spinach...

You'll Need: blender

Prep: 5 minutes

2 cups spinach leaves

1 cup frozen strawberries (no sugar added), slightly thawed

1 cup chopped pineapple

¾ cup unsweetened vanilla almond milk

2 packets natural no-calorie sweetener

⅛ teaspoon coconut extract

1 cup crushed ice (about 6 ice cubes)

1½ teaspoons unsweetened shredded coconut

1. Place all ingredients *except* shredded coconut in a blender, and blend at high speed until smooth, stopping and stirring if needed.

2. Serve topped with coconut.

MAKES 1 SERVING

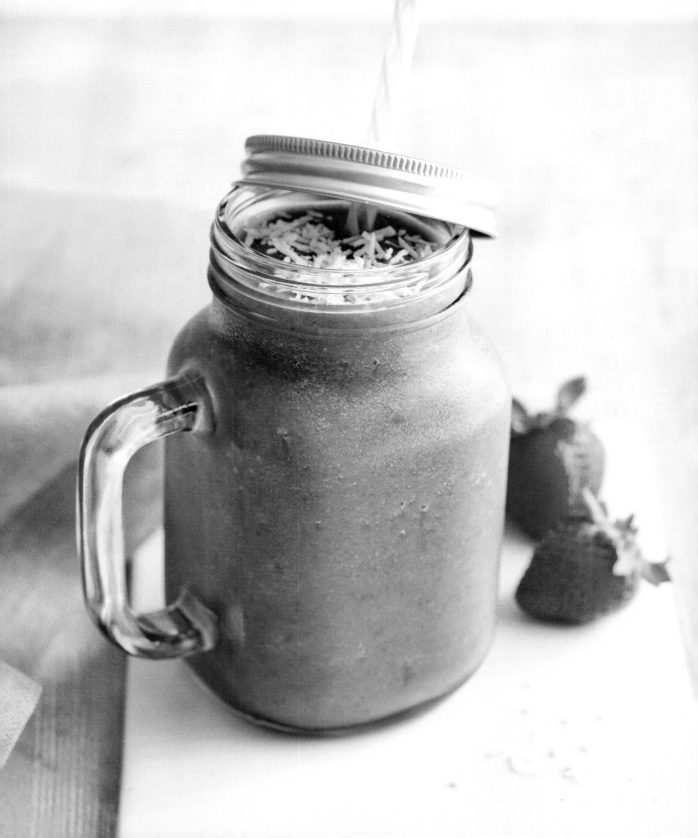

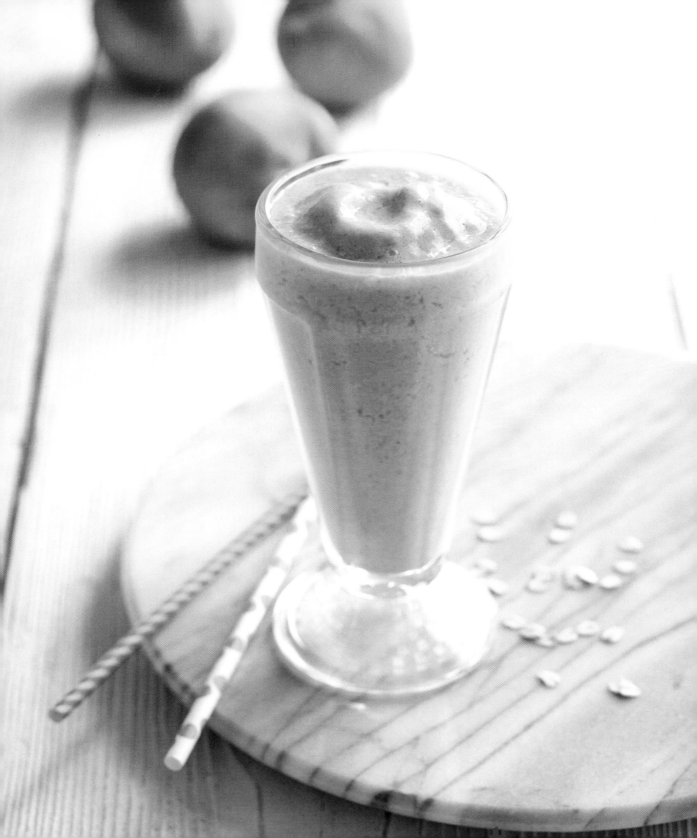

Peach Cobbler Smoothie

Entire recipe (about 14 ounces): 176 calories, 3.5g total fat (0g sat fat), 201mg sodium, 29.5g carbs, 4.5g fiber, 15g sugars, 9g protein

Never had raw oats in a smoothie? They give this smoothie a thicker consistency and bring that cobbler taste to life!

You'll Need: blender

Prep: 5 minutes

1 cup frozen peach slices (no sugar added), slightly thawed

1 cup unsweetened vanilla almond milk

¼ cup fat-free plain Greek yogurt

2 tablespoons old-fashioned oats

2 packets natural no-calorie sweetener

¼ teaspoon cinnamon

⅛ teaspoon nutmeg

⅛ teaspoon vanilla extract

½ cup crushed ice (about 3 ice cubes)

Optional: ground ginger

1. Place all ingredients in a blender. Blend at high speed until smooth, stopping and stirring if needed.

MAKES 1 SERVING

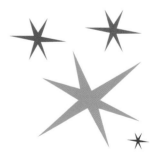

Apple Cinnamon Smoothie

Entire recipe (about 20 ounces): 128 calories, 2g total fat (0g sat fat), 156mg sodium, 22g carbs, 3g fiber, 15g sugars, 7g protein

You'll Need: blender

Prep: 5 minutes

1 cup peeled and chopped Fuji or Gala apple

¾ cup unsweetened vanilla almond milk

¼ cup fat-free plain Greek yogurt

2 packets natural no-calorie sweetener

¼ teaspoon cinnamon

¼ teaspoon vanilla extract

1 cup crushed ice (about 6 ice cubes)

1. Place all ingredients in a blender, and blend at high speed until smooth, stopping and stirring if needed.

MAKES 1 SERVING

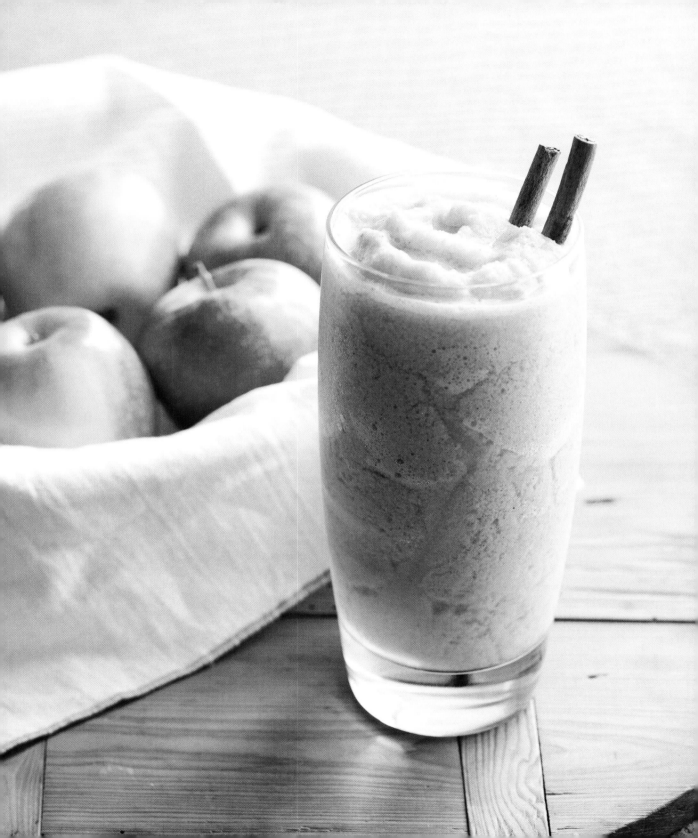

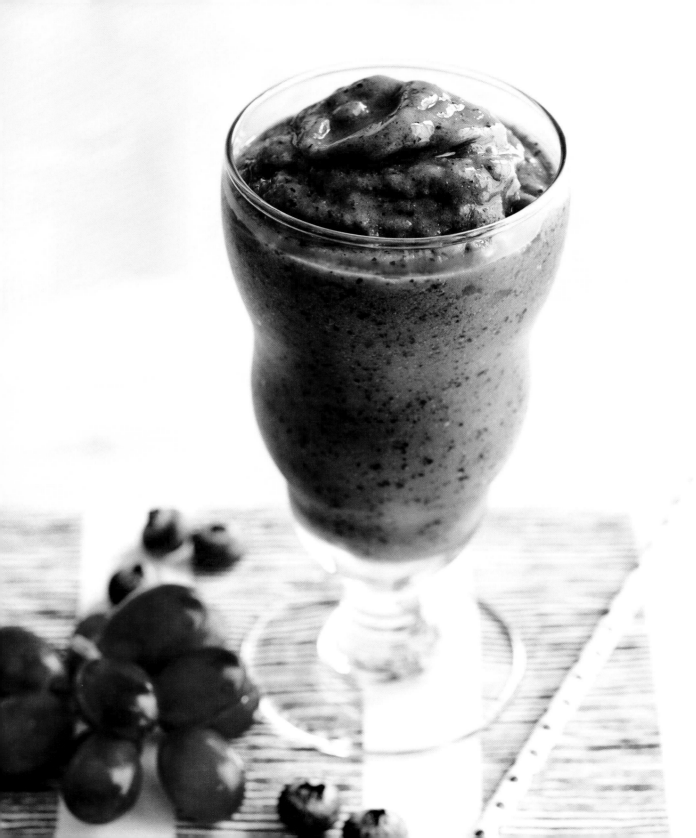

Purple Power Smoothie

Entire recipe (about 18 ounces): 163 calories, 2.5g total fat (0g sat fat), 136mg sodium, 37g carbs, 5g fiber, 24g sugars, 2g protein

The cinnamon gives this smoothie a little something extra . . . It's unexpected and delicious!

You'll Need: blender

Prep: 5 minutes

¾ **cup unsweetened vanilla almond milk**

½ **cup frozen blueberries (no sugar added)**

½ **cup seedless red grapes**

⅓ **cup sliced and frozen banana**

1 packet natural no-calorie sweetener

⅛ **teaspoon cinnamon**

1 cup crushed ice (about 6 ice cubes)

1. Place all ingredients in a blender, and blend at high speed until smooth, stopping and stirring if needed.

MAKES 1 SERVING

HG Tip
Store banana slices in your freezer at all times so you can easily whip up recipes like this!

Carrot Pineapple Smoothie

Entire recipe (about 16 ounces): 135 calories, 1.5g total fat (0g sat fat), 146mg sodium, 24.5g carbs, 2.5g fiber, 18.5g sugars, 6.5g protein

You'll Need: blender

Prep: 5 minutes

½ cup pineapple chunks packed in juice (not drained)

½ cup unsweetened vanilla almond milk

⅓ cup shredded carrot

¼ cup fat-free plain Greek yogurt

1 packet natural no-calorie sweetener

⅛ teaspoon cinnamon, or more to taste

1 cup crushed ice (about 6 ice cubes)

Optional: ground ginger

1. Place all ingredients in a blender. Blend at high speed until smooth, stopping and stirring if needed.

MAKES 1 SERVING

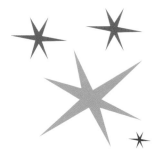

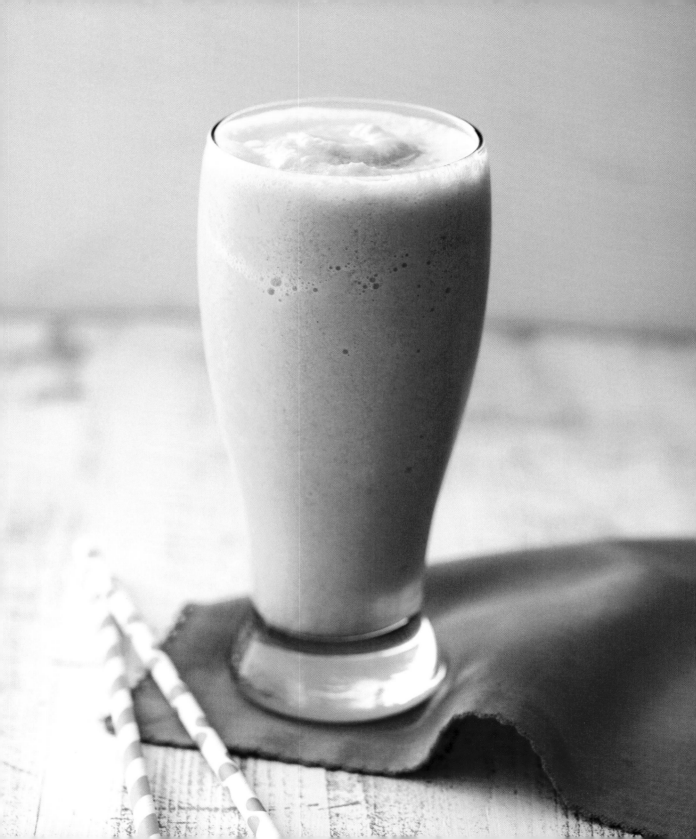

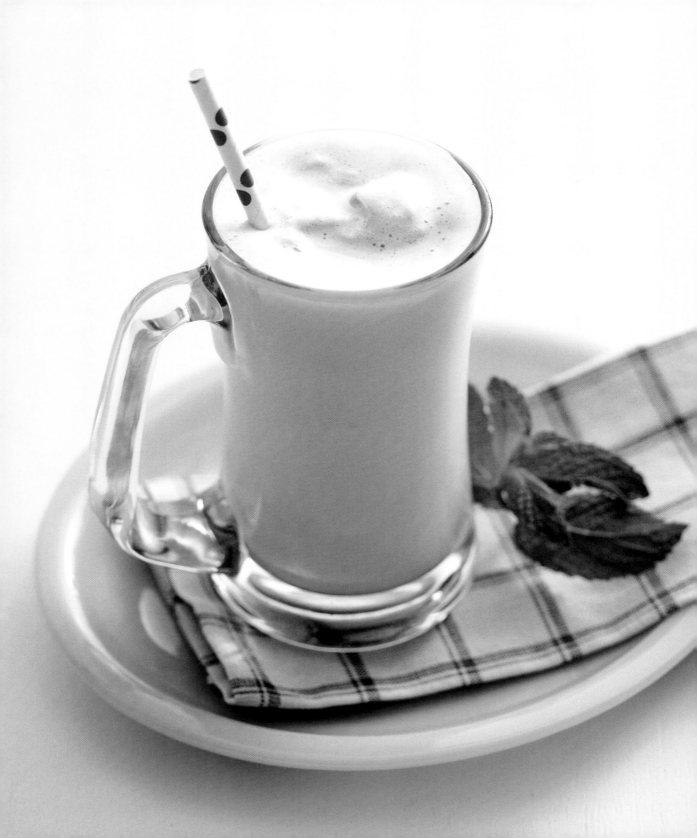

Clean & Hungry Shamrock Shake

Entire recipe (about 16 ounces): 87 calories, 3g total fat (0.5g sat fat), 165mg sodium, 4.5g carbs, 1g fiber, 1g sugars, 11g protein

You don't have to wait until St. Paddy's Day to enjoy this hint-of-mint vanilla shake. P.S. You can't taste the spinach at all . . . Promise!

You'll Need: blender

Prep: 5 minutes

¾ **cup unsweetened vanilla almond milk**

⅓ **cup spinach leaves**

3 tablespoons plain protein powder with about 100 calories per serving

2 packets natural no-calorie sweetener

¼ **teaspoon peppermint extract**

⅛ **teaspoon vanilla extract**

1¼ **cups crushed ice (about 8 ice cubes)**

1. Place all ingredients in a blender. Blend at high speed until smooth, stopping and stirring if needed.

MAKES 1 SERVING

> ## HG FYI
> A full serving of protein powder is about 6 tablespoons . . . A little goes a long way!

Piña Colada Shake

Entire recipe (about 20 ounces): 106 calories, 0.5g total fat (0.5g sat fat), 31mg sodium, 14.5g carbs, 1g fiber, 11g sugars, 10.5g protein

You'll Need: blender

Prep: 5 minutes

⅓ cup canned crushed pineapple packed in juice (not drained)

3 tablespoons plain protein powder with about 100 calories per serving

2 packets natural no-calorie sweetener

¼ teaspoon vanilla extract

⅛ teaspoon coconut extract

1 cup crushed ice (about 6 ice cubes)

1. Place all ingredients in a blender.

2. Add ⅓ cup water, and blend at high speed until smooth, stopping and stirring if needed.

MAKES 1 SERVING

For more healthy recipes, plus the latest food news, tips & tricks, and more, **sign up for free daily emails at Hungry-Girl.com!**

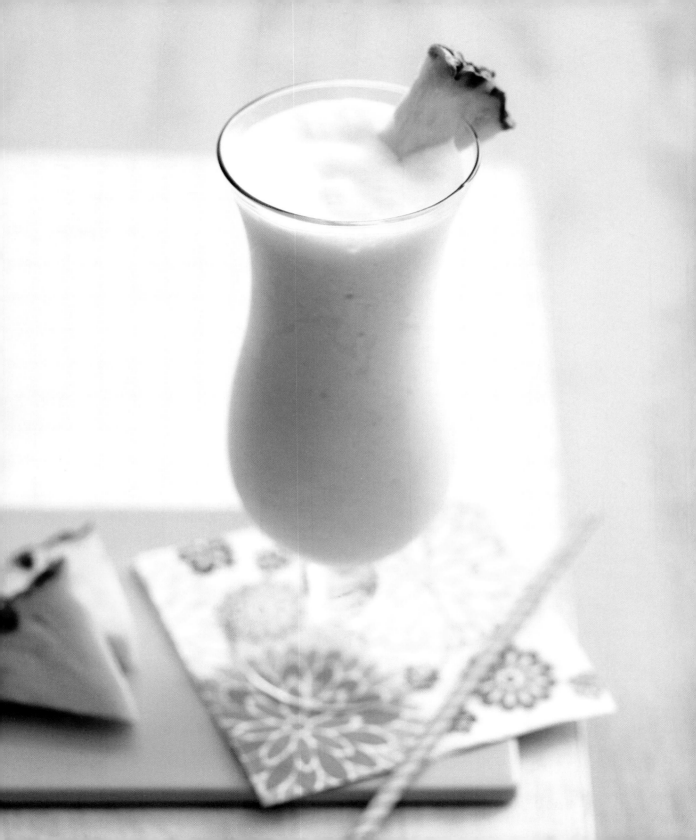

5

Slow-Cooker Soups, Stews & More

Slow-cooker recipes are some of the most popular Hungry Girl recipes in existence . . . Not surprising, considering how easy and amazing they are!

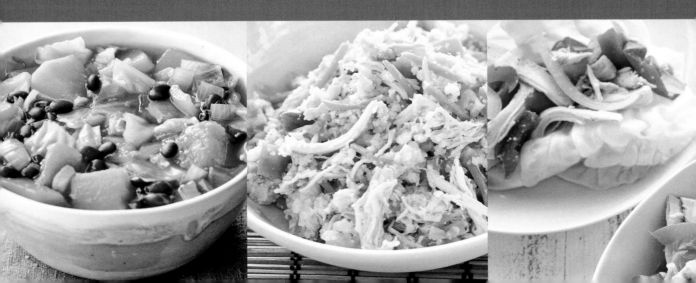

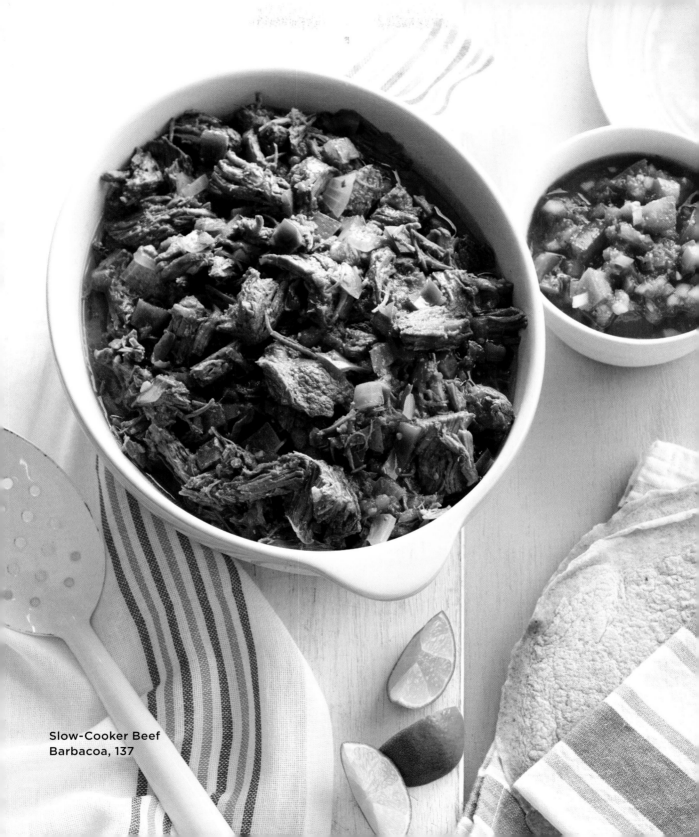

Slow-Cooker Beef
Barbacoa, 137

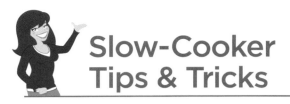

Slow-Cooker
Tips & Tricks

You'll need a slow cooker with at least a 4-quart capacity. This is a pretty standard size, but larger slow cookers will work too.

The soups and stews freeze and thaw fantastically well. First, let them cool completely. Then distribute single servings into sealable microwave-safe containers. Freeze away; then heat 'n eat!

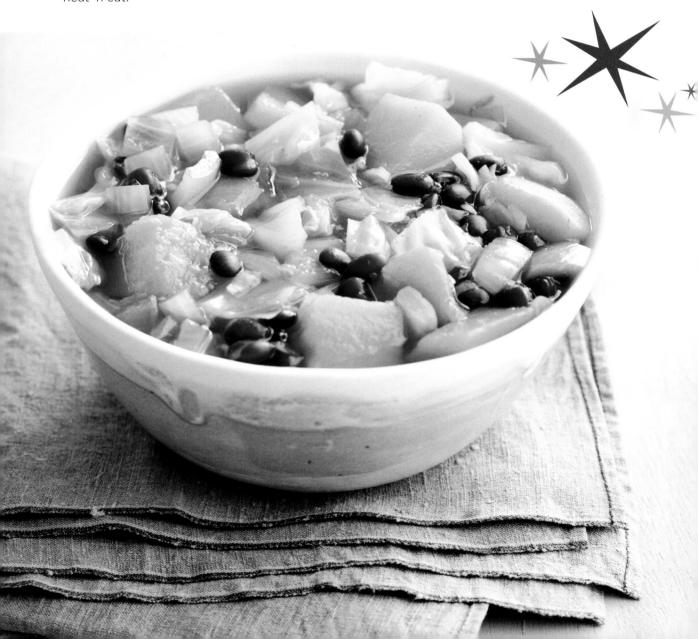

Black Bean & Butternut Soup

⅙ᵗʰ of recipe (about 1¼ cups): 115 calories, 0.5g total fat (0g sat fat), 639mg sodium, 24g carbs, 5.5g fiber, 5g sugars, 5g protein

You'll Need: slow cooker

Prep: 10 minutes • **Cook:** 3 to 4 hours *or* 7 to 8 hours

3 cups butternut squash cut into 1-inch chunks (about half of a medium squash)

One 15-ounce can black beans, drained and rinsed

1 cup chopped onion

1 cup chopped cabbage

1 teaspoon chopped garlic

¼ teaspoon ground cumin

¼ teaspoon cayenne pepper

4 cups vegetable broth

Optional seasonings: salt and black pepper

1. Combine all ingredients *except* broth in a slow cooker. Add broth, and mix well.

2. Cover and cook on high for 3 to 4 hours *or* on low for 7 to 8 hours, until veggies are soft.

MAKES 6 SERVINGS

Cauliflower & Corn Soup

⅙th of recipe (about 1⅓ cups): 120 calories, 1g total fat (0g sat fat), 519mg sodium, 24.5g carbs, 4.5g fiber, 7.5g sugars, 5.5g protein

The chicken broth gives this soup lots of flavor, but for a vegetarian soup, veggie broth works!

You'll Need: slow cooker

Prep: 15 minutes • **Cook:** 3 to 4 hours *or* 7 to 8 hours

5 cups roughly chopped cauliflower

2 cups frozen sweet corn kernels

1 cup chopped red bell pepper

1 cup chopped onion

6 ounces (about 5) baby red potatoes, chopped

1 teaspoon chopped garlic

1 teaspoon ground cumin

¼ teaspoon each salt and black pepper

4 cups reduced-sodium chicken broth

½ cup unsweetened plain almond milk

2 tablespoons chopped fresh cilantro

1. In a slow cooker, combine all ingredients *except* broth, almond milk, and cilantro. Add broth and almond milk, and mix well.

2. Cover and cook on high for 3 to 4 hours *or* on low for 7 to 8 hours, until veggies are soft.

3. Stir in cilantro.

MAKES 6 SERVINGS

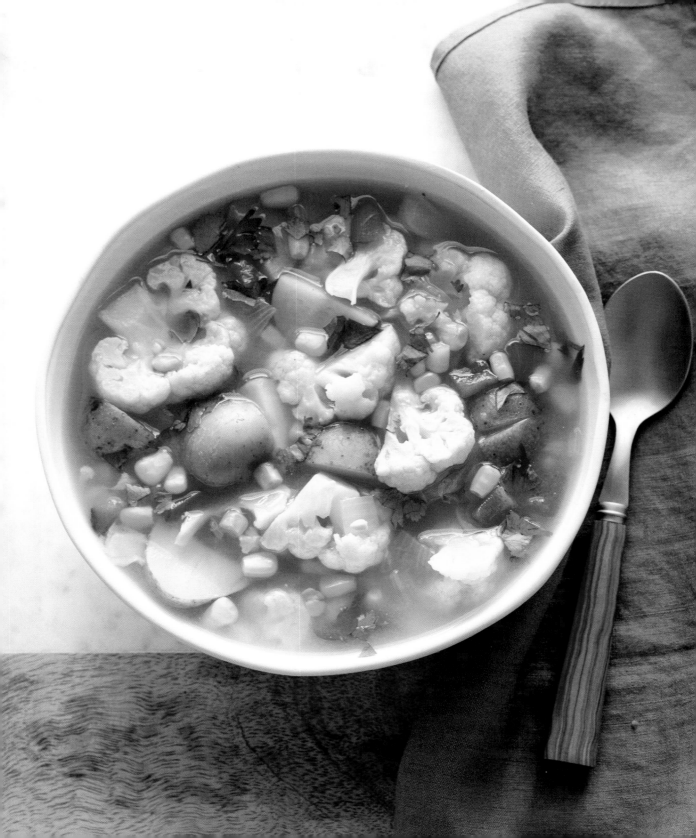

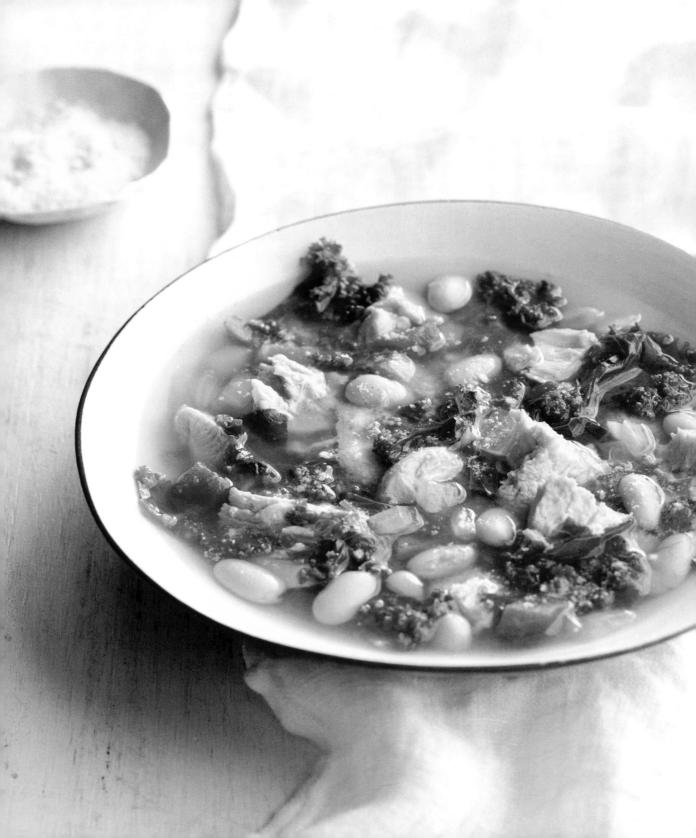

Chicken, Kale & Cannellini Broth Bowl

⅕th of recipe (about 1½ cups): 273 calories, 4.5g total fat (1g sat fat), 604mg sodium, 23g carbs, 6g fiber, 5g sugars, 34g protein

This one eats like a meal ... LOVE IT.

You'll Need: slow cooker

Prep: 15 minutes • **Cook:** 3 to 4 hours *or* 7 to 8 hours, plus 30 minutes

2 cups reduced-sodium chicken broth

One 14.5-ounce can diced tomatoes, drained

2 teaspoons ground thyme

1½ teaspoons chopped garlic

2 dried bay leaves

1¼ pounds raw boneless skinless chicken breasts

One 15-ounce can cannellini (white kidney) beans, drained and rinsed

1 cup chopped onion

3 cups roughly chopped kale leaves

5 teaspoons grated Parmesan cheese

Optional seasonings: salt and black pepper

1. In a slow cooker, combine chicken broth, drained tomatoes, thyme, garlic, and bay leaves. Add 2 cups water, and mix until uniform.

2. Add chicken, cannellini beans, and onion, and stir to mix.

3. Cover and cook on high for 3 to 4 hours *or* on low for 7 to 8 hours, until chicken is cooked through.

4. Transfer chicken to a cutting board, and roughly chop.

5. Remove bay leaves from the slow cooker, and discard.

6. Return chopped chicken to the slow cooker. Add kale, and stir to mix.

7. If cooking at low heat, increase heat to high.

8. Cover and cook for 30 minutes, or until kale is tender.

9. Top each serving with 1 teaspoon Parm.

MAKES 5 SERVINGS

White Chicken Chili

⅛th of recipe (about 1 cup): 254 calories, 3g total fat (0.5g sat fat), 507mg sodium, 27.5g carbs, 7.5g fiber, 5.5g sugars, 29.5g protein

You'll Need: large microwave-safe bowl, blender or food processor, slow cooker, large bowl

Prep: 30 minutes • **Cook:** 3 to 4 hours *or* 7 to 8 hours, plus 5 minutes

4 cups roughly chopped cauliflower

½ cup fat-free plain Greek yogurt

2 teaspoons chopped garlic

3 cups reduced-sodium chicken broth

1½ pounds raw boneless skinless chicken breasts, halved

¼ teaspoon each salt and black pepper

Two 15.5-ounce cans cannellini (white kidney) beans, drained and rinsed

1 cup chopped red and green bell peppers

1 cup chopped onion

1 cup frozen sweet corn kernels

1 teaspoon chili powder

1 teaspoon ground cumin

¼ teaspoon cayenne pepper

1. Place cauliflower in a large microwave-safe bowl. Add 3 tablespoons water. Cover and microwave for 5 minutes, or until soft.

2. In a blender or food processor, combine cooked cauliflower, yogurt, and garlic. Add 1 cup broth, and blend on high speed until smooth and uniform.

3. Place chicken in a slow cooker, and season with salt and black pepper. Add blended cauliflower mixture and all remaining ingredients, including remaining 2 cups broth. Stir to mix.

4. Cover and cook on high for 3 to 4 hours *or* on low for 7 to 8 hours, until chicken is fully cooked.

5. Transfer chicken to a large bowl. Shred with two forks—one to hold the chicken in place and the other to scrape across and shred it.

6. Return shredded chicken to the slow cooker, and mix well.

MAKES 8 SERVINGS

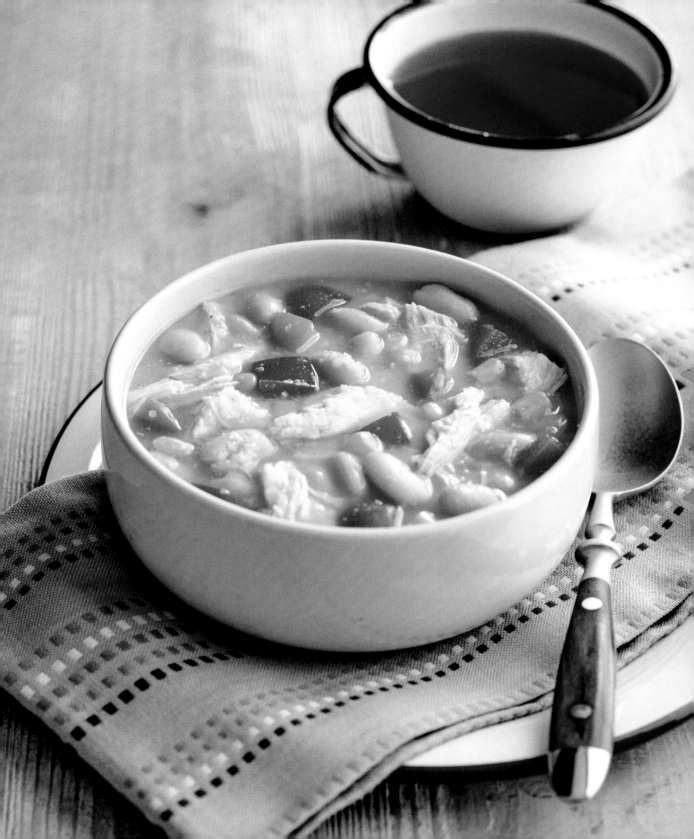

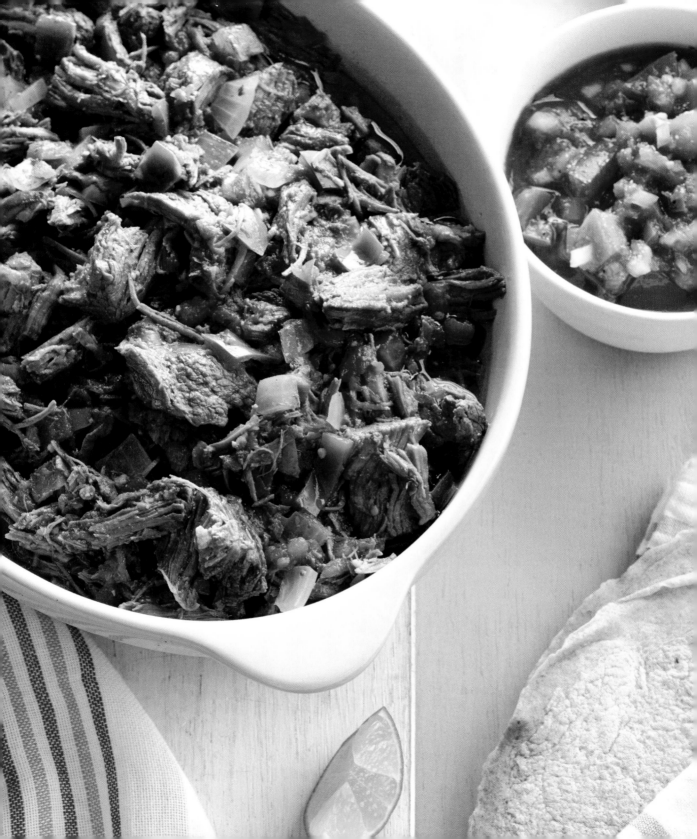

Slow-Cooker Beef Barbacoa

¹⁄₁₂ᵗʰ of recipe (about ½ cup): 173 calories, 7g total fat (3g sat fat), 285mg sodium, 3.5g carbs, 1g fiber, 1.5g sugars, 24.5g protein

This recipe takes a little longer than the average slow-cooker meal, but it's worth it . . . Promise! Try it wrapped in my Clean & Hungry Whole-Wheat Tortillas (recipe and store-bought alternatives on page 25).

You'll Need: slow cooker, large bowl

Prep: 20 minutes • **Cook:** 4 to 5 hours *or* 8 to 9 hours

3 pounds raw boneless chuck beef roast, trimmed of excess fat, cut into large chunks

½ teaspoon salt

¼ teaspoon black pepper

One 10-ounce can diced tomatoes with green chiles (not drained)

1 cup chopped onion

½ cup seeded and chopped jalapeño peppers

½ cup beef broth

2 tablespoons apple cider vinegar

1 tablespoon chopped garlic

1 teaspoon ground cumin

1 teaspoon ground chipotle pepper

½ teaspoon oregano

1 dried bay leaf

Optional topping: chopped fresh cilantro

1. Place beef in a slow cooker, and season with salt and black pepper. Add all remaining ingredients, and stir to mix.

2. Cook on high for 4 to 5 hours *or* on low for 8 to 9 hours, until beef is cooked through.

3. Transfer beef to a large bowl. Shred with two forks—one to hold the beef in place and the other to scrape across and shred it.

4. Remove bay leaf from the slow cooker, and discard.

5. Return shredded beef to the slow cooker, and mix well.

MAKES 12 SERVINGS

HG Alternative

Like your barbacoa extra spicy? Leave in the seeds when you chop up your jalapeños. Hot stuff!

Hawaiian Chicken with Cauliflower Rice

¼th of recipe (about 1¾ cups): 241 calories, 3.5g total fat (0.5g sat fat), 596mg sodium, 23.5g carbs, 5.5g fiber, 14g sugars, 29.5g protein

Instead of calorie-dense grains, this dish contains riced cauliflower. For more cauliflower rice recipes and information, flip to Chapter 9!

You'll Need: slow cooker, large bowl, blender

Prep: 20 minutes • **Cook:** 3 to 4 hours *or* 7 to 8 hours, plus 45 minutes

1 pound raw boneless skinless chicken breasts, halved

¼ teaspoon each salt and black pepper

2 cups shredded carrots

1 cup chopped green bell pepper

1 cup crushed pineapple packed in juice (not drained)

1 cup reduced-sodium chicken broth

½ cup Clean & Hungry Teriyaki Sauce (recipe and store-bought alternatives on page 23)

2 teaspoons chopped garlic

1 packet natural no-calorie sweetener

4 cups roughly chopped cauliflower

1. Place chicken in a slow cooker, and season with salt and black pepper. Add all remaining ingredients *except* cauliflower. Stir to mix.

2. Cover and cook on high for 3 to 4 hours *or* on low for 7 to 8 hours, until chicken is fully cooked.

3. Transfer chicken to a large bowl. Shred with two forks—one to hold the chicken in place and the other to scrape across and shred it. Return shredded chicken to the slow cooker, and mix well.

4. Pulse cauliflower in a blender until reduced to rice-sized pieces, working in batches as needed. Add cauliflower rice to the slow cooker, and stir to mix.

5. If cooking at low heat, increase heat to high.

6. Cover and cook for 45 minutes, or until cauliflower rice is tender.

MAKES 4 SERVINGS

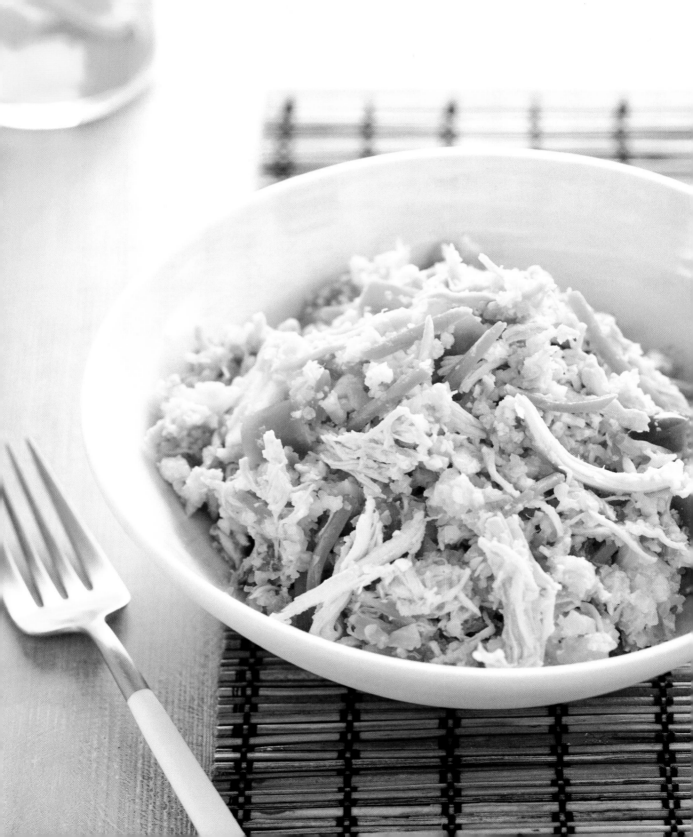

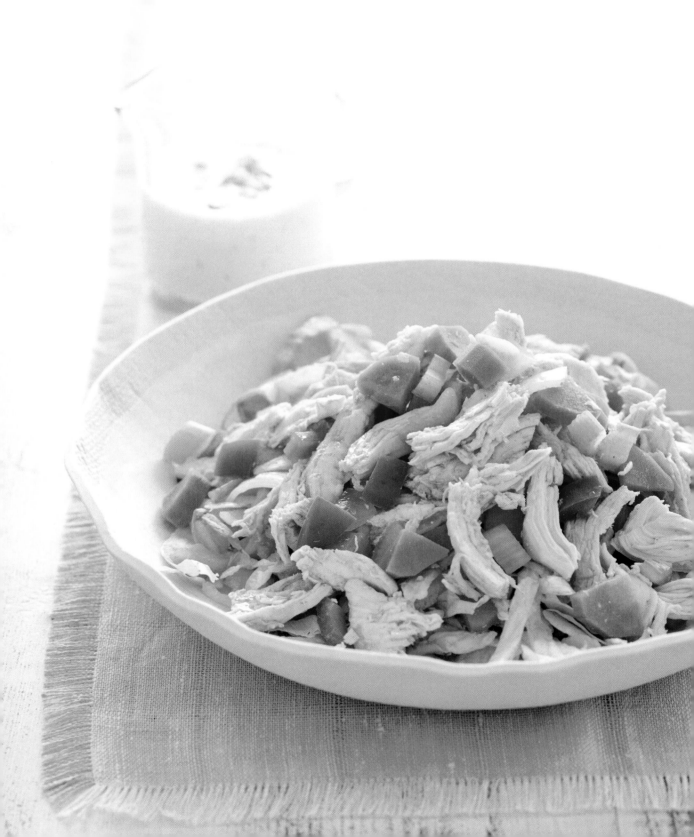

Slow-Cooker Buffalo Chicken

⅙ᵗʰ of recipe (about 1 cup): 175 calories, 3g total fat (0.5g sat fat), 627mg sodium, 9g carbs, 2.5g fiber, 4g sugars, 26.5g protein

Yup—Frank's RedHot is completely clean: It contains only cayenne peppers, vinegar, water, salt, and garlic powder. And if you love Buffalo chicken, don't miss the Buffalo Chicken Stuffed Portabellas (page 153), Buffalo Turkey Meatloaf (page 175), and Big Buffalo Cauliflower Bites (page 247).

You'll Need: slow cooker, large bowl, slotted spoon

Prep: 15 minutes • **Cook:** 3 to 4 hours *or* 7 to 8 hours

1½ pounds raw boneless skinless chicken breasts, halved

2 cups chopped celery

2 cups chopped carrots

1 cup chopped onion

1 cup low-sodium chicken broth

½ cup seeded and chopped jalapeño peppers

⅓ cup Frank's RedHot Original Cayenne Pepper Sauce

1½ teaspoons chopped garlic

¼ teaspoon cayenne pepper

Optional topping: Clean & Hungry Chunky Blue Cheese Dressing (recipe and store-bought alternatives on page 22)

1. Place chicken in a slow cooker. Top with remaining ingredients. Add 1 cup water, and stir to mix.

2. Cover and cook on high for 3 to 4 hours *or* on low for 7 to 8 hours, until chicken is fully cooked and veggies are tender.

3. Transfer chicken to a large bowl. Shred with two forks—one to hold the chicken in place and the other to scrape across and shred it.

4. Return shredded chicken to the slow cooker, and mix well.

5. Serve with a slotted spoon, draining the broth.

MAKES 6 SERVINGS

Slow-Cooker Chicken Fajitas

⅛ᵗʰ of recipe (about ¾ cup): 128 calories, 2.5g total fat (0.5g sat fat), 328mg sodium, 5g carbs, 1g fiber, 2.5g sugars, 20g protein

This flavorful shredded chicken is SO versatile. Top off your salads, pile it into corn tortillas, or just add a fork!

You'll Need: slow cooker, large bowl, slotted spoon

Prep: 15 minutes • **Cook:** 3 to 4 hours *or* 7 to 8 hours

1½ pounds raw boneless skinless chicken breasts, halved

½ teaspoon each salt and black pepper

2 cups sliced red and green bell peppers

2 cups sliced onion

1 teaspoon chili powder

1 teaspoon ground cumin

1 teaspoon garlic powder

½ teaspoon onion powder

⅛ teaspoon cayenne pepper

2 cups reduced-sodium chicken broth

1. Place chicken in a slow cooker, and season with salt and black pepper. Add peppers, onion, and seasonings. Top with broth, and stir to mix.

2. Cover and cook on high for 3 to 4 hours *or* on low for 7 to 8 hours, until chicken is fully cooked.

3. Transfer chicken to a large bowl. Shred with two forks—one to hold the chicken in place and the other to scrape across and shred it.

4. Return shredded chicken to the slow cooker, and mix well.

5. Serve with a slotted spoon, draining the broth.

MAKES 8 SERVINGS

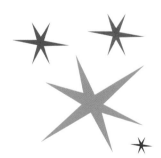

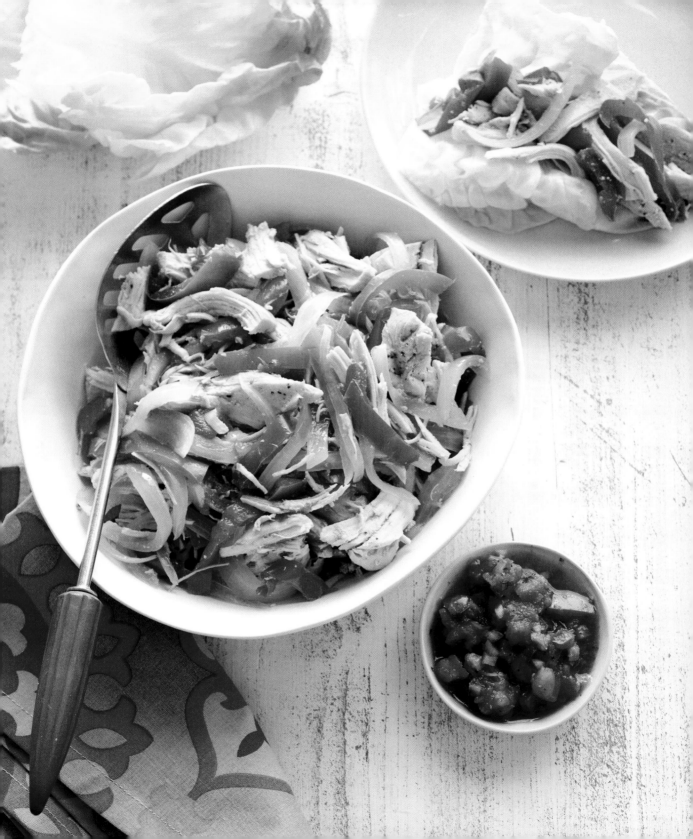

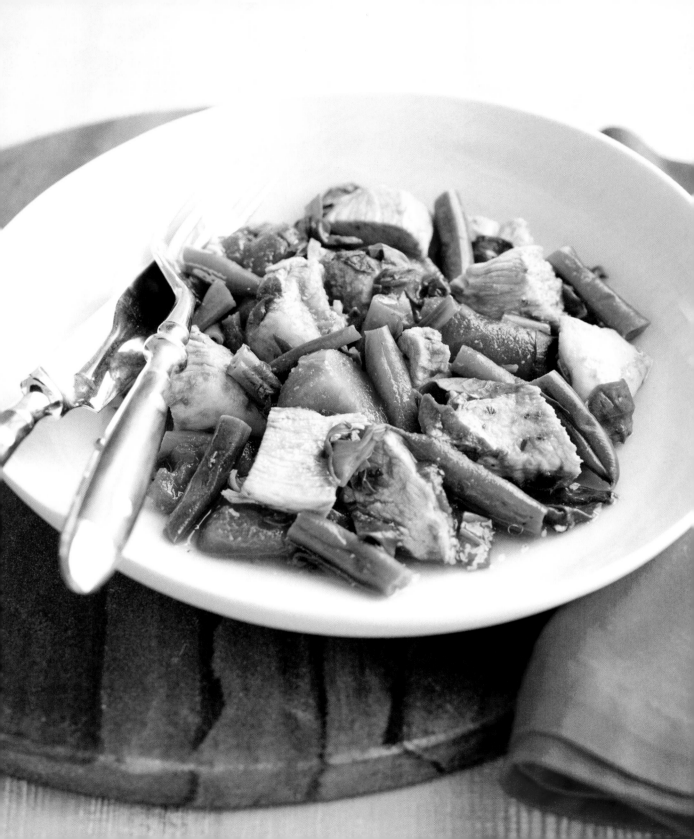

Mama Shelley's Slow-Cooker Chicken

¼th of recipe (about 1¾ cups): 270 calories, 4g total fat
(1g sat fat), 663mg sodium, 21.5g carbs, 5g fiber, 12g sugars,
35.5g protein

Mama Shelley is the mother-in-law of longtime HG staffer Jamie. Yay, Shelley!

You'll Need: slow cooker

Prep: 20 minutes • **Cook:** 3 to 4 hours *or* 7 to 8 hours, plus 5 minutes

Two 14.5-ounce cans stewed tomatoes (not drained)

⅓ cup balsamic vinegar

2 teaspoons garlic powder

1 teaspoon dried oregano

1 teaspoon dried basil

1¼ pounds raw boneless skinless chicken breasts

¼ teaspoon each salt and black pepper

1½ cups green beans, trimmed and cut into 1-inch pieces

6 cups roughly chopped spinach leaves

1. In a slow cooker, combine tomatoes, balsamic vinegar, garlic powder, oregano, and basil. Mix until uniform.

2. Season chicken with salt and pepper, and add to the slow cooker.

3. Add green beans, and mix well.

4. Cover and cook on high for 3 to 4 hours *or* on low for 7 to 8 hours, until chicken is cooked through and green beans are tender.

5. Turn off slow cooker, and transfer chicken to a cutting board. Roughly chop, and return to the slow cooker.

6. Stir in spinach, re-cover, and let sit for 5 minutes, or until spinach has wilted.

MAKES 4 SERVINGS

6

Foil Packs

Foil packs—a.k.a. foods baked in a packet made out of aluminum foil—are a revelation. The food is cooked to perfection, and cleanup is a breeze . . .

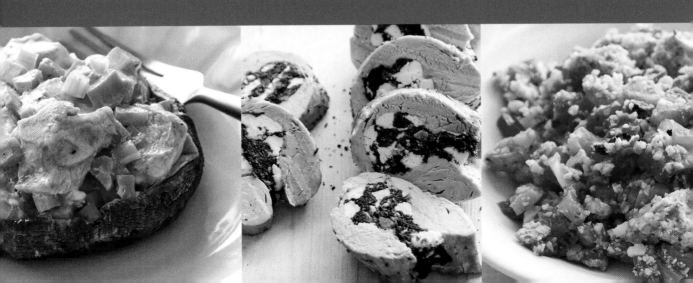

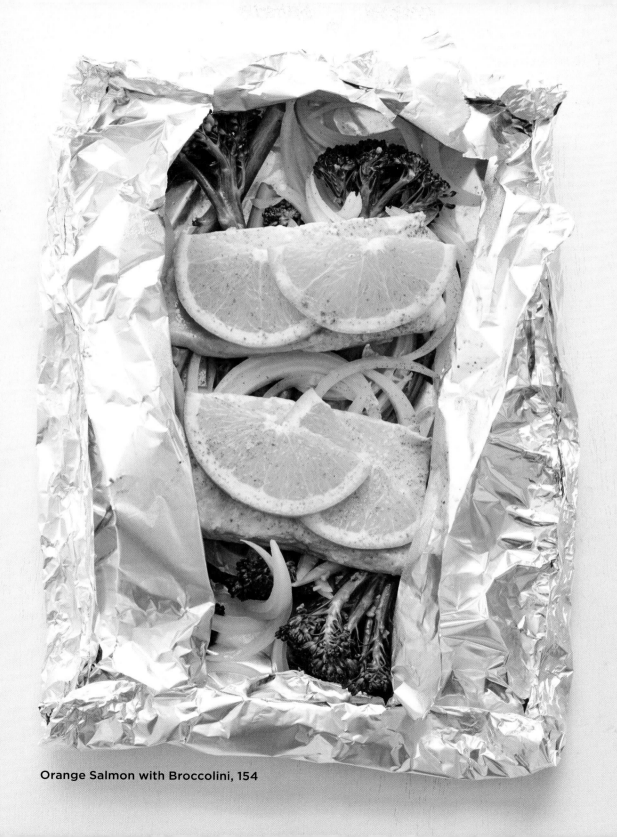

Orange Salmon with Broccolini, 154

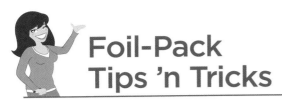

Foil-Pack
Tips 'n Tricks

Heavy-duty foil is essential. You need the good sturdy stuff.

When you fold your foil, form a tightly sealed package. Don't let any of that steam escape. Also leave a little extra room at the top for steaming to take place.

The hot steam will be released when you open your foil pack. So let it cool for a few minutes, and then cut the foil to release some of the steam before opening it.

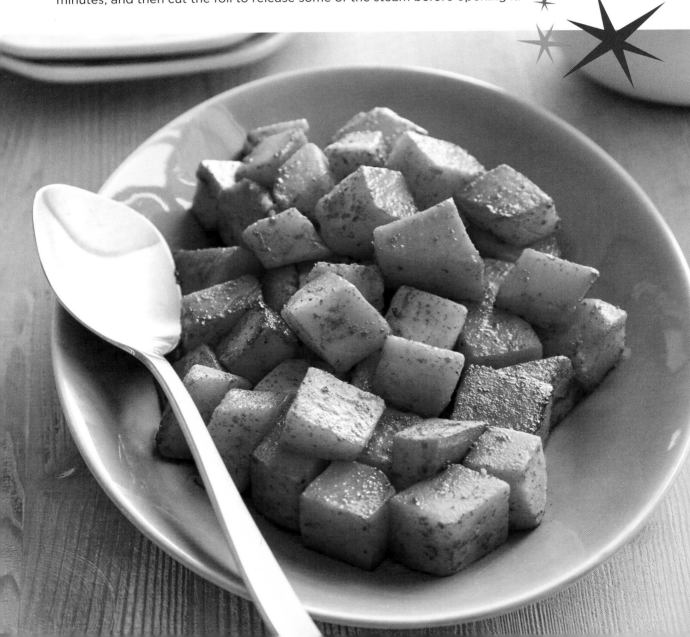

Spicy Sweet Potato 'n Squash

¼th of recipe (about ¾ cup): 112 calories, 3.5g total fat (0.5g sat fat), 331mg sodium, 20g carbs, 3.5g fiber, 4g sugars, 1.5g protein

You'll Need: heavy-duty aluminum foil, baking sheet, nonstick spray, large bowl

Prep: 10 minutes • **Cook:** 30 minutes

1 tablespoon olive oil

1 packet natural no-calorie sweetener

1 teaspoon chili powder

½ teaspoon salt

¼ teaspoon cayenne pepper

2 cups butternut squash cut into 1-inch chunks

8 ounces sweet potato (about 1 medium potato), peeled and cut into 1-inch chunks

1. Preheat oven to 400 degrees. Lay a large piece of heavy-duty foil on a baking sheet and spray with nonstick spray.

2. In a large bowl, combine olive oil, sweetener, chili powder, salt, and cayenne pepper. Mix well. Add squash and potato, and toss to coat.

3. Distribute mixture onto the center of the foil. Cover with another large piece of foil. Fold together and seal all four edges of the foil pieces, forming a well-sealed packet.

4. Bake for 30 minutes, or until squash and potato are soft.

5. Cut packet to release hot steam before opening entirely.

MAKES 4 SERVINGS

Peanut Chicken with Green Beans

Entire recipe: 319 calories, 6g total fat (1g sat fat), 433mg sodium, 28.5g carbs, 6.5g fiber, 13g sugars, 39.5g protein

You'll Need: heavy-duty aluminum foil, baking sheet, nonstick spray, small bowl

Prep: 15 minutes   •   **Cook:** 20 minutes

¼ **cup unsweetened plain almond milk**

1½ **tablespoons powdered peanut butter or defatted peanut flour**

1 **teaspoon honey**

½ **teaspoon lime juice**

¼ **teaspoon crushed garlic**

Dash cayenne pepper

1 **cup green beans, trimmed and cut into 1-inch pieces**

1 **cup sliced onion**

One 5-ounce raw boneless skinless chicken breast cutlet, pounded to ¼-inch thickness

⅛ **teaspoon each salt and black pepper**

1. Preheat oven to 375 degrees. Lay a large piece of heavy-duty foil on a baking sheet and spray with nonstick spray.

2. To make the sauce, in a small bowl, combine almond milk with powdered peanut butter/peanut flour; mix until smooth and uniform. Add honey, lime juice, garlic, and cayenne pepper. Mix until uniform.

3. Distribute green beans and onion onto the center of the foil. Season chicken with salt and black pepper, and place over the veggies. Top with sauce.

4. Cover with another large piece of foil. Fold together and seal all four edges of the foil pieces, forming a well-sealed packet.

5. Bake for 20 minutes, or until chicken is cooked through and veggies are tender.

6. Cut packet to release hot steam before opening entirely.

MAKES 1 SERVING

Ingredient FYI

Powdered peanut butter (a.k.a. defatted peanut flour) has less than half the calories of traditional PB! Flip to page 4 for shopping tips . . .

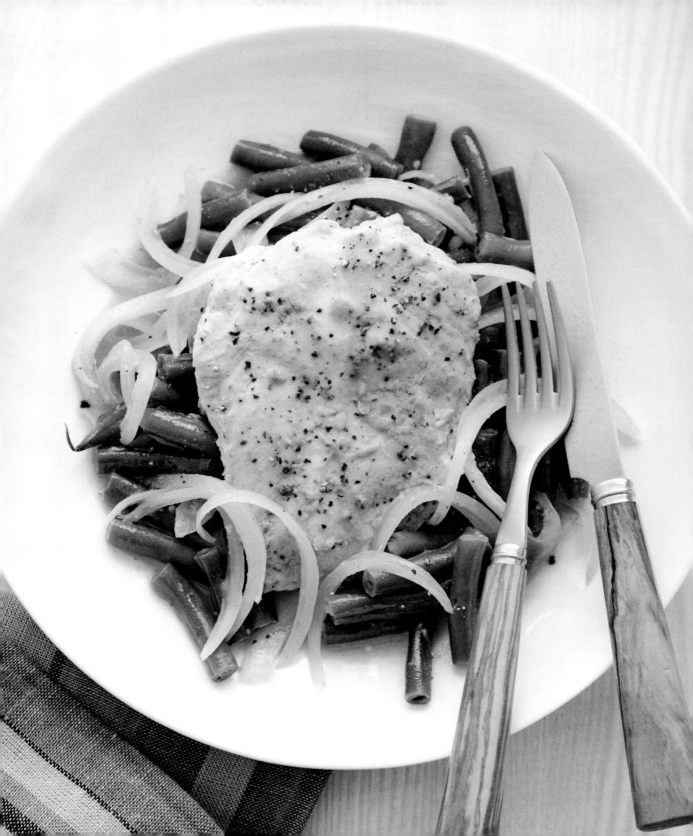

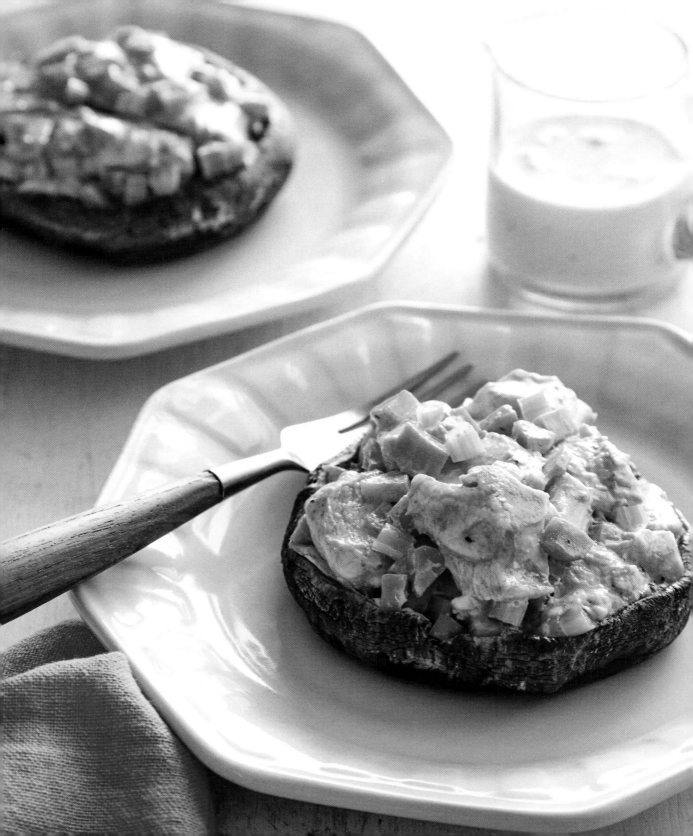

Buffalo Chicken Stuffed Portabellas

½ of recipe (1 stuffed mushroom): 228 calories, 6g total fat (2.5g sat fat), 564mg sodium, 9.5g carbs, 2.5g fiber, 4g sugars, 34g protein

This recipe is INCREDIBLE. Fans of Buffalo chicken should also check out the Slow-Cooker Buffalo Chicken (page 141), Buffalo Turkey Meatloaf (page 175), and Big Buffalo Cauliflower Bites (page 247).

You'll Need: heavy-duty aluminum foil, baking sheet, nonstick spray, medium bowl

Prep: 10 minutes • **Cook:** 25 minutes

2 teaspoons Frank's RedHot Original Cayenne Pepper Sauce

1 tablespoon fat-free plain Greek yogurt

Dash each salt and black pepper

8 ounces raw boneless skinless chicken breast, cut into bite-sized pieces

¼ cup finely chopped celery

¼ cup finely chopped carrots

2 large portabella mushroom caps (stems removed)

¼ cup Clean & Hungry Chunky Blue Cheese Dressing (recipe and store-bought alternatives on page 22)

1. Preheat oven to 375 degrees. Lay a large piece of heavy-duty foil on a baking sheet and spray with nonstick spray.

2. In a medium bowl, combine hot sauce, yogurt, salt, and pepper. Add chicken, celery, and carrots. Stir to coat.

3. Place mushroom caps on the foil, rounded sides down. Evenly divide chicken mixture between the mushroom caps.

4. Cover with another large piece of foil. Fold together and seal all four edges of the foil pieces, forming a well-sealed packet.

5. Bake for 25 minutes, or until chicken is cooked through and mushroom caps are soft.

6. Cut packet to release hot steam before opening entirely.

7. Top with blue cheese dressing.

MAKES 2 SERVINGS

Orange Salmon with Broccolini

½ of recipe (1 fillet with veggies): 276 calories, 12.5g total fat (4g sat fat), 411mg sodium, 14.5g carbs, 2g fiber, 7g sugars, 26g protein

This is one of the best salmon recipes to ever come out of the Hungry Girl Kitchen. Try it!

You'll Need: heavy-duty aluminum foil, baking sheet, nonstick spray, small microwave-safe bowl

Prep: 10 minutes • **Cook:** 25 minutes

1 large orange

1 tablespoon whipped butter

1 teaspoon chopped garlic

¼ teaspoon salt

8 stalks broccolini

1 cup sliced onion

Two 4-ounce raw skinless salmon fillets

2 dashes paprika

1. Preheat oven to 375 degrees. Lay a large piece of heavy-duty foil on a baking sheet and spray with nonstick spray.

2. Cut orange in half widthwise. Cut 2 thin slices from the cut side of each half, yielding 4 slices. Squeeze ¼ cup of juice from the remaining orange halves into a small microwave-safe bowl.

3. Add butter to the bowl. Microwave for 25 seconds, or until melted. Add garlic and ⅛ teaspoon salt, and mix until uniform.

4. Distribute broccolini and onion onto the center of the foil.

5. Lay salmon fillets over the veggies, and sprinkle with remaining ⅛ teaspoon salt. Drizzle salmon and veggies with orange juice mixture, and top each fillet with 2 orange slices. Sprinkle with paprika.

6. Cover with another large piece of foil. Fold together and seal all four edges of the foil pieces, forming a well-sealed packet.

7. Bake for 20 minutes, or until salmon is cooked through and veggies are tender.

8. Cut packet to release hot steam before opening entirely.

MAKES 2 SERVINGS

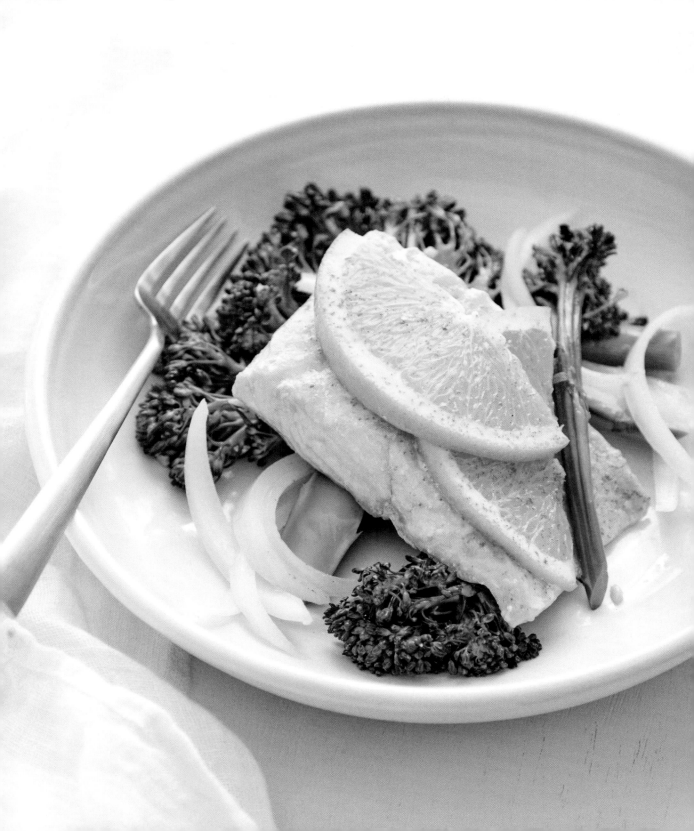

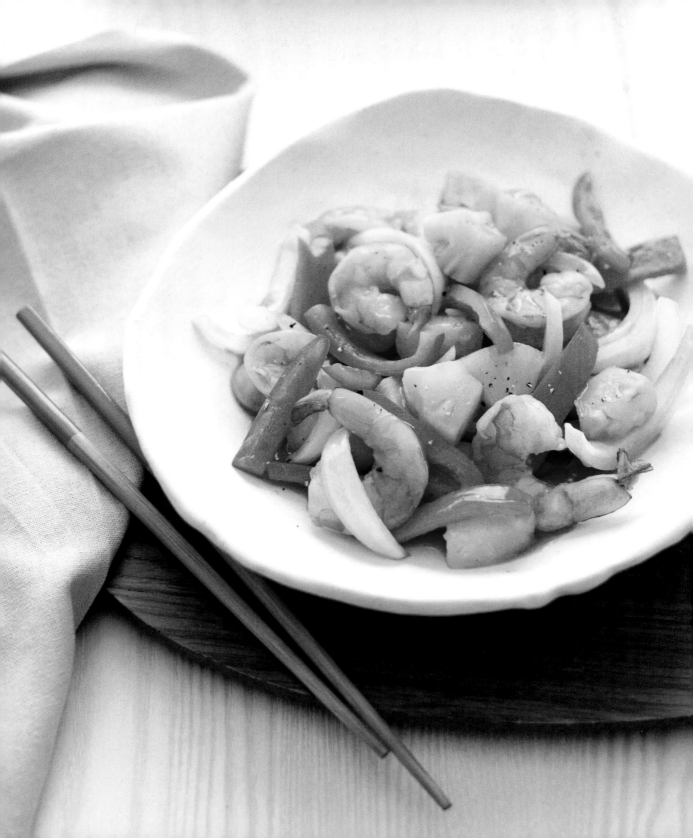

Shrimp Teriyaki

½ of recipe (about 1¾ cups): 190 calories, 1.5g total fat (0.5g sat fat), 525mg sodium, 21.5g carbs, 3g fiber, 13g sugars, 23g protein

You'll Need: heavy-duty aluminum foil, baking sheet, nonstick spray, small bowl

Prep: 10 minutes • **Cook:** 20 minutes

¼ **cup Clean & Hungry Teriyaki Sauce (recipe and store-bought alternatives on page 23)**

1 packet natural no-calorie sweetener

1 cup sliced red bell pepper

1 cup sliced onion

1 cup pineapple chunks (fresh or previously packed in juice)

8 ounces (about 16) raw large shrimp, peeled, tails removed, deveined

Optional seasonings: salt and black pepper

1. Preheat oven to 375 degrees. Lay a large piece of heavy-duty foil on a baking sheet and spray with nonstick spray.

2. In a small bowl, stir sweetener into teriyaki sauce.

3. Distribute bell pepper, onion, and pineapple onto the center of the foil. Top with shrimp.

4. Drizzle sweetened teriyaki sauce over the shrimp, veggies, and pineapple.

5. Cover with another large piece of foil. Fold together and seal all four edges of the foil pieces, forming a well-sealed packet.

6. Bake for 20 minutes, or until shrimp are cooked through and veggies are tender.

7. Cut packet to release hot steam before opening entirely.

MAKES 2 SERVINGS

Z'paghetti Marinara with Shrimp

½ of recipe (about 2½ cups): 266 calories, 5g total fat (2g sat fat), 871mg sodium, 25.5g carbs, 7g fiber, 15.5g sugars, 32g protein

What's "z'paghetti"? It's the Hungry Girl name for zucchini noodles, and it's a *fantastic* swap for ordinary pasta. For more z'paghetti recipes, don't miss Chapter 8: Z'paghetti, Spaghetti Squash & More Veggie-Noodle Dishes.

You'll Need: heavy-duty aluminum foil, baking sheet, nonstick spray, spiral vegetable slicer (or vegetable peeler), large bowl

Prep: 15 minutes • **Cook:** 25 minutes

28 ounces (about 4 medium) zucchini

8 ounces (about 16) raw large shrimp, peeled, tails removed, deveined

¼ teaspoon Italian seasoning

¼ teaspoon garlic powder

⅛ teaspoon black pepper

1 cup Clean & Hungry Marinara Sauce (recipe and store-bought alternatives on page 20)

2 tablespoons grated Parmesan cheese

1. Preheat oven to 375 degrees. Lay a large piece of heavy-duty foil on a baking sheet and spray with nonstick spray.

2. Using a spiral vegetable slicer, cut zucchini into spaghetti-like noodles. (If you don't have a spiral veggie slicer, peel zucchini into super-thin strips, rotating the zucchini after each strip.) Roughly chop for shorter noodles.

3. Place zucchini noodles in the center of the foil and top with shrimp. Sprinkle with seasonings. Top with marinara sauce and Parm.

4. Cover with another large piece of foil. Fold together and seal all four edges of the foil pieces, forming a well-sealed packet.

5. Bake for 25 minutes, or until zucchini noodles have softened and shrimp are fully cooked.

6. Cut packet to release hot steam before opening entirely.

7. Transfer packet contents to a large bowl, and toss to mix.

MAKES 2 SERVINGS

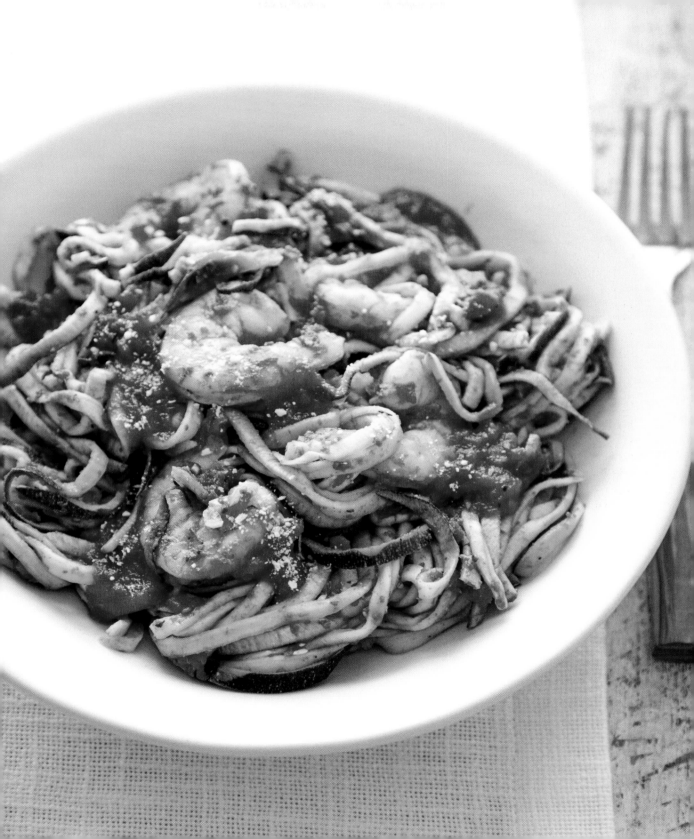

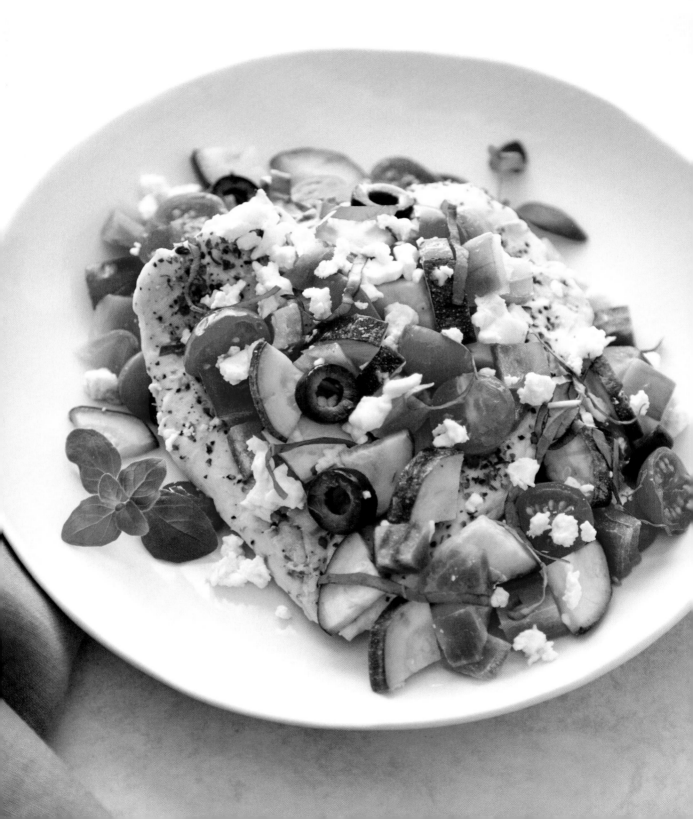

Mediterranean Chicken

Entire recipe: 304 calories, 9.5g total fat (4g sat fat),
678mg sodium, 15g carbs, 3g fiber, 7.5g sugars, 37.5g protein

You'll Need: heavy-duty aluminum foil, baking sheet, nonstick spray

Prep: 15 minutes • **Cook:** 25 minutes

One 5-ounce raw boneless
skinless chicken breast cutlet,
pounded to ¼-inch thickness

⅛ teaspoon oregano

⅛ teaspoon each salt and
black pepper

½ cup chopped zucchini

½ cup chopped red onion

½ cup cherry tomatoes, halved

1 tablespoon sliced black olives

1 tablespoon chopped fresh basil

1½ teaspoons lemon juice

3 tablespoons crumbled feta
cheese

1. Preheat oven to 375 degrees. Lay a large piece of
heavy-duty foil on a baking sheet and spray with
nonstick spray.

2. Season chicken with oregano, salt, and pepper, and
place in the center of the foil. Top with veggies,
olives, and basil. Drizzle with lemon juice, and
sprinkle with cheese.

3. Cover with another large piece of foil. Fold together
and seal all four edges of the foil pieces, forming a
well-sealed packet.

4. Bake for 25 minutes, or until chicken is cooked
through and veggies are tender.

5. Cut packet to release hot steam before opening
entirely.

MAKES 1 SERVING

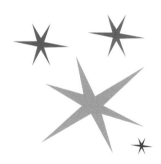

Chicken & Shrimp Jambalaya

Entire recipe: 320 calories, 3.5g total fat (0.5g sat fat), 667mg sodium, 30.5g carbs, 10g fiber, 14.5g sugars, 41.5g protein

Rather than use rice—which is pretty calorie dense—this hearty and delicious dish is made with riced cauliflower. So cool! For more recipes like this, check out Chapter 9: Cauliflower Rice & More Cauliflower Creations.

You'll Need: heavy-duty aluminum foil, baking sheet, nonstick spray, blender, large bowl

Prep: 20 minutes • **Cook:** 25 minutes

2 cups roughly chopped cauliflower

3 ounces raw boneless skinless chicken breast, cut into bite-sized pieces

3 ounces (about 6) raw large shrimp, peeled, tails removed, deveined, chopped

¼ teaspoon paprika

¼ teaspoon cayenne pepper

¼ teaspoon onion powder

¼ teaspoon oregano

¼ teaspoon black pepper

½ cup canned fire-roasted diced tomatoes (not drained)

½ cup chopped tomatoes

¼ cup chopped onion

¼ cup chopped green bell pepper

¼ cup chopped celery

1 teaspoon chopped garlic

Optional seasonings: salt and additional black pepper

1. Preheat oven to 400 degrees. Lay a large piece of heavy-duty foil on a baking sheet and spray with nonstick spray.

2. Pulse cauliflower in a blender until reduced to rice-sized pieces.

3. In a large bowl, combine chicken with shrimp. Season with ⅛ teaspoon of each seasoning.

4. Add cauliflower rice and all remaining ingredients, including the remaining ⅛ teaspoon of each seasoning. Mix well. Distribute mixture onto the center of the foil.

5. Cover with another large piece of foil. Fold together and seal all four edges of the foil pieces, forming a well-sealed packet.

6. Bake for 25 minutes, or until chicken and shrimp are cooked through and veggies are tender.

7. Cut packet to release hot steam before opening entirely.

MAKES 1 SERVING

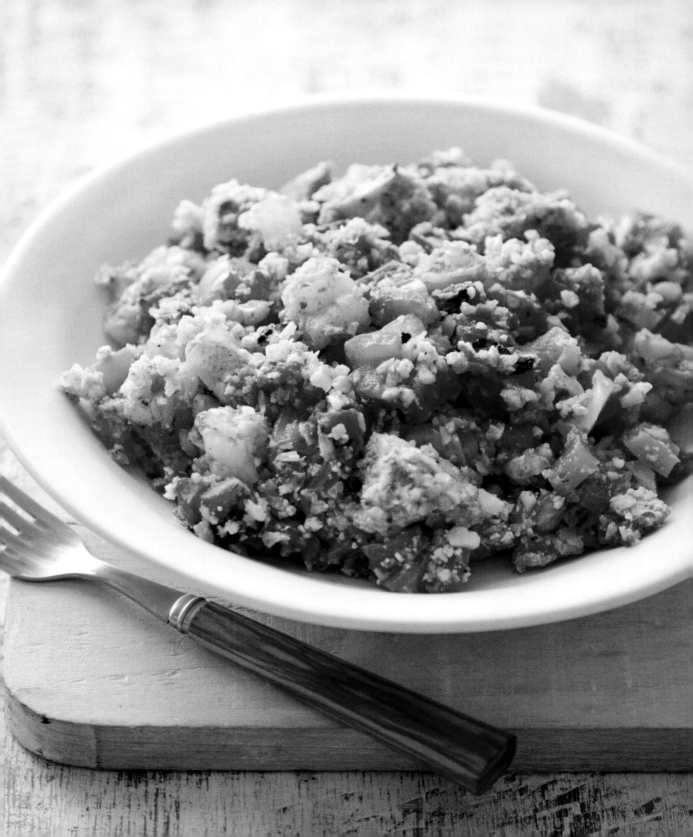

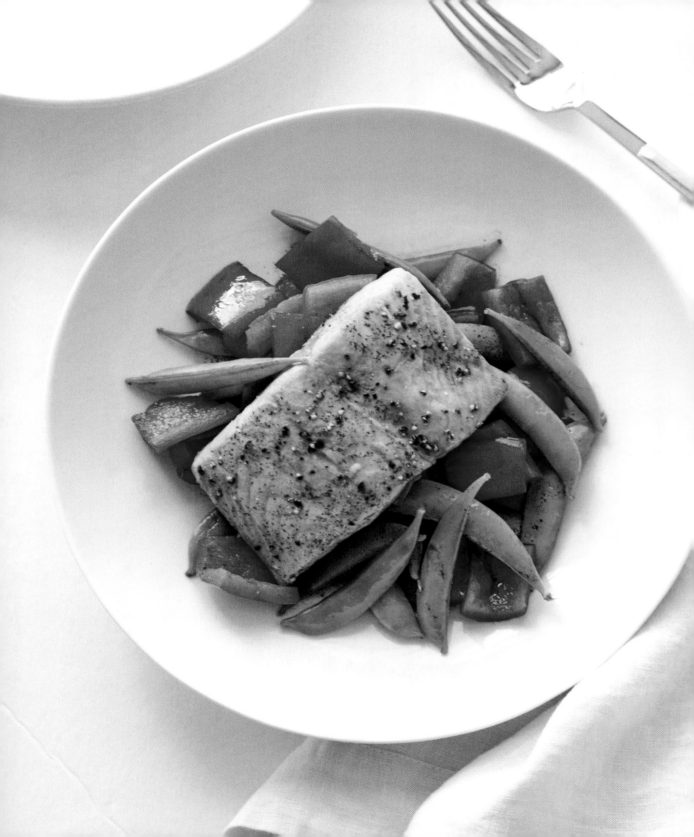

Balsamic Honey Salmon 'n Veggies

Entire recipe: 340 calories, 9.5g total fat (2g sat fat), 379mg sodium, 37.5g carbs, 4g fiber, 31g sugars, 26.5g protein

You'll Need: heavy-duty aluminum foil, baking sheet, nonstick spray, medium bowl, whisk

Prep: 10 minutes • **Cook:** 20 minutes

3 tablespoons balsamic vinegar

1 tablespoon honey

1 cup red bell pepper cut into 1-inch chunks

1 cup sugar snap peas

One 4-ounce raw skinless salmon fillet

⅛ teaspoon each salt and black pepper

1. Preheat oven to 375 degrees. Lay a large piece of heavy-duty foil on a baking sheet and spray with nonstick spray.

2. In a medium bowl, whisk balsamic vinegar with honey until uniform.

3. Lay bell pepper and snap peas on the center of the foil. Season salmon with salt and black pepper, and place over the veggies. Drizzle with vinegar mixture.

4. Cover with another large piece of foil. Fold together and seal all four edges of the foil pieces, forming a well-sealed packet.

5. Bake for 20 minutes, or until fish is cooked through and veggies are tender.

6. Cut packet to release hot steam before opening entirely.

MAKES 1 SERVING

Kale & Feta Stuffed Pork

¼ᵗʰ of recipe (2 medallions, each about 1 inch thick):
182 calories, 5.5g total fat (3g sat fat), 543mg sodium, 4.5g carbs,
1g fiber, <0.5g sugars, 27.5g protein

This dish seems fancy, but it's so easy to make. And so delicious! Feta and pork bring out the best in each other . . .

You'll Need: heavy-duty aluminum foil, baking sheet, nonstick spray, large microwave-safe bowl, meat mallet, toothpicks

Prep: 20 minutes • **Cook:** 40 minutes

4 cups roughly chopped kale leaves

½ cup crumbled feta cheese

2 teaspoons chopped garlic

One 1-pound raw pork tenderloin, trimmed of excess fat

½ teaspoon each salt and black pepper

1. Preheat oven to 425 degrees. Lay a large piece of heavy-duty foil on a baking sheet and spray with nonstick spray.

2. In a large microwave-safe bowl, microwave kale for 2 minutes, or until wilted. Blot away excess moisture. Add feta and garlic, and mix well.

3. Season pork with salt and pepper. Slice like a hot dog bun—midway through the thickest part of the length, stopping about three-quarters of the way through.

4. Pound pork with a meat mallet to ½-inch thickness. Distribute kale-feta mixture lengthwise along the center of the tenderloin.

5. Roll up tenderloin widthwise over the mixture. Secure with toothpicks.

6. Carefully transfer tenderloin to the center of the foil. Cover with another large piece of foil. Fold together and seal all four edges of the foil pieces, forming a well-sealed packet.

7. Bake for 30 minutes, or until pork is cooked through.

8. Cut packet to release hot steam before opening entirely. Let pork rest for 5 minutes.

9. Slice into 8 medallions.

MAKES 4 SERVINGS

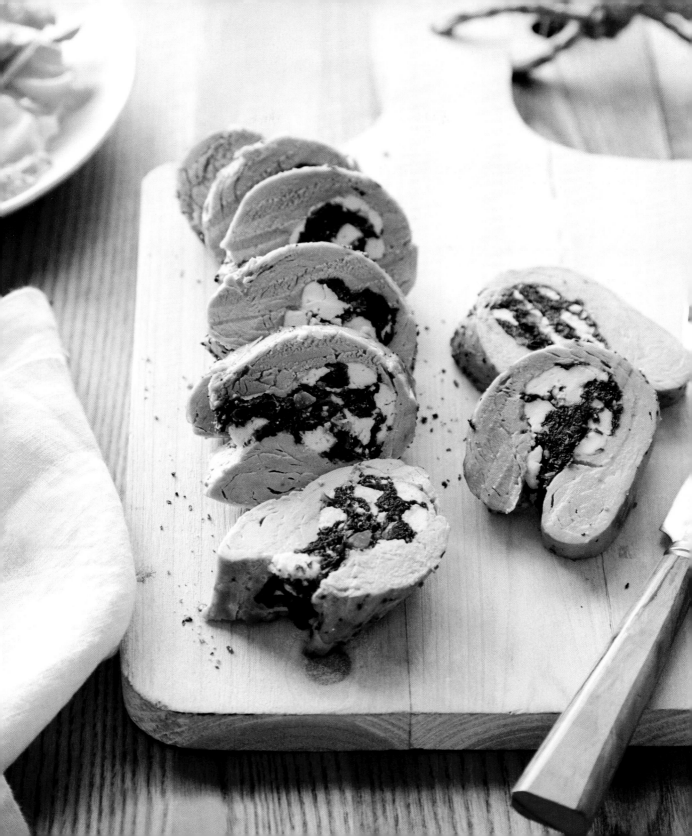

7

Meatloaf & Casseroles

This chapter's a MUST if you're looking
for family-friendly, multi-serving meals.
So many incredibly tasty dishes!

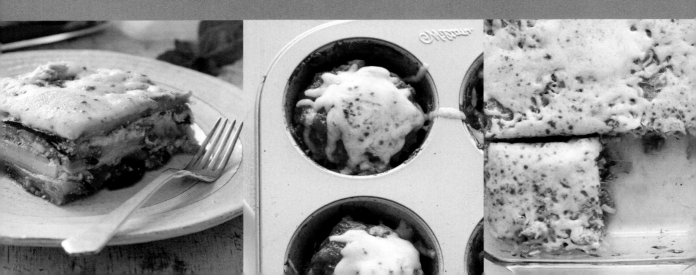

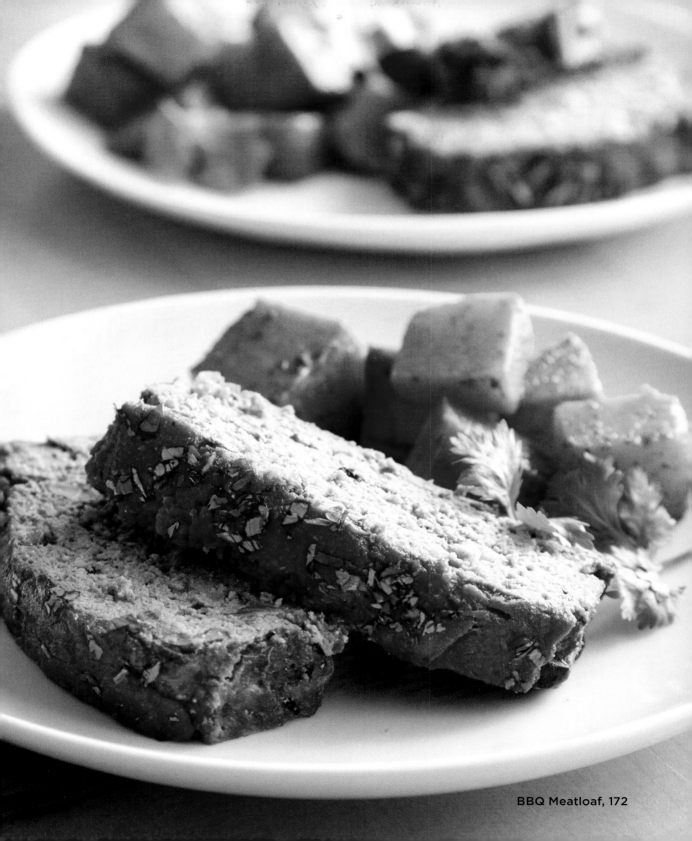

BBQ Meatloaf, 172

Meatball-Style Mini Meatloaves

¹⁄₁₂ᵗʰ of recipe (1 mini meatloaf): 94 calories, 3g total fat (1.5g sat fat), 235mg sodium, 4.5g carbs, 1g fiber, 1.5g sugars, 11.5g protein

You'll Need: 12-cup muffin pan, nonstick spray, large bowl

Prep: 15 minutes • **Cook:** 40 minutes

1 pound raw extra-lean ground beef (4% fat or less)

1 cup finely chopped onion

1 cup finely chopped mushrooms

¼ cup whole-wheat panko breadcrumbs

¼ cup (about 2 large) egg whites

1 teaspoon Italian seasoning

½ teaspoon garlic powder

½ teaspoon each salt and black pepper

¾ cup Clean & Hungry Marinara Sauce (recipe and store-bought alternatives on page 20)

¾ cup shredded part-skim mozzarella cheese

1 tablespoon grated Parmesan cheese

1. Preheat oven to 375 degrees. Spray a 12-cup muffin pan with nonstick spray.

2. In a large bowl, mix all ingredients *except* marinara sauce, mozzarella, and Parm. Evenly distribute mixture among the muffin cups, and smooth out the tops. Evenly top with marinara sauce.

3. Bake until firm with lightly browned edges, about 35 minutes.

4. Sprinkle with mozzarella and Parm. Bake until melted, about 5 minutes.

MAKES 12 SERVINGS

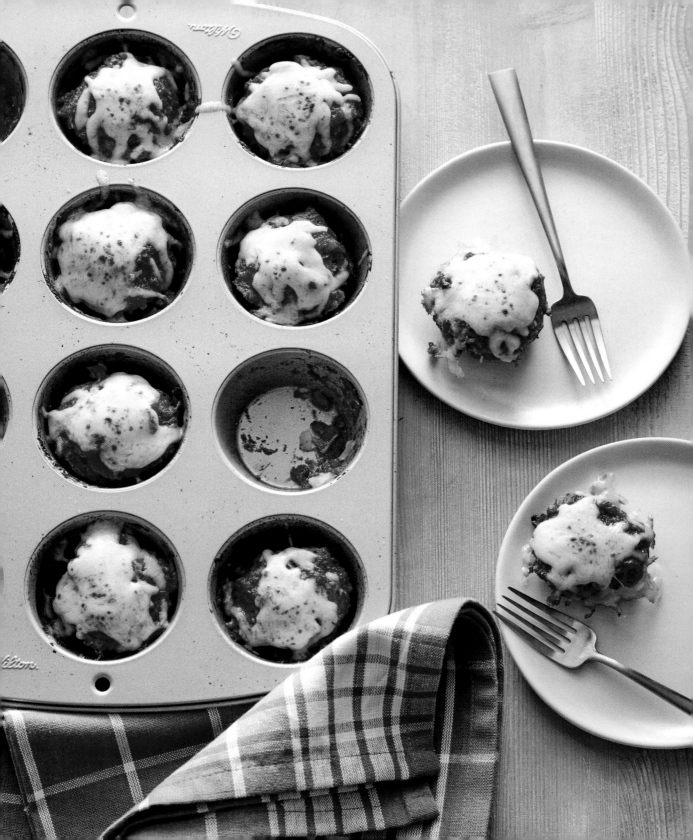

BBQ Meatloaf

⅕th of meatloaf (2 slices, each about ¾ inch thick): 196 calories, 5.5g total fat (2g sat fat), 481mg sodium, 13.5g carbs, 2g fiber, 6.5g sugars, 22g protein

You'll Need: 9-inch by 5-inch loaf pan, nonstick spray, skillet, large bowl

Prep: 15 minutes • **Cook:** 1 hour and 15 minutes

2 cups sliced onion

1 tablespoon whipped butter

½ teaspoon plus 1 dash salt

¼ teaspoon plus 1 dash black pepper

1½ cups chopped portabella mushrooms

1 pound raw extra-lean ground beef (4% fat or less)

¼ cup whole-wheat panko breadcrumbs

¼ cup (about 2 large) egg whites

¼ teaspoon onion powder

¼ teaspoon garlic powder

½ cup Clean & Hungry BBQ Sauce (recipe and store-bought alternatives on page 19)

2 tablespoons chopped fresh cilantro

1. Preheat oven to 400 degrees. Spray a 9-inch by 5-inch loaf pan with nonstick spray.

2. Bring a skillet sprayed with nonstick spray to medium-low heat. Add onion and butter. Cook and stir until onion has caramelized, about 20 minutes.

3. Roughly chop caramelized onions. Transfer to a large bowl, and stir in a dash each salt and pepper.

4. Remove skillet from heat; clean, if needed. Re-spray and bring to medium heat. Cook and stir mushrooms until soft, about 5 minutes. Remove from heat and, once cool enough to handle, blot away excess moisture. Transfer to the large bowl.

5. Add beef, breadcrumbs, egg whites, onion powder, garlic powder, remaining ½ teaspoon salt, and remaining ¼ teaspoon pepper. Add ¼ cup BBQ sauce, and mix thoroughly.

6. Transfer mixture to the loaf pan, and smooth out the top. Evenly top with remaining ¼ cup BBQ sauce, and sprinkle with cilantro.

7. Bake until cooked through, about 50 minutes.

MAKES 5 SERVINGS

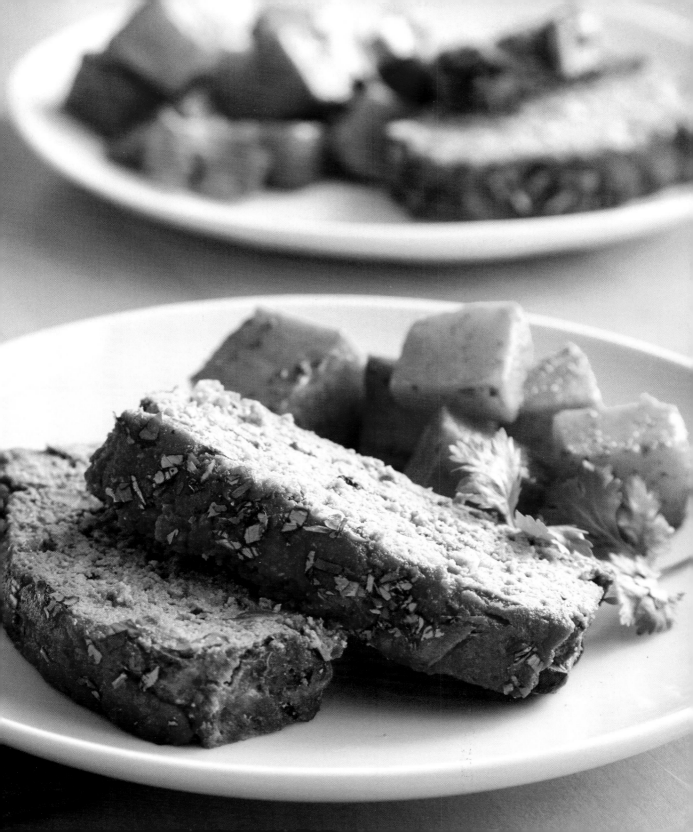

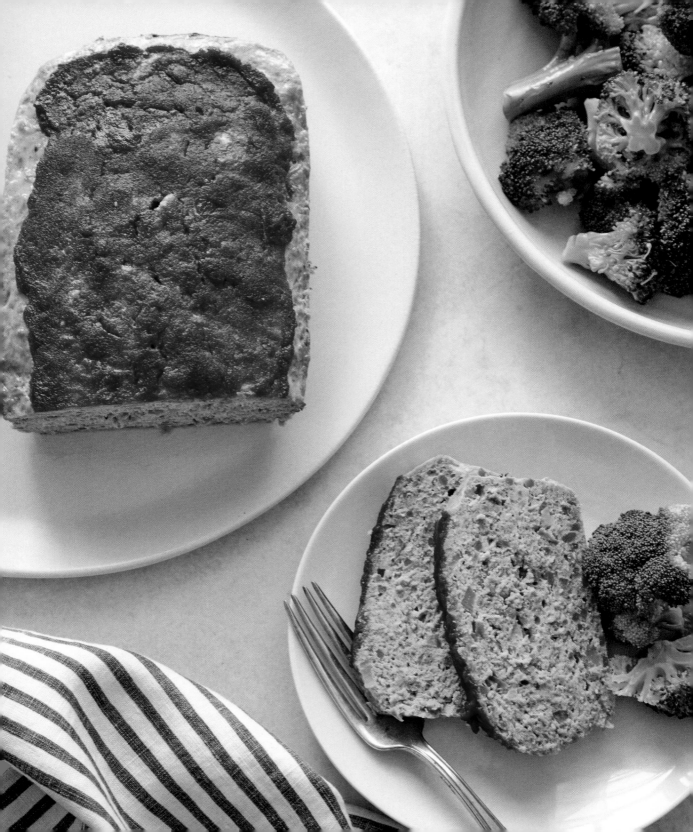

Buffalo Turkey Meatloaf

⅕th of meatloaf (2 slices, each about ¾ inch thick): 200 calories, 8g total fat (2.5g sat fat), 629mg sodium, 7.5g carbs, 1.5g fiber, 2.5g sugars, 25g protein

So much flavor! For more Buffalo-sauced deliciousness, check out the Slow-Cooker Buffalo Chicken (page 141), Buffalo Chicken Stuffed Portabellas (page 153), and Big Buffalo Cauliflower Bites (page 247).

You'll Need: 9-inch by 5-inch loaf pan, nonstick spray, skillet, large bowl, small bowl

Prep: 20 minutes • **Cook:** 1 hour

½ cup shredded carrots, finely chopped

½ cup finely chopped celery

½ cup finely chopped onion

1 teaspoon chopped garlic

1¼ pounds raw lean ground turkey (7% fat or less)

¼ cup whole-wheat panko breadcrumbs

¼ cup (about 2 large) egg whites

⅛ teaspoon black pepper

⅛ teaspoon cayenne pepper

¼ cup Frank's RedHot Original Cayenne Pepper Sauce

2 tablespoons Clean & Hungry Ketchup (recipe and store-bought alternatives on page 24)

Optional topping: Clean & Hungry Chunky Blue Cheese Dressing (recipe and store-bought alternatives on page 22)

1. Preheat oven to 400 degrees. Spray a 9-inch by 5-inch loaf pan with nonstick spray.

2. Bring a skillet sprayed with nonstick spray to medium-high heat. Add veggies and ¼ cup water. Cover and cook until veggies have mostly softened and water has evaporated, about 5 minutes. Add garlic, and cook and stir until fragrant, about 1 minute. Transfer to a large bowl.

3. To the large bowl, add turkey, breadcrumbs, egg whites, black pepper, and cayenne pepper. Add 3 tablespoons hot sauce, and mix thoroughly.

4. Transfer mixture to the loaf pan, and smooth out the top.

5. In a small bowl, combine ketchup with remaining 1 tablespoon hot sauce. Mix until uniform. Spread over meatloaf.

6. Bake until cooked through, about 50 minutes.

MAKES 5 SERVINGS

⅛th of pan (about 4½ inches by 4½ inches): 249 calories, 6g total fat (3g sat fat), 611mg sodium, 22g carbs, 5g fiber, 10g sugars, 28g protein

(GF)

This life-changing casserole recipe comes from Melisa, an American Airlines flight attendant who I met on board a flight from Boston to Los Angeles. She recognized me and told me she'd lost over 100 POUNDS with Hungry Girl's help! We became pals and she shared one of her favorite personal recipes with me and now it's a favorite of MINE! Thanks, Melisa!

You'll Need: 9-inch by 13-inch baking pan, nonstick spray, extra-large skillet, spiral vegetable slicer (or vegetable peeler), large bowl

Prep: 25 minutes • **Cook:** 1 hour • **Cool:** 10 minutes

Plus prep and cook times for spaghetti squash (page 198) if not made in advance.

1 pound raw boneless skinless chicken breast cutlets, pounded to ½-inch thickness

½ teaspoon each salt and black pepper

14 ounces (about 2 medium) zucchini

3 cups chopped mushrooms

1½ cups chopped onion

1 tablespoon chopped garlic

4 cups cooked spaghetti squash, drained of excess moisture

1¾ cups Clean & Hungry Marinara Sauce (recipe and store-bought alternatives on page 20)

½ cup (about 4 large) egg whites

1 tablespoon Italian seasoning

1 cup shredded part-skim mozzarella cheese

1. Preheat oven to 375 degrees. Spray a 9-inch by 13-inch baking pan with nonstick spray.

2. Bring an extra-large skillet sprayed with nonstick spray to medium heat. Season chicken with ¼ teaspoon each salt and pepper. Cook for about 4 minutes per side, until cooked through. Transfer to a cutting board.

3. Using a spiral vegetable slicer, cut zucchini into spaghetti-like noodles. (If you don't have a spiral veggie slicer, peel zucchini into super-thin strips, rotating the zucchini after each strip.) Roughly chop for shorter noodles. Transfer to a large bowl.

4. Clean skillet, if needed. Re-spray, and bring to medium-high heat. Add mushrooms, onion, and garlic. Cook and stir until slightly softened and lightly browned, about 4 minutes.

5. Transfer skillet contents to the large bowl. Add spaghetti squash, marinara sauce, egg whites, Italian seasoning, and remaining ¼ teaspoon each salt and pepper.

6. Chop chicken, and add to the large bowl. Mix thoroughly.

7. Transfer mixture to the baking pan, and smooth out the surface. Top with cheese.

8. Bake until entire dish is hot and bubbly, cheese has melted and lightly browned, and any liquid on top has evaporated, about 45 minutes.

9. Let cool for 10 minutes. If needed, blot away excess moisture.

MAKES 6 SERVINGS

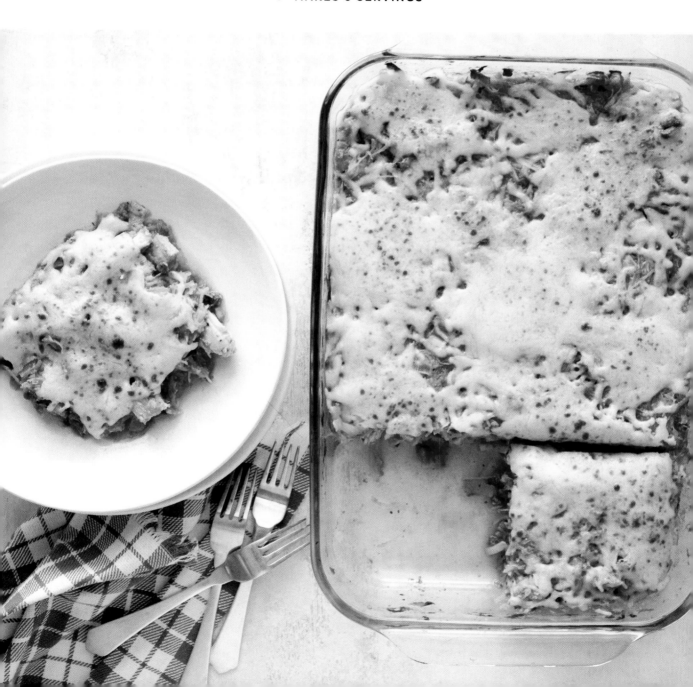

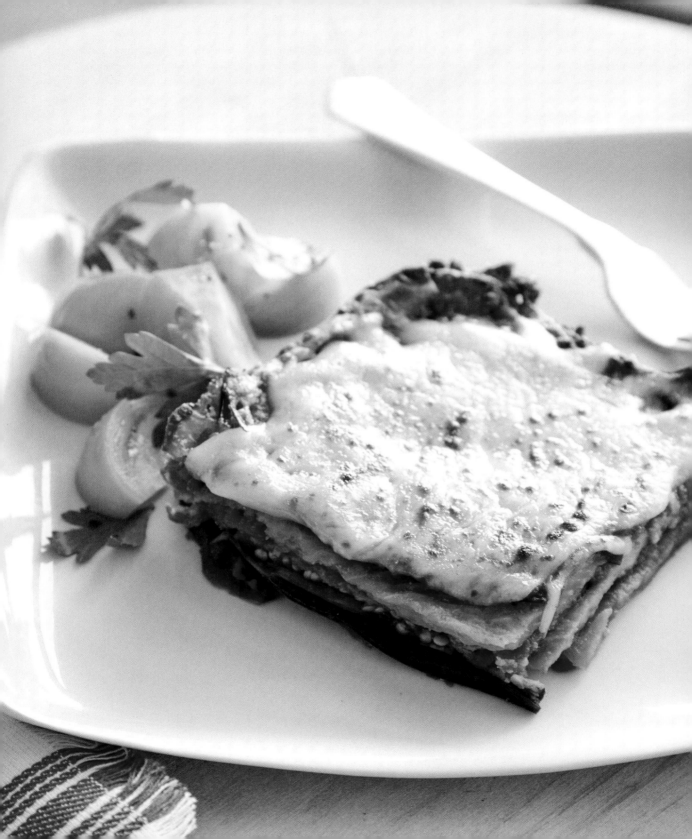

Naked Eggplant Parm

¼th of pan (about 4 inches by 4 inches): 182 calories, 8g total fat (5g sat fat), 659mg sodium, 15g carbs, 6.5g fiber, 6.5g sugars, 14g protein

This recipe will soon become a family favorite. You NEED to try this one...

You'll Need: baking sheet, 8-inch by 8-inch baking pan, nonstick spray, aluminum foil

Prep: 15 minutes • **Cook:** 1 hour and 5 minutes • **Cool:** 10 minutes

1 large eggplant (about 20 ounces), ends removed

½ teaspoon garlic powder

½ teaspoon onion powder

¼ teaspoon salt

1 cup Clean & Hungry Marinara Sauce (recipe and store-bought alternatives on page 20)

1 cup shredded part-skim mozzarella cheese

¼ cup grated Parmesan cheese

1. Preheat oven to 400 degrees. Spray a baking sheet and an 8-inch by 8-inch baking pan with nonstick spray.

2. Cut eggplant lengthwise into ½-inch slices. Sprinkle with seasonings, and lay on the baking sheet.

3. Bake for 20 minutes.

4. Flip eggplant. Bake until lightly browned, and slightly softened, about 10 minutes. Remove sheet, but leave oven on.

5. Evenly layer the following ingredients in the baking pan: ¼ cup sauce, half of the eggplant slices, ¼ cup sauce, ½ cup mozzarella cheese, 2 tablespoons Parm, and ¼ cup sauce.

6. Continue layering with remaining eggplant slices, ¼ cup sauce, ½ cup mozzarella cheese, and 2 tablespoons Parm.

7. Cover pan with foil, and bake for 30 minutes, or until hot and bubbly.

8. Uncover and bake until cheese has melted, about 5 minutes.

9. Let cool for 10 minutes before slicing.

MAKES 4 SERVINGS

No-Noodle Veggie Lasagna

¼ᵗʰ of pan (about 4 inches by 4 inches): 266 calories, 11g total fat (7g sat fat), 753mg sodium, 23.5g carbs, 8g fiber, 13g sugars, 21.5g protein

This is a cleaned-up version of a Hungry Girl classic. Instead of pasta sheets, it's made with sliced eggplant and zucchini!

You'll Need: 2 baking sheets, 8-inch by 8-inch baking pan, nonstick spray, medium bowl, aluminum foil

Prep: 25 minutes • **Cook:** 1 hour • **Cool:** 10 minutes

20 ounces (2 to 3 medium) zucchini, ends removed

1 large eggplant (about 20 ounces), ends removed

1 teaspoon garlic powder

1 teaspoon onion powder

¼ teaspoon salt

1 cup light/low-fat ricotta cheese

1 tablespoon chopped fresh basil

1 teaspoon chopped garlic

1 cup Clean & Hungry Marinara Sauce (recipe and store-bought alternatives on page 20)

1 cup shredded part-skim mozzarella cheese

¼ cup grated Parmesan cheese

1. Preheat oven to 375 degrees. Spray 2 baking sheets and an 8-inch by 8-inch baking pan with nonstick spray.

2. Slice zucchini in half widthwise, and then slice each half lengthwise into ¼-inch-thick strips. Cut eggplant lengthwise into ¼-inch-thick slices.

3. Sprinkle veggie slices with seasonings, and evenly place on the baking sheets, slightly overlapping if needed.

4. Bake for 10 minutes.

5. Flip veggie slices. Bake until softened, about 10 more minutes.

6. Thoroughly blot veggies dry.

7. Increase oven temperature to 400 degrees.

8. In a medium bowl, combine ricotta, basil, and chopped garlic. Mix until uniform.

9. Evenly layer the following ingredients in the baking pan: ¼ cup sauce, half of the veggies, half of the seasoned ricotta, ¼ cup sauce, ½ cup mozzarella cheese, 2 tablespoons Parm, and ¼ cup sauce.

10. Continue layering with remaining veggies, seasoned ricotta, ¼ cup sauce, ½ cup mozzarella cheese, and 2 tablespoons Parm.

11. Cover pan with foil, and bake for 30 minutes, or until hot and bubbly.

12. Uncover and bake until cheese has lightly browned, about 5 minutes.

13. Let cool for 10 minutes before slicing.

MAKES 4 SERVINGS

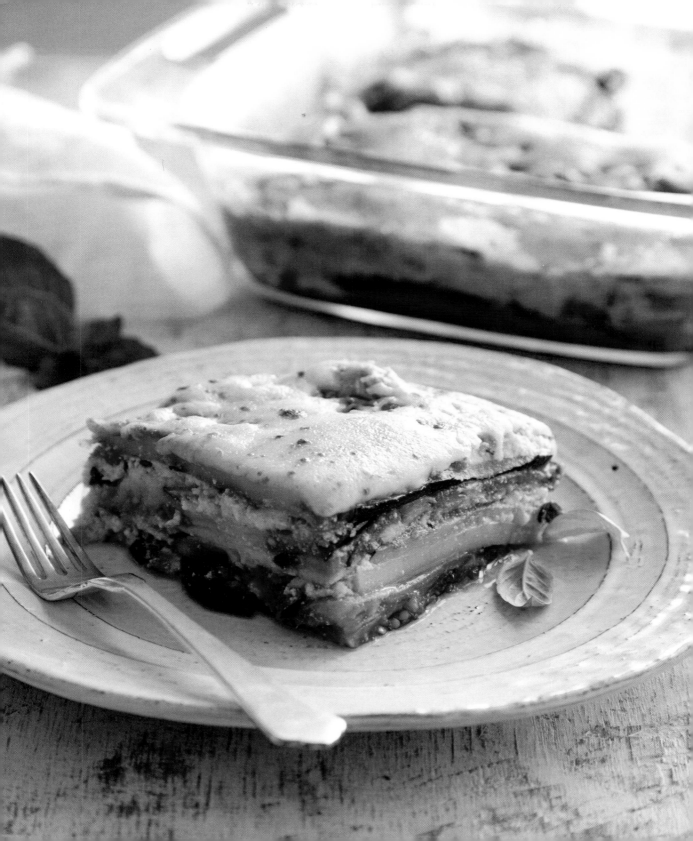

8

Z'paghetti, Spaghetti Squash & More Veggie-Noodle Dishes

Traditional pasta dishes can be high in calories and carbs. Not these veggie-based creations! P.S. Eight out of nine of 'em are completely gluten-free. Dig in . . .

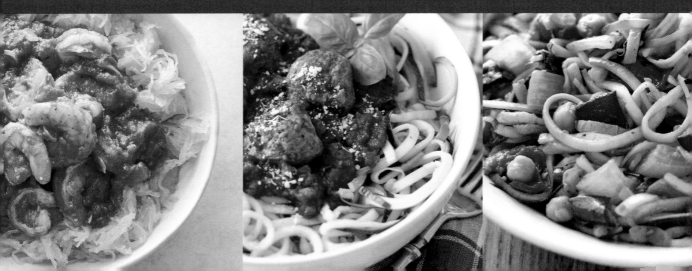

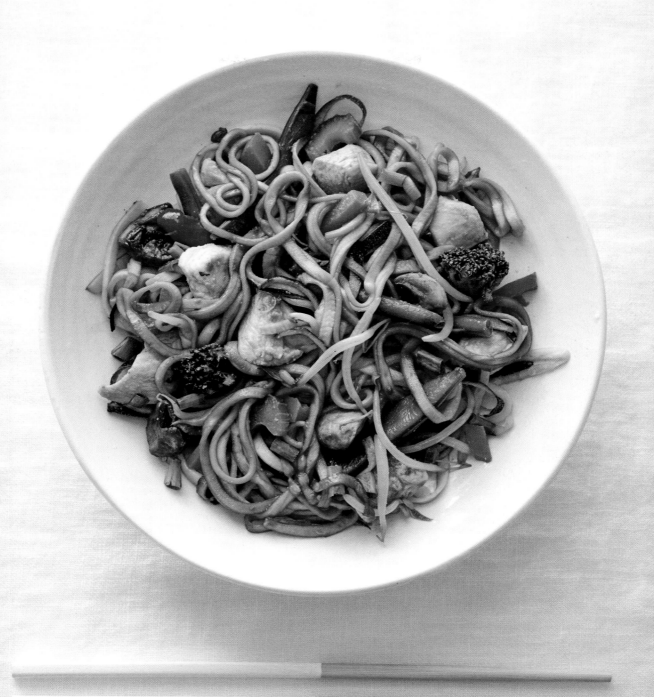

Chicken Zucchini So Low Mein, 195

All About Z'paghetti, a.k.a. Zucchini Noodles

When sliced into skinny noodle-like strands, zucchini becomes an *amazing* pasta swap. You may never look at the summer squash the same way again . . .

You'll wanna get yourself a spiralizer. While there are fancy versions of this handy kitchen tool, a basic (read: inexpensive) model works perfectly. You can find them online and at stores like Bed Bath & Beyond. The Veggetti is the Hungry Girl top pick . . .

Alternatively, zucchini noodles can be made with a standard veggie peeler. Just peel the zucchini into super-thin strips, rotating the zucchini after each strip. This will give you wider noodles—more like "z'ettuccine"—but the results will be just as delicious.

HG tip: If using a handheld spiralizer like the Veggetti, wrap a paper towel around the stem end of the zucchini. This will help you to firmly grip the zucchini and create as many noodles as possible.

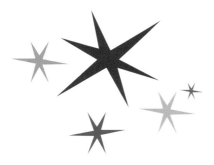

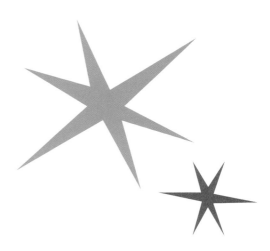

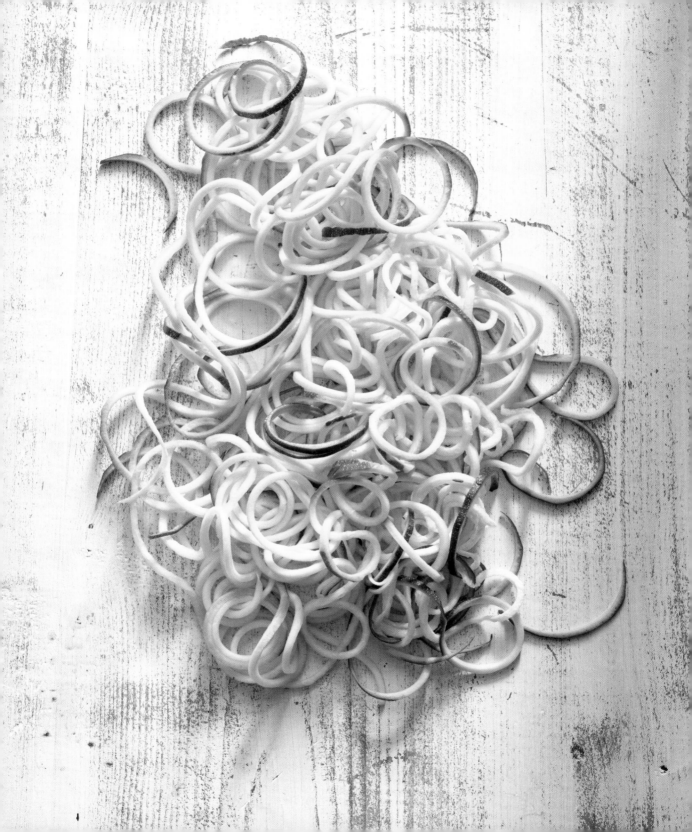

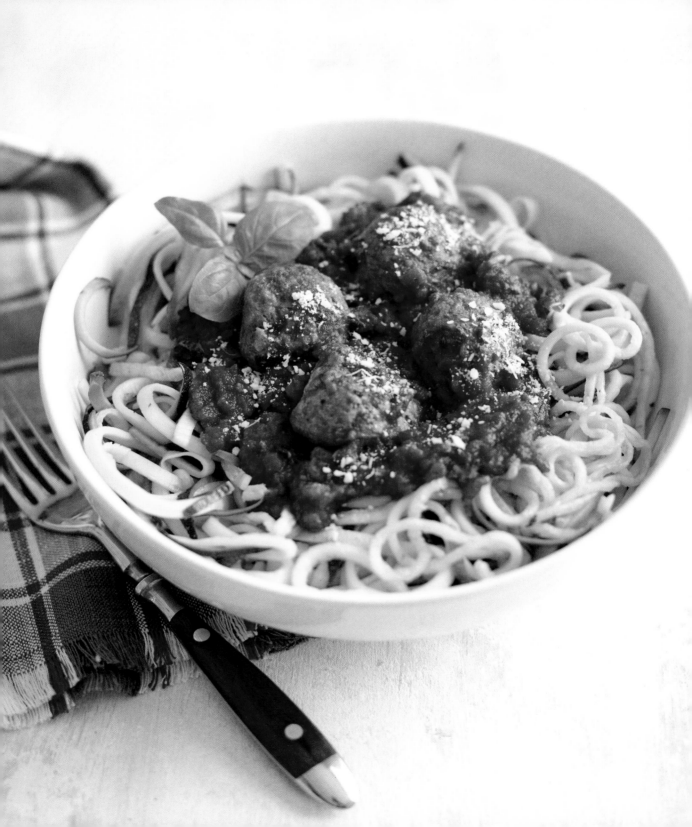

Z'paghetti & Meatballs

½ of recipe (about 1½ cups zucchini noodles with 4 meatballs): 299 calories, 7.5g total fat (3g sat fat), 766mg sodium, 29.5g carbs, 7.5g fiber, 16g sugars, 31g protein

Everyone's favorite comfort food got a lean 'n clean makeover. For a gluten-free version, just leave out the breadcrumbs . . .

You'll Need: baking sheet, nonstick spray, medium bowl, spiral vegetable slicer (or vegetable peeler), extra-large skillet, strainer, large bowl

Prep: 15 minutes • **Cook:** 20 minutes

6 ounces raw extra-lean ground beef (4% fat or less)

2 tablespoons whole-wheat panko breadcrumbs

2 tablespoons (about 1 large) egg white

⅛ teaspoon each salt and black pepper

1½ teaspoons chopped garlic

½ teaspoon Italian seasoning

28 ounces (about 4 medium) zucchini

1 cup Clean & Hungry Marinara Sauce (recipe and store-bought alternatives on page 20)

2 tablespoons chopped fresh basil

2 tablespoons grated Parmesan cheese

1. Preheat oven to 400 degrees. Spray a baking sheet with nonstick spray.

2. In a medium bowl, combine beef, breadcrumbs, egg white, salt, pepper, ½ teaspoon garlic, and ¼ teaspoon Italian seasoning. Mix thoroughly. Evenly form into 8 meatballs and place on the baking sheet, evenly spaced.

3. Bake until cooked through, about 10 minutes.

4. Meanwhile, using a spiral vegetable slicer, cut zucchini into spaghetti-like noodles. (If you don't have a spiral veggie slicer, peel zucchini into super-thin strips, rotating the zucchini after each strip.) Roughly chop for shorter noodles.

5. Bring an extra-large skillet sprayed with nonstick spray to medium-high heat. Cook and stir zucchini noodles until hot and slightly softened, about 3 minutes.

6. Transfer noodles to a strainer, and thoroughly drain excess liquid. Transfer to a large bowl, and cover to keep warm.

7. Remove skillet from heat; clean, if needed. Re-spray, and return to medium-high heat. Carefully add sauce, basil, remaining 1 teaspoon garlic, and remaining ¼ teaspoon Italian seasoning. Stir well. Add meatballs, and stir to coat. Cook until hot, about 3 minutes.

8. Spoon sauce and meatballs over the zucchini noodles, and sprinkle with Parm.

MAKES 2 SERVINGS

Shrimp & Avocado Z'paghetti

Entire recipe: 300 calories, 10.5g total fat (2.5g sat fat), 780mg sodium, 22g carbs, 7g fiber, 12g sugars, 33.5g protein

You'll Need: small bowl, spiral vegetable slicer (or vegetable peeler), large skillet, nonstick spray, medium bowl

Prep: 10 minutes • **Cook:** 5 minutes

1½ ounces (about 3 tablespoons) mashed avocado

3 tablespoons fat-free plain Greek yogurt

⅛ teaspoon each salt and black pepper

2 teaspoons grated Parmesan cheese

14 ounces (about 2 medium) zucchini

4 ounces (about 8) raw large shrimp, peeled, tails removed, deveined

⅛ teaspoon onion powder

⅛ teaspoon garlic powder

1½ teaspoons chopped garlic

Optional seasonings: additional salt and black pepper

1. In a small bowl, combine avocado, yogurt, salt, pepper, and 1 teaspoon Parm. Mix until smooth and uniform.

2. Using a spiral vegetable slicer, cut zucchini into spaghetti-like noodles. (If you don't have a spiral veggie slicer, peel zucchini into super-thin strips, rotating the zucchini after each strip.) Roughly chop for shorter noodles.

3. Bring a large skillet sprayed with nonstick spray to medium-high heat. Add shrimp, and season with onion powder and garlic powder. Cook and stir for 1 minute.

4. Add zucchini noodles and chopped garlic to the skillet. Cook and stir until shrimp are cooked through, zucchini noodles are hot and slightly softened, and garlic is fragrant, about 3 minutes.

5. Remove skillet from heat. Transfer to a medium bowl, and blot away excess moisture. Add avocado mixture, and stir to coat.

6. Serve sprinkled with remaining 1 teaspoon Parm.

MAKES 1 SERVING

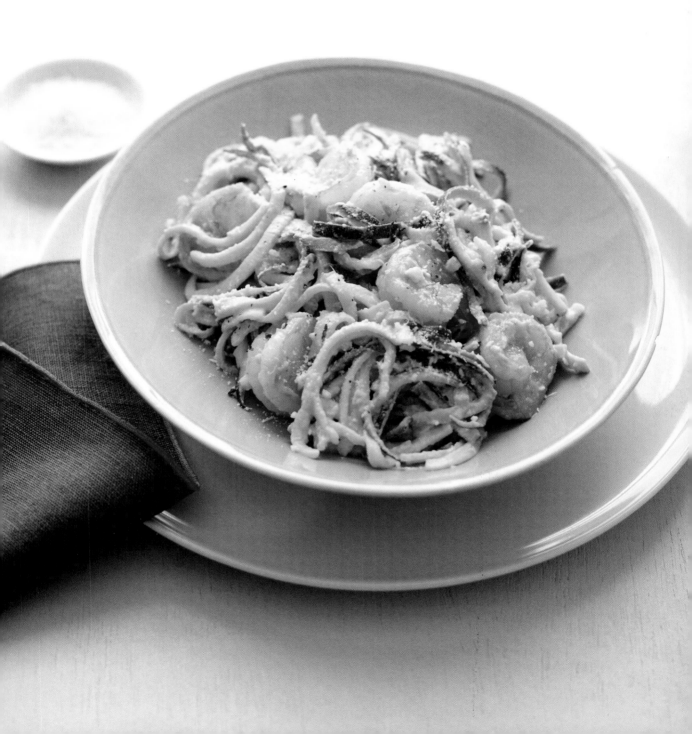

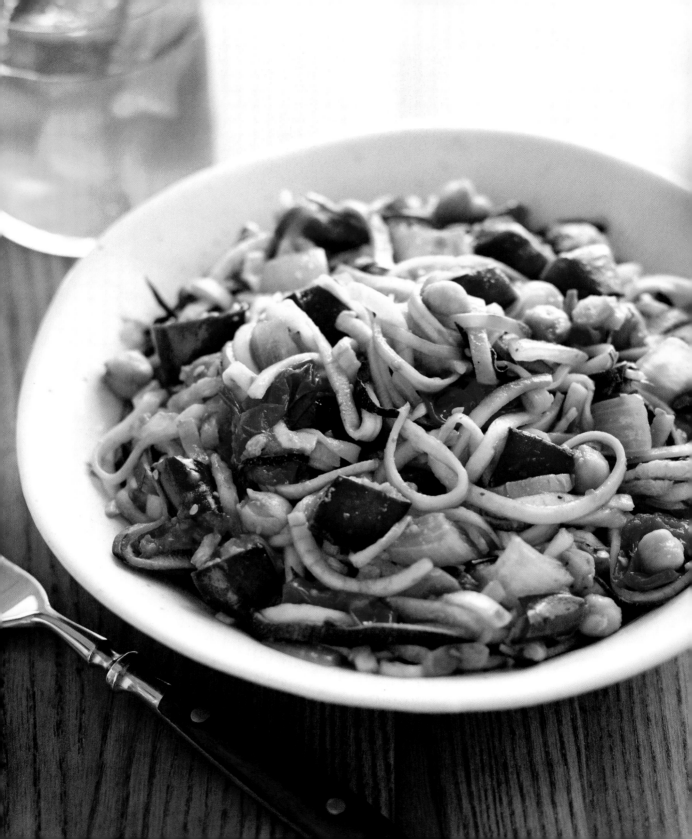

Ratatouille Z'paghetti with Chickpeas

½ of recipe (about 3¾ cups): 315 calories, 6g total fat (1g sat fat), 546mg sodium, 60g carbs, 19g fiber, 24g sugars, 15.5g protein

You'll Need: baking sheet, nonstick spray, medium bowl, spiral vegetable slicer (or vegetable peeler), medium-large bowl, large skillet

Prep: 10 minutes • **Cook:** 30 minutes

2 cups cherry tomatoes

1 teaspoon olive oil

4 cups cubed eggplant

1 cup roughly chopped onion

¼ teaspoon each salt and black pepper

28 ounces (about 4 medium) zucchini

1 cup canned chickpeas (garbanzo beans), drained and rinsed

2 tablespoons tomato paste

1. Preheat oven to 450 degrees. Spray a baking sheet with nonstick spray.

2. In a medium bowl, top tomatoes with olive oil, and toss to coat.

3. Lay tomatoes on one half of the baking sheet, and lay eggplant and onion on the other half. Mist eggplant and onion with nonstick spray. Sprinkle everything with ⅛ teaspoon each salt and pepper.

4. Bake until tomatoes burst and all veggies have softened and slightly blackened, 20 to 25 minutes.

5. Meanwhile, using a spiral vegetable slicer, cut zucchini into spaghetti-like noodles. (If you don't have a spiral veggie slicer, peel zucchini into super-thin strips, rotating the zucchini after each strip.) Roughly chop for shorter noodles.

6. Transfer cooked veggies (including any juices from the tomatoes) to a medium-large bowl. Add chickpeas and tomato paste, and stir until evenly mixed.

7. Bring a large skillet sprayed with nonstick spray to medium-high heat. Add zucchini noodles, and sprinkle with remaining ⅛ teaspoon each salt and pepper. Cook and stir for 2 minutes.

8. Add veggie-chickpea mixture to the skillet. Cook and stir until noodles have slightly softened and entire dish is hot and well mixed, about 2 more minutes.

MAKES 2 SERVINGS

Pesto Z'paghetti with Chicken

½ of recipe (about 1½ cups of zucchini noodles with 3 ounces chicken): 311 calories, 10.5g total fat (3.5g sat fat), 822mg sodium, 19.5g carbs, 4.5g fiber, 13g sugars, 38.5g protein

You'll Need: spiral vegetable slicer (or vegetable peeler), small blender or food processor, large skillet, nonstick spray, strainer

Prep: 20 minutes • **Cook:** 20 minutes

28 ounces (about 4 medium) zucchini

½ cup light/low-fat ricotta cheese

1 tablespoon grated Parmesan cheese

¼ ounce (about 2 teaspoons) pine nuts

¼ cup plus 2 tablespoons chopped fresh basil

1 tablespoon chopped garlic

½ teaspoon each salt and black pepper

8 ounces raw boneless skinless chicken breast cutlets, pounded to ½-inch thickness

HG FYI

In order to thoroughly blend the sauce, you'll need a small blender or food processor—the Magic Bullet is the top Hungry Girl pick.

Z'paghetti fans!

Check out the Z'paghetti Marinara with Shrimp on page 158 . . . It's z'paghetti in a foil pack!

1. Using a spiral vegetable slicer, cut zucchini into spaghetti-like noodles. (If you don't have a spiral veggie slicer, peel zucchini into super-thin strips, rotating the zucchini after each strip.) Roughly chop for shorter noodles.

2. To make the sauce, combine the following ingredients in a small blender or food processor: ricotta cheese, Parm, pine nuts, ¼ cup basil, 1½ teaspoons chopped garlic, and ¼ teaspoon each salt and pepper. Add 3 tablespoons water. Blend until uniform.

3. Bring a large skillet sprayed with nonstick spray to medium heat. Season chicken with remaining ¼ teaspoon each salt and pepper. Cook for about 4 minutes per side, until cooked through. Transfer to a cutting board.

4. Remove skillet from heat; clean, if needed. Re-spray, and bring to medium-high heat. Add zucchini noodles and remaining 1½ teaspoons chopped garlic to the skillet. Cook and stir until zucchini noodles are hot and slightly softened, and garlic is fragrant, about 3 minutes.

5. Transfer noodles to a strainer, and thoroughly drain excess liquid.

6. Remove skillet from heat, re-spray, and return to medium-high heat. Return noodles to the skillet. Add sauce, and cook and stir until sauce is evenly distributed and mixture is hot, about 2 minutes.

7. Slice chicken, and serve over noodles. Top with remaining 2 tablespoons chopped basil.

MAKES 2 SERVINGS

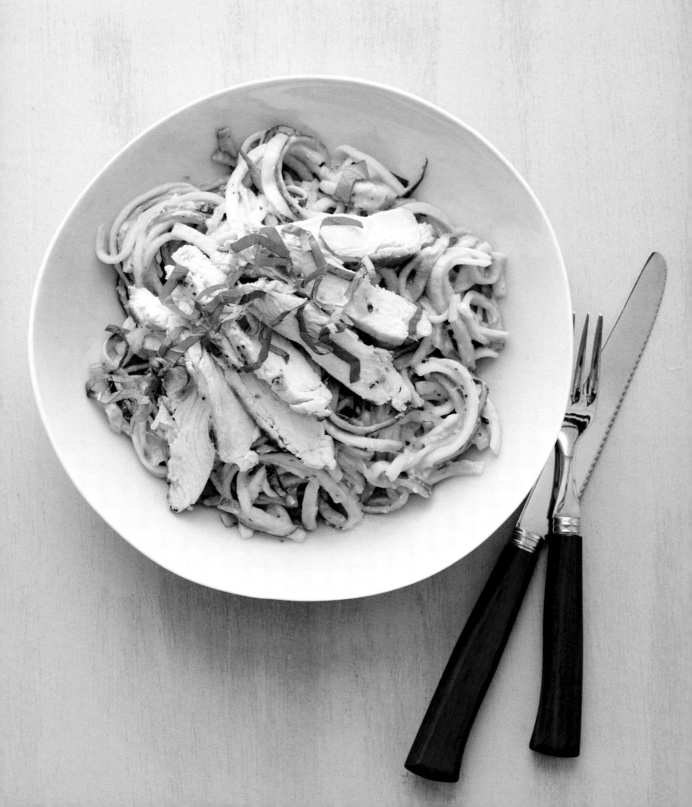

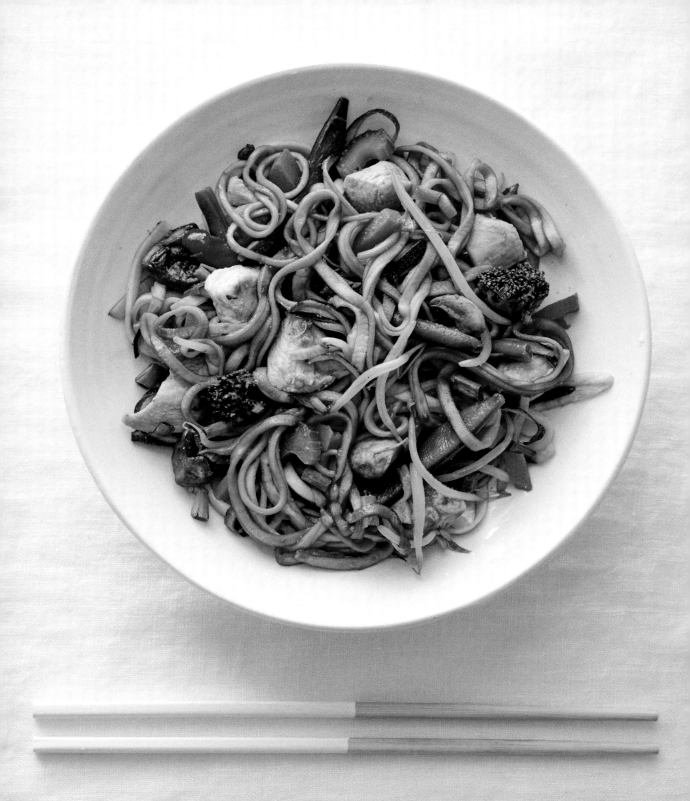

Chicken Zucchini So Low Mein

½ of recipe (about 2 cups): 266 calories, 6.5g total fat (1g sat fat), 633mg sodium, 21.5g carbs, 5.5g fiber, 12.5g sugars, 34g protein

Fans of Chinese food: This one's for you. It's the ultimate swap...

You'll Need: small bowl, spiral vegetable slicer (or vegetable peeler), wok (or large skillet), nonstick spray, strainer

Prep: 15 minutes • **Cook:** 15 minutes

2 tablespoons reduced-sodium/lite soy sauce

1 packet natural no-calorie sweetener

1 teaspoon sesame oil

½ teaspoon crushed garlic

½ teaspoon onion powder

20 ounces (2 to 3 medium) zucchini

8 ounces raw boneless skinless chicken breast, cut into bite-sized pieces

¼ teaspoon garlic powder

1 cup frozen Asian-style stir-fry vegetables

1 cup bean sprouts

1 cup quartered mushrooms

¼ cup chopped scallions

1. To make the sauce, in a small bowl, combine soy sauce, sweetener, sesame oil, crushed garlic, and ¼ teaspoon onion powder. Mix well.

2. Using a spiral vegetable slicer, cut zucchini into spaghetti-like noodles. (If you don't have a spiral veggie slicer, peel zucchini into super-thin strips, rotating the zucchini after each strip.) Roughly chop for shorter noodles.

3. Bring a wok (or large skillet) sprayed with nonstick spray to medium-high heat. Add chicken pieces, and sprinkle with garlic powder and remaining ¼ teaspoon onion powder. Add frozen veggies, bean sprouts, and mushrooms. Cook and stir for about 5 minutes, until chicken is cooked through and veggies are hot and tender.

4. Add zucchini noodles and scallions. Cook and stir until hot and slightly softened, about 3 minutes.

5. Transfer wok contents to a strainer, and thoroughly drain excess liquid.

6. Return wok to medium-high heat, and return drained mixture to the wok. Add sauce, and cook and stir until sauce is evenly distributed and mostly absorbed, about 2 minutes.

MAKES 2 SERVINGS

Gluten FYI

Certain brands add gluten to their soy sauce. If you avoid gluten, read labels carefully. Or grab a specially marked product like Kikkoman Gluten-Free Soy Sauce.

Cold Sesame Zucchini Noodles

Entire recipe: 137 calories, 7.5g total fat (1g sat fat), 576mg sodium, 15g carbs, 4g fiber, 8.5g sugars, 7g protein

These peanutty noodles don't even need to be cooked. Have this dish as a snack, or add a little protein (shrimp rocks!) to make it a meal!

You'll Need: small bowl, spiral vegetable slicer (or vegetable peeler), medium bowl

Prep: 10 minutes • **Chill:** 15 minutes

1 tablespoon reduced-sodium/lite soy sauce

1½ teaspoons plain rice vinegar

1½ teaspoons powdered peanut butter/defatted peanut flour

1 teaspoon sesame oil

Half a packet natural no-calorie sweetener

¼ teaspoon crushed garlic

⅛ teaspoon ground ginger

10 ounces (about 1 large) zucchini

2 tablespoons chopped scallions

1 teaspoon sesame seeds

Optional topping: red pepper flakes

1. To make the sauce, in a small bowl, combine soy sauce, rice vinegar, powdered peanut butter/peanut flour, sesame oil, sweetener, garlic, and ginger. Using a fork, whisk until uniform.

2. Using a spiral vegetable slicer, cut zucchini into spaghetti-like noodles. (If you don't have a spiral veggie slicer, peel zucchini into super-thin strips, rotating the zucchini after each strip.) Roughly chop for shorter noodles.

3. Place zucchini noodles in a medium bowl. Add sauce, and toss to coat. Cover and refrigerate until chilled, at least 15 minutes.

4. Give mixture a stir, and top with scallions and sesame seeds.

MAKES 1 SERVING

Gluten FYI

Certain brands add gluten to their soy sauce. If you avoid gluten, read labels carefully. Or grab a specially marked product like Kikkoman Gluten-Free Soy Sauce.

Ingredient FYI

Powdered peanut butter and defatted peanut flour have less than half the calories of regular peanut butter. Check out page 4 for shopping tips.

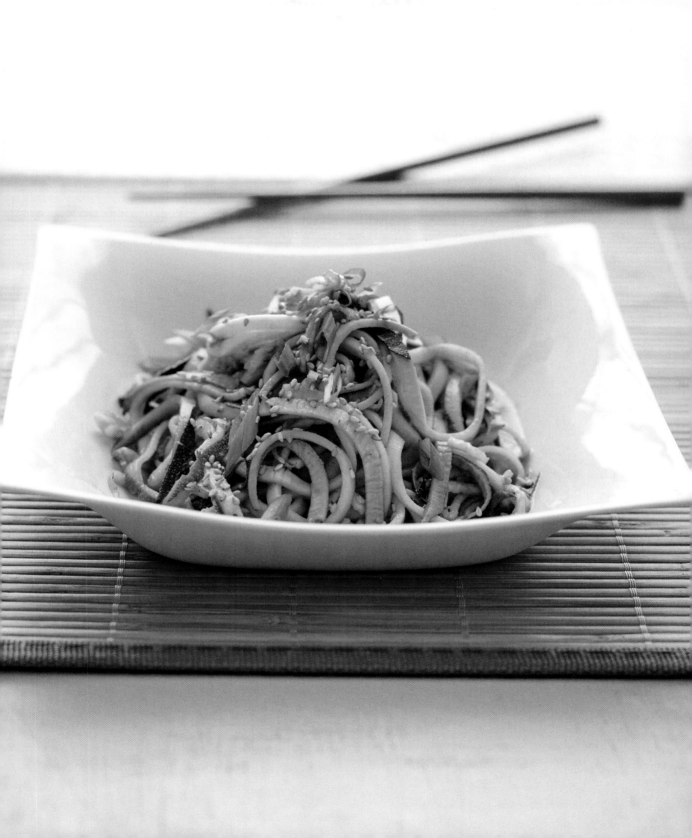

Three Easy Ways to Cook Spaghetti Squash

Choose your method, and then use the cooked spaghetti squash in the recipes on the following pages! And don't miss That Flight Attendant's Dish on page 176 . . .

easiest **IN A SLOW COOKER:**

You'll Need: slow cooker, strainer

Prep: 10 minutes • **Cook:** 2½ hours

Place whole squash in a slow cooker with ½ cup water. Cover and cook on high for 2½ hours, or until squash is soft. Slice squash in half lengthwise; scoop out and discard seeds.

fastest **IN A MICROWAVE:**

You'll Need: extra-large microwave-safe bowl, strainer

Prep: 15 minutes • **Cook:** 20 minutes

1. Microwave squash for 6 minutes, or until soft enough to cut. Once cool enough to handle, halve lengthwise; scoop out and discard seeds.

2. Place one half in an extra-large microwave-safe bowl, cut side down. Add ¼ cup water. Cover and cook for 7 minutes, or until soft. Repeat with remaining squash half.

classic **IN THE OVEN:**

You'll Need: large baking pan, strainer

Prep: 15 minutes • **Cook:** 50 minutes

1. Preheat oven to 400 degrees.

2. Microwave squash for 6 minutes, or until soft enough to cut. Once cool enough to handle, halve lengthwise; scoop out and discard seeds.

3. Fill a large baking pan with ½ inch water, and place squash halves in the pan, cut sides down. Bake until tender, about 40 minutes.

Once your squash is cooked . . .

1. Use a fork to scrape out spaghetti squash strands. Place in a strainer to drain excess moisture. Thoroughly blot dry, removing as much moisture as possible.

2. If not eating immediately, let cool completely. Cover and refrigerate.

HG FYI:

A 4-pound squash yields about 5 cups cooked squash . . . sometimes more!

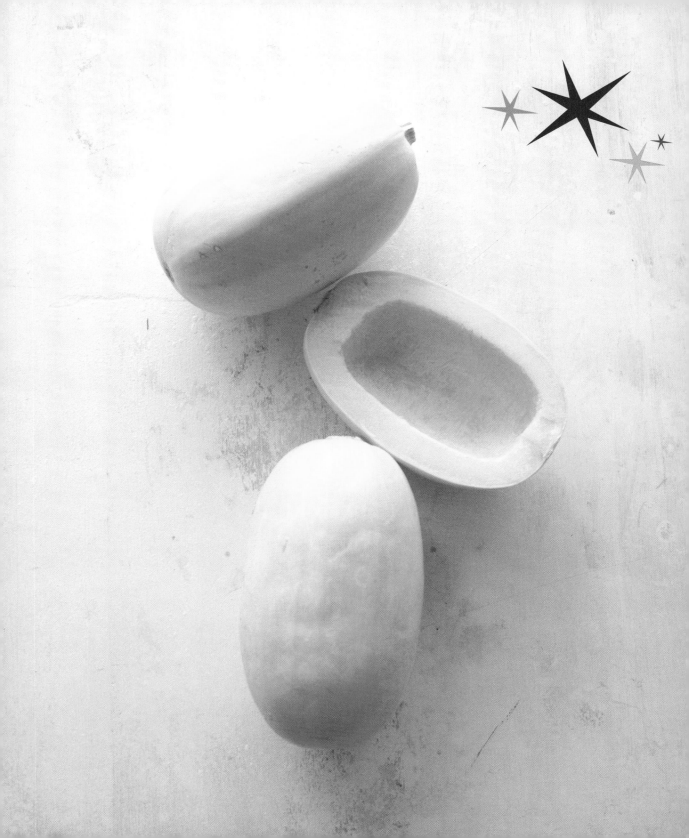

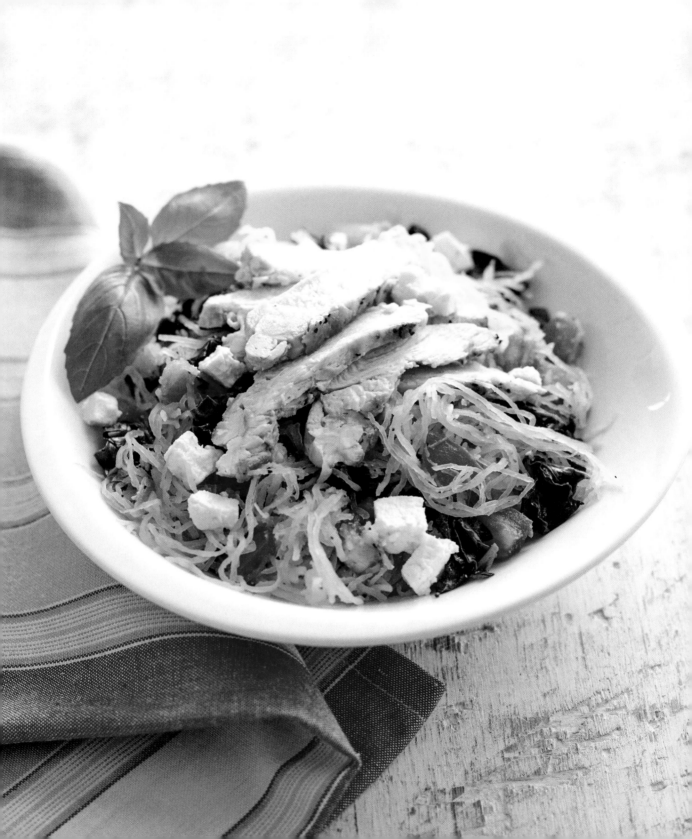

Mediterranean Spaghetti Squash with Chicken

¼ᵗʰ of recipe (about 1⅔ cups veggies with 3½ ounces chicken): 254 calories, 6.5g total fat (3g sat fat), 587mg sodium, 18.5g carbs, 5g fiber, 7.5g sugars, 31g protein

You'll Need: extra-large skillet, nonstick spray, large bowl

Prep: 20 minutes • **Cook:** 20 minutes

Plus prep and cook times for spaghetti squash (page 198) if not made in advance.

1 pound raw boneless skinless chicken breast cutlets, pounded to ½-inch thickness

1 teaspoon garlic powder

1 teaspoon onion powder

½ teaspoon each salt and black pepper

6 cups roughly chopped spinach leaves

5 cups cooked spaghetti squash, drained of excess moisture

1½ cups chopped tomato

¼ cup chopped fresh basil

½ cup crumbled feta cheese

Optional seasonings: additional salt and black pepper

1. Bring an extra-large skillet sprayed with nonstick spray to medium heat. Season chicken with ½ teaspoon garlic powder, ½ teaspoon onion powder, and ¼ teaspoon each salt and pepper. Cook for about 4 minutes per side, until cooked through. Transfer to a cutting board.

2. Remove skillet from heat; clean, if needed. Re-spray, and return to medium heat. Cook and stir spinach until slightly wilted, about 2 minutes. Add spaghetti squash, tomato, and basil. Sprinkle with remaining ½ teaspoon garlic powder, ½ teaspoon onion powder, and ¼ teaspoon each salt and pepper. Cook and stir until hot and well mixed, about 5 minutes.

3. Transfer skillet contents to a large bowl. Sprinkle with feta.

4. Slice chicken, and serve over cheese-topped veggies.

MAKES 4 SERVINGS

Spaghetti Squash Amore

¼th of recipe (about 1¾ cups): 169 calories, 3.5g total fat (1.5g sat fat), 630mg sodium, 27g carbs, 7g fiber, 13g sugars, 10.5g protein

Why amore? Because you'll fall in love with the creamy tomato sauce, garlic, and flavorful veggies in this Italian-style noodle dish . . .

You'll Need: large microwave-safe bowl, medium bowl, large skillet, nonstick spray

Prep: 15 minutes   •   **Cook:** 15 minutes

Plus prep and cook times for spaghetti squash (page 198) if not made in advance.

5 cups cooked spaghetti squash, drained of excess moisture

1 cup canned crushed tomatoes

¼ cup grated Parmesan cheese

¼ cup chopped fresh basil

½ teaspoon Italian seasoning

½ teaspoon salt

2 cups chopped portabella mushrooms

2 cups chopped zucchini

1 cup chopped red bell pepper

1 teaspoon chopped garlic

⅔ cup frozen peas

¼ cup fat-free plain Greek yogurt

1. Place spaghetti squash in a large microwave-safe bowl. Reheat, if needed, and cover to keep warm.

2. In a medium bowl, combine crushed tomatoes, Parm, basil, Italian seasoning, and salt. Mix well.

3. Bring a large skillet sprayed with nonstick spray to medium-high heat. Add mushrooms, zucchini, and bell pepper. Cook and stir for 5 minutes.

4. Add garlic to the skillet. Cook and stir until veggies have softened and garlic is fragrant, about 2 minutes.

5. Reduce heat to low. Add peas and seasoned crushed tomatoes. Cook and stir until hot and well mixed, about 3 minutes.

6. Remove from heat, and stir in yogurt.

7. Add skillet contents to the large bowl of spaghetti squash, and mix well.

MAKES 4 SERVINGS

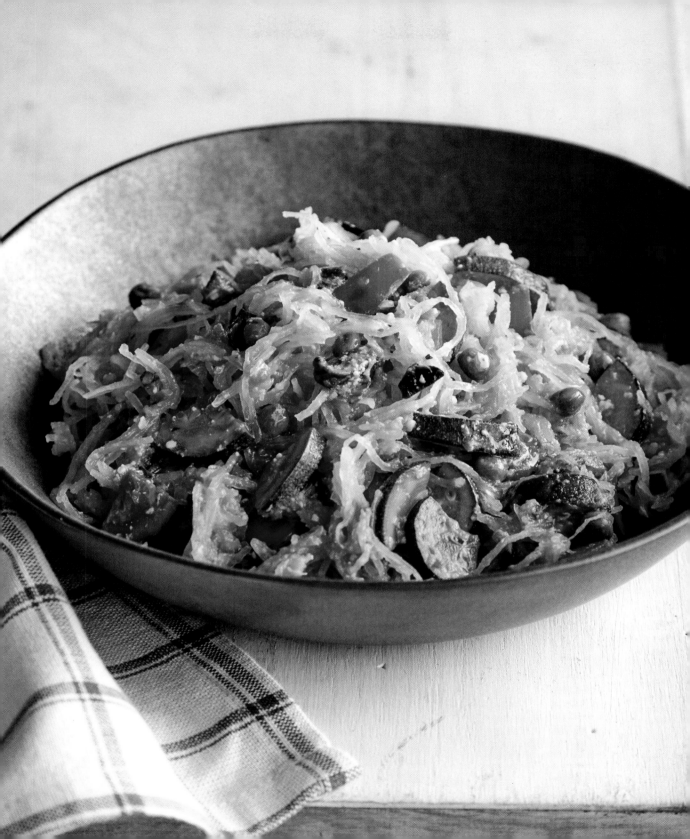

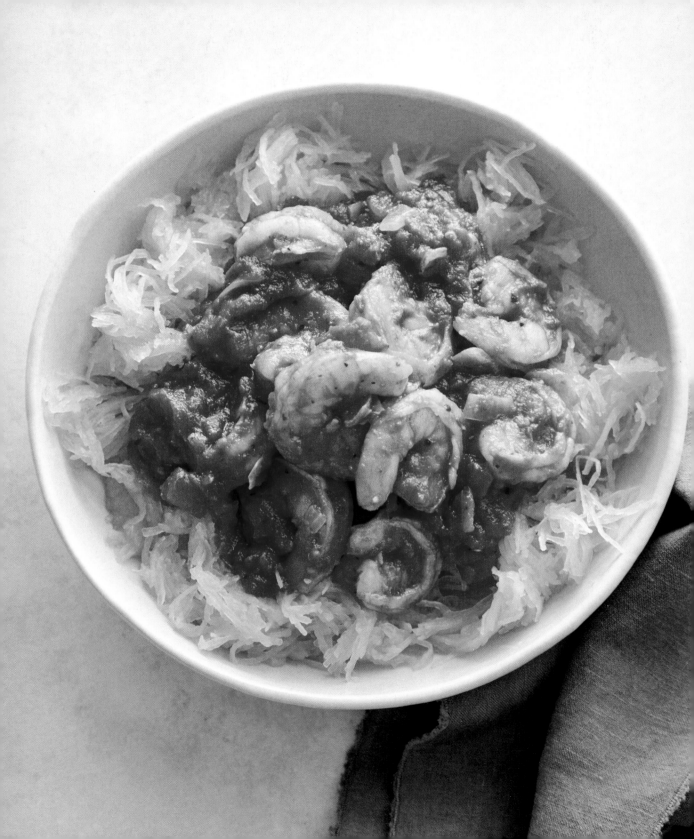

Shrimp Fra Diavolo Spaghetti Squash

¼th of recipe (about 1¼ cups squash with 1¼ cups sauce and shrimp):
255 calories, 1.5g total fat (0.5g sat fat), 803mg sodium, 34g carbs, 7.5g fiber, 15g sugars, 26g protein

You'll Need: 2 large bowls (1 microwave-safe), extra-large skillet, nonstick spray
Prep: 15 minutes • **Cook:** 15 minutes
Plus prep and cook times for spaghetti squash (page 198) if not made in advance.

5 cups cooked spaghetti squash, drained of excess moisture

2 cups canned crushed tomatoes

One 14.5-ounce can diced tomatoes, drained

¼ cup tomato paste

2 teaspoons Italian seasoning

1½ teaspoons lemon juice

1 teaspoon red pepper flakes

1 cup chopped onion

1 pound (about 32) raw large shrimp, peeled, tails removed, deveined

1 tablespoon chopped garlic

1. Place spaghetti squash in a large microwave-safe bowl. Reheat if needed, and cover to keep warm.

2. In another large bowl, combine crushed tomatoes, drained diced tomatoes, tomato paste, Italian seasoning, lemon juice, and red pepper flakes. Mix until uniform.

3. Bring an extra-large skillet sprayed with nonstick spray to medium-high heat. Cook and stir onion until partially softened, about 4 minutes.

4. Add shrimp and garlic to the skillet. Cook and stir until onion has mostly softened and shrimp are cooked through, about 4 more minutes.

5. Reduce heat to medium low. Add tomato mixture. Cook and stir until hot, about 3 minutes.

6. Serve saucy shrimp over spaghetti squash.

MAKES 4 SERVINGS

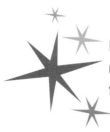

For more healthy recipes, plus the latest food news, tips & tricks, and more, sign up for free daily emails at Hungry-Girl.com!

9

Cauliflower Rice & More Cauliflower Creations

The things cauliflower can do are UNREAL (not to mention delicious!). From rice dish do-overs to low-carb pizza crust, the cruciferous superstar will make magic happen in your kitchen . . .

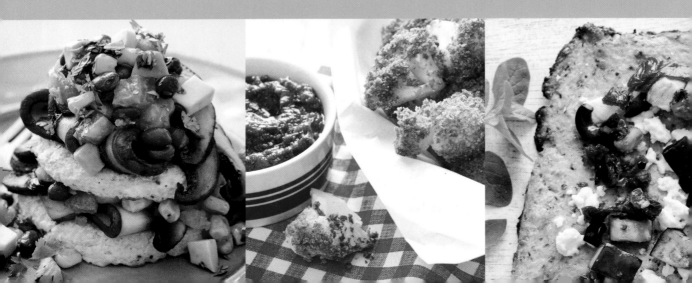

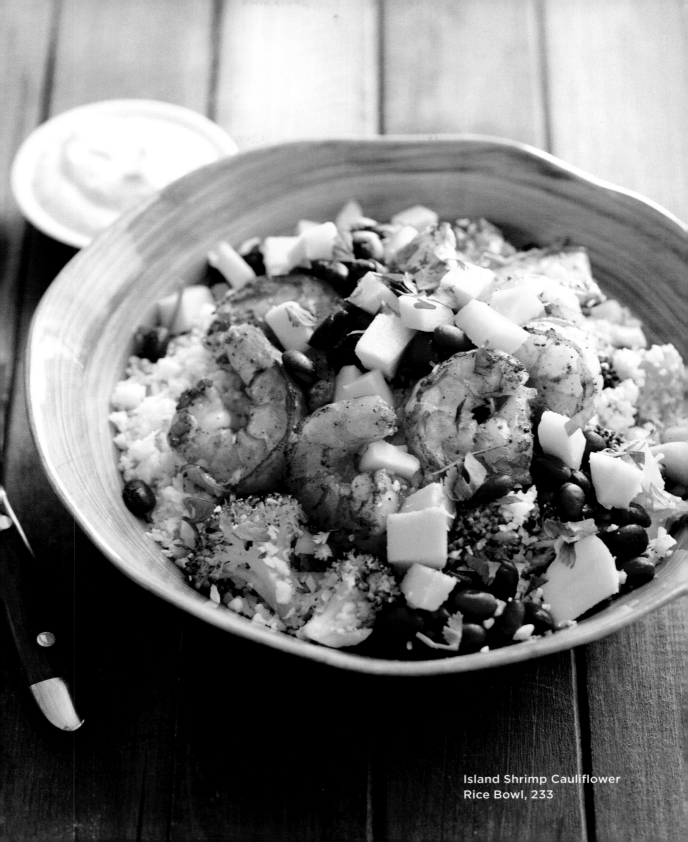

Island Shrimp Cauliflower
Rice Bowl, 233

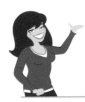

All About Cauliflower

Why cauliflower? It's the perfect swap for starchy carbs like rice, potatoes, and breadcrumbs. While there's nothing wrong with those foods, they're more calorie dense—often, they don't give you a lot of bang for your calorie buck. For example, one cup of cooked white rice has around 200 calories and 40g carbs, and it only has about 4g protein and almost no fiber. You could have TWO cups of cauliflower rice for about 60 calories, 13g carbs, 5g protein, and 6g fiber.

The average head of cauliflower yields about 6 cups of roughly chopped cauliflower. Want to save time? Buy pre-cut florets and give 'em a rough chop.

There are two main ways to prepare cauliflower in these recipes: as cauliflower crumbs and as cauliflower rice. For the crumb 411, see the section below. For more about making cauliflower rice, flip to page 229.

Cauliflower Crumbs 101

For the recipes on the following pages, you'll be reducing the cauliflower to a crumb-like consistency. Here's some need-to-know info . . .

Break out the food processor. A standard blender won't reduce the cauliflower enough; a food processor is the perfect tool for the job.

After the crumbs are cooked, you'll want to remove as much moisture as possible. This step is crucial. The more liquid you remove (there will be A LOT!), the better your recipe results will be. Using a clean dish towel (or paper towels, in a pinch), firmly press out the moisture through the fine-mesh strainer. Repeat, as needed, until you can't squeeze out any more liquid.

A fine-mesh strainer is a necessity. These strainers are fairly inexpensive and definitely worth picking up. After all, we're talkin' healthy hash browns and low-calorie pizza crusts!

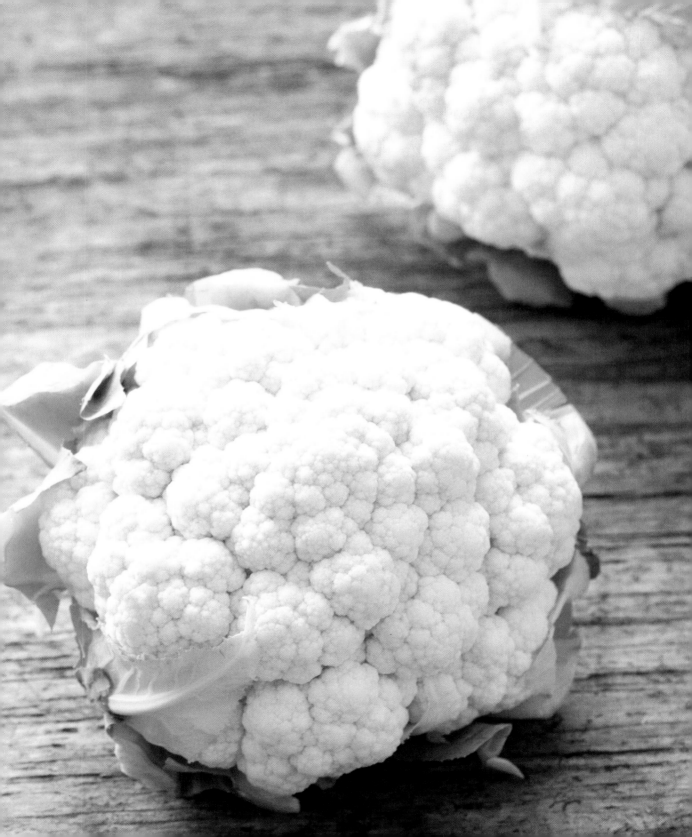

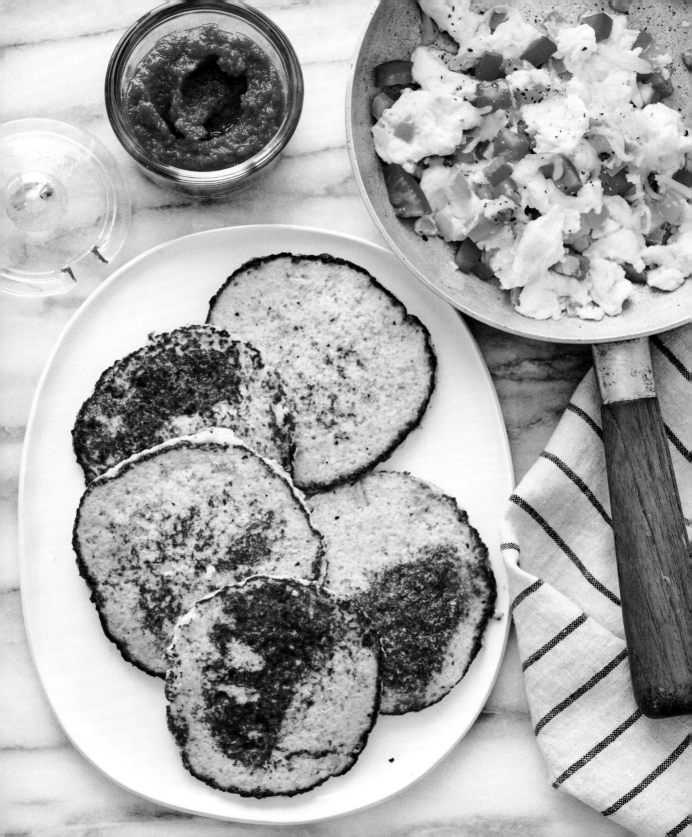

Cauliflower Hash Browns

⅙ᵗʰ of recipe (1 hash brown): 54 calories, 2.5g total fat (<0.5g sat fat), 152mg sodium, 5.5g carbs, 2g fiber, 2.5g sugars, 3.5g protein

You'll Need: food processor, large microwave-safe bowl, fine-mesh strainer, clean dish towel (optional), large skillet, nonstick spray

Prep: 15 minutes • **Cook:** 20 minutes • **Cool:** 10 minutes

4 cups roughly chopped cauliflower

½ cup finely chopped onion

½ cup (about 4 large) egg whites

¼ teaspoon each salt and black pepper

¼ teaspoon paprika

1 tablespoon olive oil

1. Pulse cauliflower in a food processor until reduced to the consistency of coarse breadcrumbs, working in batches as needed.

2. Place cauliflower crumbs in a large microwave-safe bowl; cover and microwave for 3½ minutes.

3. Uncover and stir. Re-cover and microwave for another 3½ minutes, or until hot and soft.

4. Transfer cauliflower crumbs to a fine-mesh strainer to drain. Let cool for 10 minutes, or until cool enough to handle.

5. Using a clean dish towel (or paper towels), firmly press out as much liquid as possible from the cauliflower crumbs in the strainer—there will be a lot of liquid!

6. Return cauliflower crumbs to the large bowl.

7. Add all remaining ingredients *except* olive oil. Mix until uniform. Firmly form into 6 patties, each about ¼ inch thick.

8. Spray a large skillet with nonstick spray, and drizzle with ½ tablespoon olive oil. Bring to medium heat. Carefully lay 3 patties in the skillet. Cook until slightly crispy, golden brown, and cooked through, about 3 minutes per side, flipping carefully.

9. Repeat with remaining ½ tablespoon olive oil and remaining 3 patties, adding the oil carefully to avoid splattering.

MAKES 6 SERVINGS

Cheesy Cauliflower Tater Tots

¼th of recipe (7 tater tots): 68 calories, 2g total fat (1g sat fat), 291mg sodium, 6.5g carbs, 2g fiber, 2g sugars, 6g protein

These tasty nuggets are incredible dipped in Clean & Hungry BBQ Sauce or Clean & Hungry Ketchup . . . Recipes and store-bought alternatives on pages 19 and 24!

You'll Need: baking sheet, parchment paper, food processor, large microwave-safe bowl, fine-mesh strainer, clean dish towel (optional)

Prep: 20 minutes • **Cook:** 30 minutes • **Cool:** 10 minutes

2 cups roughly chopped cauliflower

¼ cup (about 2 large) egg whites

¼ cup whole-wheat panko breadcrumbs

2 tablespoons grated Parmesan cheese

2 tablespoons shredded part-skim mozzarella cheese

¼ teaspoon garlic powder

¼ teaspoon onion powder

¼ teaspoon salt

⅛ teaspoon black pepper

1. Preheat oven to 400 degrees. Line a baking sheet with parchment paper.

2. Pulse cauliflower in a food processor until reduced to the consistency of coarse breadcrumbs.

3. Place cauliflower crumbs in a large microwave-safe bowl; cover and microwave for 2 minutes.

4. Uncover and stir. Re-cover and microwave for another 2 minutes, or until hot and soft.

5. Transfer cauliflower crumbs to a fine-mesh strainer to drain. Let cool for 10 minutes, or until cool enough to handle.

6. Using a clean dish towel (or paper towels), firmly press out as much liquid as possible from the cauliflower crumbs in the strainer—there will be a lot of liquid!

7. Return cauliflower crumbs to the large bowl. Add all remaining ingredients, and mix thoroughly.

8. Firmly and evenly form into 28 nuggets, each about 1 inch long, ½ inch wide, and ½ thick. Place them on the baking sheet, evenly spaced.

9. Bake for 10 minutes.

10. Carefully flip. Bake until golden brown and crispy, 10 to 12 minutes.

MAKES 4 SERVINGS

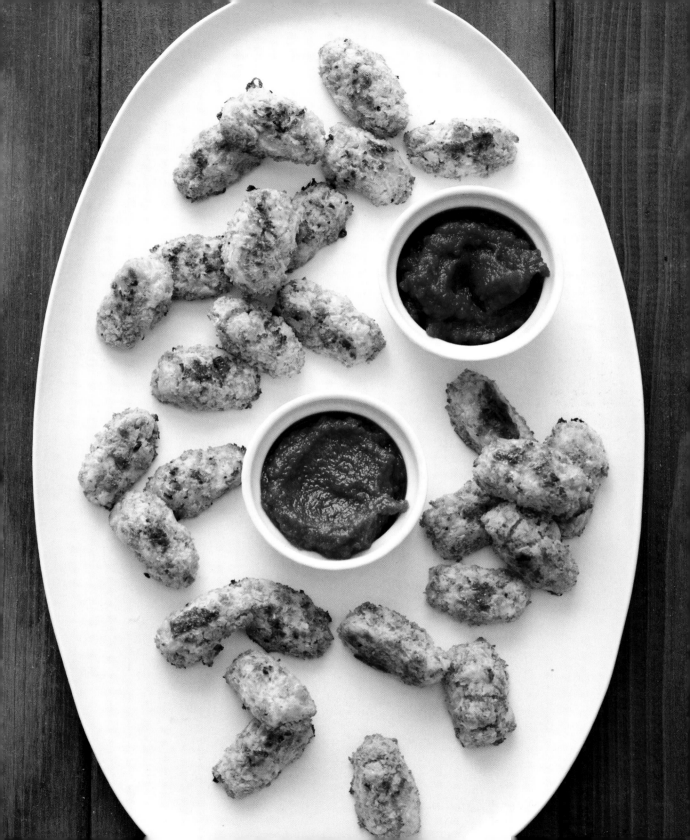

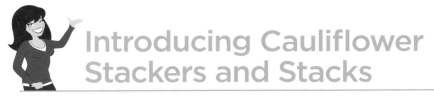

Introducing Cauliflower Stackers and Stacks

On the next few pages, you'll find a bunch of recipes I'm super proud to call Hungry Girl creations. Read on to get the full 411. Then let the stacking begin!

What are Cauliflower Stackers? They're delicious patties that taste like potato pancakes but are actually made from (you guessed it!) cauliflower.

So what are Stacks? When the snack-worthy Cauliflower Stackers were first created, it immediately became clear they'd be fantastic in mini meals. Enter these recipes: The Breakfast Stack, The Italian Stack, and The Mexican Stack.

A batch of Stackers makes six and lasts several days in the fridge. Snack on 'em straight, use them in the Stack recipes . . . or do both!

If you're not eating them immediately, let the Stackers cool completely. Then cover and refrigerate until ready to eat. (Be careful . . . They're fragile.)

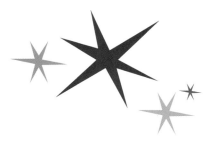

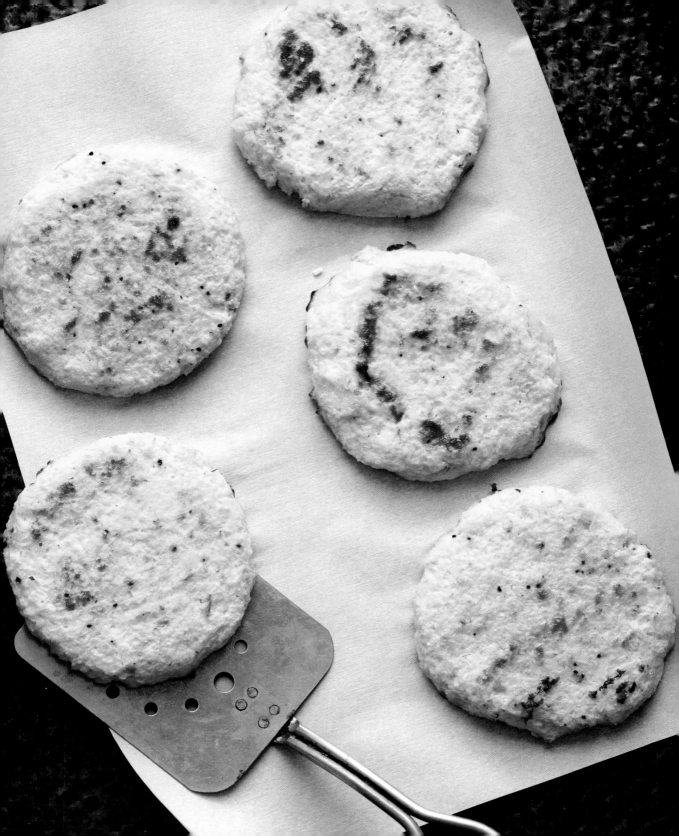

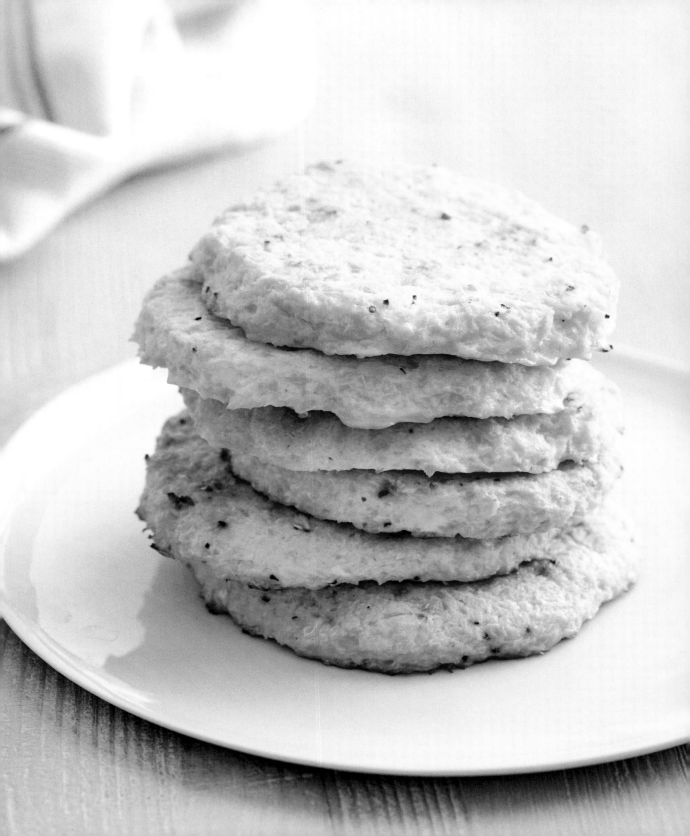

Cauliflower Stackers

⅙th of recipe (1 stacker): 56 calories, 2g total fat (1g sat fat), 203mg sodium, 4.5g carbs, 2g fiber, 2g sugars, 6g protein

You'll Need: baking sheet, parchment paper, food processor, large microwave-safe bowl, fine-mesh strainer, clean dish towel (optional)

Prep: 15 minutes • **Cook:** 30 minutes • **Cool:** 10 minutes

4 cups roughly chopped cauliflower

½ cup (about 4 large) egg whites

¼ cup grated Parmesan cheese

½ teaspoon garlic powder

½ teaspoon onion powder

⅛ teaspoon each salt and black pepper

1. Preheat oven to 375 degrees. Line a baking sheet with parchment paper.

2. Pulse cauliflower in a food processor until reduced to the consistency of coarse breadcrumbs, working in batches as needed.

3. Place cauliflower crumbs in a large microwave-safe bowl; cover and microwave for 3½ minutes.

4. Uncover and stir. Re-cover and microwave for another 3½ minutes, or until hot and soft.

5. Transfer cauliflower crumbs to a fine-mesh strainer to drain. Let cool for 10 minutes, or until cool enough to handle.

6. Using a clean dish towel (or paper towels), firmly press out as much liquid as possible from the cauliflower crumbs in the strainer—there will be a lot of liquid!

7. Return cauliflower crumbs to the large bowl. Add all remaining ingredients, and mix thoroughly.

8. Evenly distribute mixture into 6 mounds on the baking sheet, about ¼ cup each. Flatten into 6 patties, each about ½ inch thick.

9. Bake for 10 minutes.

10. Carefully flip. Bake until golden brown, 10 to 12 minutes.

MAKES 6 SERVINGS

The Breakfast Stack

Entire recipe: 209 calories, 4g total fat (2g sat fat), 741mg sodium, 17.5g carbs, 5.5g fiber, 9g sugars, 26.5g protein

You'll Need: large microwave-safe mug, nonstick spray, microwave-safe plate

Prep: 5 minutes • **Cook:** 5 minutes

Plus prep and cook times for Cauliflower Stackers (page 217) if not made in advance.

¼ **cup chopped bell pepper**

2 **tablespoons chopped onion**

½ **cup (about 4 large) egg whites**

Dash onion powder

Dash garlic powder

Dash black pepper

2 **Cauliflower Stackers (recipe on page 217)**

¼ **cup Clean & Hungry Salsa (recipe and store-bought alternatives on page 18)**

1. In a large microwave-safe mug sprayed with nonstick spray, microwave bell pepper and onion for 1½ minutes, or until softened.

2. Blot away excess moisture. Add egg whites and seasonings. Stir, and microwave for 1 minute.

3. Stir and microwave for 1 more minute, or until set.

4. Gently place cauliflower stackers on a microwave-safe plate. If needed, microwave until hot.

5. Top one stacker with half of the egg scramble and 2 tablespoons salsa. Repeat layering with remaining stacker and 2 tablespoons salsa.

MAKES 1 SERVING

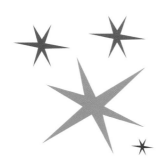

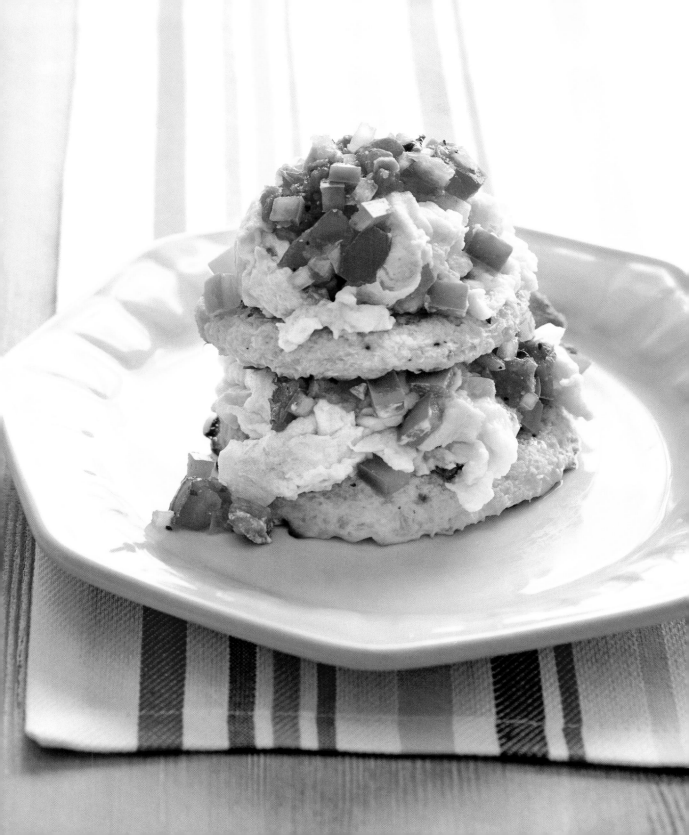

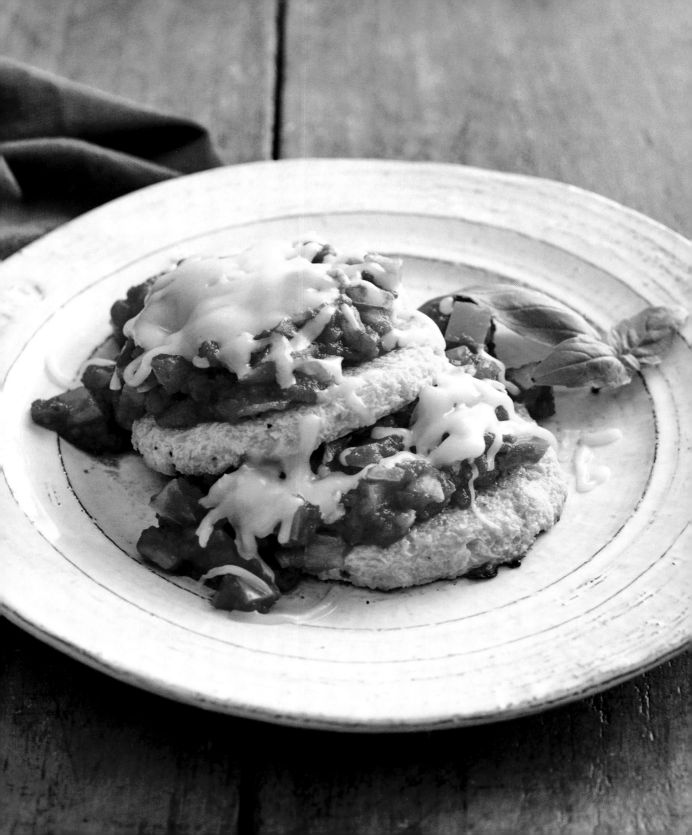

The Italian Stack

Entire recipe: 251 calories, 7.5g total fat (4.5g sat fat), 900mg sodium, 26.5g carbs, 8g fiber, 13g sugars, 21.5g protein

You'll Need: skillet, nonstick spray, microwave-safe plate

Prep: 5 minutes • **Cook:** 5 minutes

Plus prep and cook times for Cauliflower Stackers (page 217) if not made in advance.

⅓ **cup chopped green bell pepper**

¼ **cup chopped onion**

½ **cup Clean & Hungry Marinara Sauce (recipe and store-bought alternatives on page 20)**

2 Cauliflower Stackers (recipe on page 217)

3 tablespoons shredded part-skim mozzarella cheese

1. Bring a skillet sprayed with nonstick spray to medium-high heat. Add pepper and onion. Cook and stir until veggies have softened and lightly browned, about 4 minutes.

2. Remove from heat, add marinara sauce, and mix well.

3. Gently place cauliflower stackers on a microwave-safe plate. If needed, microwave until hot.

4. Top one cauliflower stacker with half of the sauce mixture. Repeat layering with remaining cauliflower stacker and sauce mixture.

5. Sprinkle with cheese. Microwave for 30 seconds, or until cheese has melted.

MAKES 1 SERVING

Entire recipe: 247 calories, 6.5g total fat (2.5g sat fat), 629mg sodium, 31.5g carbs, 10g fiber, 9g sugars, 20g protein

You'll Need: skillet, nonstick spray, plate, microwave-safe plate

Prep: 5 minutes • **Cook:** 10 minutes

Plus prep and cook times for Cauliflower Stackers (page 217) if not made in advance.

1 portabella mushroom cap (stem removed), sliced

Dash ground cumin

Dash garlic powder

Dash chili powder

2 tablespoons frozen sweet corn kernels

¼ cup canned black beans, drained and rinsed

2 tablespoons Clean & Hungry Salsa (recipe and store-bought alternatives on page 18)

2 Cauliflower Stackers (recipe on page 217)

½ ounce (about 1 tablespoon) chopped avocado

1 tablespoon finely chopped fresh cilantro

1. Bring a skillet sprayed with nonstick spray to medium-high heat. Add mushroom slices, and sprinkle with seasonings. Cook and stir until softened and browned, about 5 minutes. Transfer to a plate, and cover to keep warm.

2. Remove skillet from heat; clean, if needed. Re-spray, and return to medium-high heat. Cook and stir corn until hot and slightly blackened, 1 to 2 minutes.

3. Add beans and salsa to the skillet. Cook and stir until hot and well mixed, another 1 to 2 minutes.

4. Gently place cauliflower stackers on a microwave-safe plate. If needed, microwave until hot.

5. Top one stacker with half of the mushroom slices and half of the salsa mixture. Repeat layering with remaining stacker, mushroom slices, and salsa mixture. Top with avocado and cilantro.

MAKES 1 SERVING

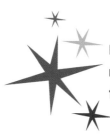

For more healthy recipes, plus the latest food news, tips & tricks, and more, **sign up for free daily emails at Hungry-Girl.com!**

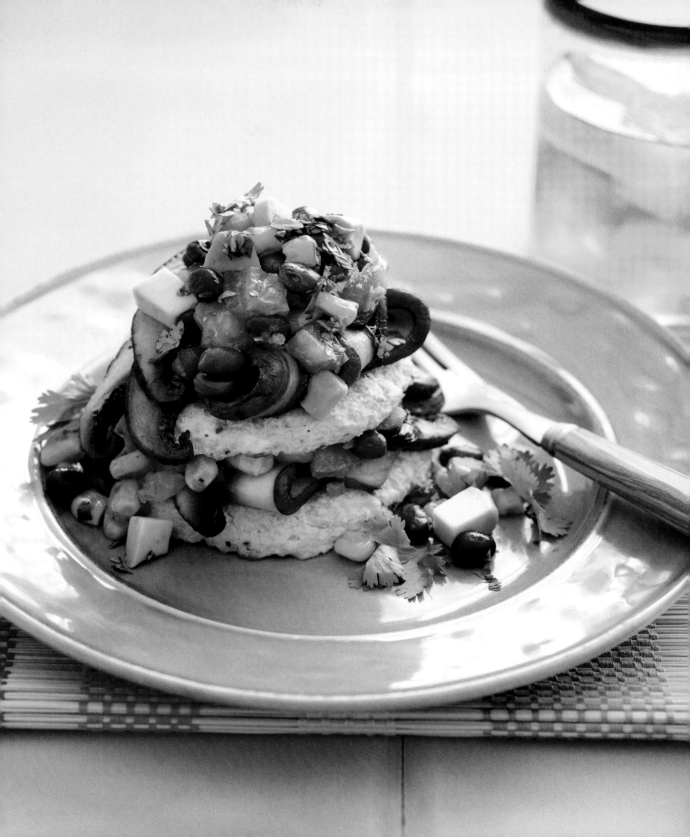

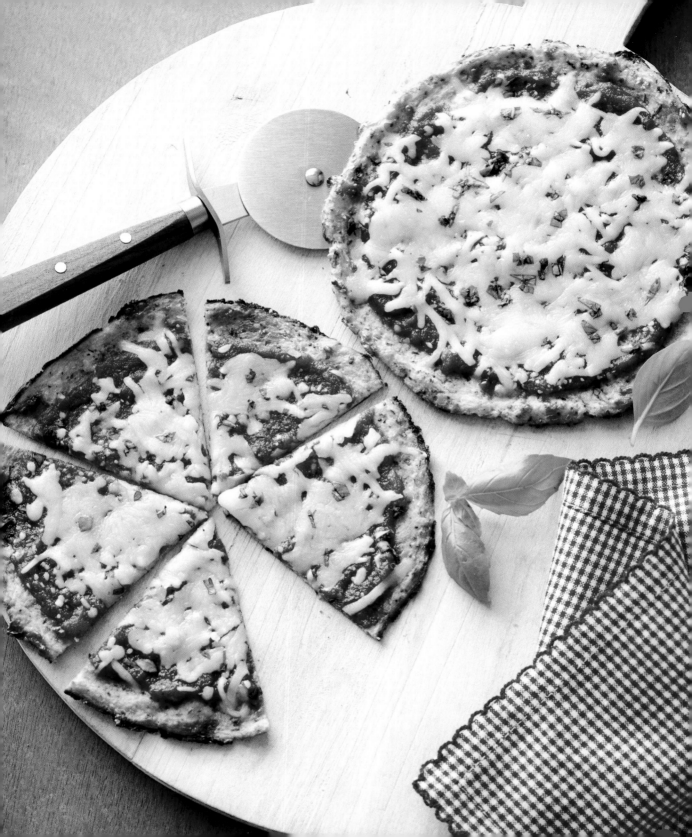

Cauliflower Crust Pizza

½ of recipe (1 pizza): 269 calories, 11g total fat (6.5g sat fat), 826mg sodium, 21.5g carbs, 8g fiber, 9.5g sugars, 24.5g protein

That's right—crispy, gluten-free pizza crust made from cauliflower. And pizza fans: Don't miss the Fork 'n Knife Skillet Pizza on page 288 . . .

You'll Need: baking sheet, parchment paper, food processor, large microwave-safe bowl, fine-mesh strainer, clean dish towel (optional), medium bowl

Prep: 25 minutes • **Cook:** 50 minutes • **Cool:** 10 minutes

Crust

5 cups roughly chopped cauliflower

¼ cup (about 2 large) egg whites

¼ cup shredded part-skim mozzarella cheese

2 tablespoons grated Parmesan cheese

1 teaspoon Italian seasoning

¼ teaspoon black pepper

⅛ teaspoon salt

Topping

½ cup canned crushed tomatoes

½ teaspoon garlic powder

½ teaspoon onion powder

½ teaspoon Italian seasoning

½ cup shredded part-skim mozzarella cheese

2 tablespoons finely chopped fresh basil

1. Preheat oven to 400 degrees. Line a baking sheet with parchment paper.

2. Pulse cauliflower in a food processor until reduced to the consistency of coarse breadcrumbs, working in batches as needed.

3. Place cauliflower crumbs in a large microwave-safe bowl; cover and microwave for 3½ minutes.

4. Uncover and stir. Re-cover and microwave for another 3½ minutes, or until hot and soft.

5. Transfer cauliflower crumbs to a fine-mesh strainer to drain. Let cool for 10 minutes, or until cool enough to handle.

6. Using a clean dish towel (or paper towels), firmly press out as much liquid as possible from the cauliflower crumbs in the strainer—there will be a lot of liquid!

7. Return cauliflower crumbs to the large bowl, and add all remaining crust ingredients. Mix thoroughly.

8. To form the crusts, evenly divide cauliflower mixture into two circles on the parchment-lined baking sheet, each about ¼ inch thick and 7 inches in diameter.

9. Bake until the tops have browned, about 35 minutes.

10. Meanwhile, in a medium bowl, combine crushed tomatoes, garlic powder, onion powder, and Italian seasoning. Mix well. Spread over each crust, leaving a ½-inch border. Sprinkle with cheese and basil.

11. Bake until cheese has melted and crust is crispy, 5 to 7 minutes.

MAKES 2 SERVINGS

Greek Cauliflower Flatbreads

½ of recipe (1 flatbread): 272 calories, 11.5g total fat (6.5g sat fat), 859mg sodium, 25g carbs, 9.5g fiber, 11.5g sugars, 21.5g protein

You'll Need: baking sheet, parchment paper, food processor, large microwave-safe bowl, fine-mesh strainer, clean dish towel (optional), skillet, nonstick spray

Prep: 25 minutes • **Cook:** 50 minutes • **Cool:** 10 minutes

Flatbread

5 cups roughly chopped cauliflower

¼ cup (about 2 large) egg whites

¼ cup shredded part-skim mozzarella cheese

2 tablespoons grated Parmesan cheese

1 teaspoon Italian seasoning

¼ teaspoon black pepper

⅛ teaspoon salt

Topping

1 cup chopped eggplant

¼ teaspoon garlic powder

¼ teaspoon onion powder

⅓ cup crumbled feta cheese

3 tablespoons bagged sun-dried tomatoes (not packed in oil), chopped

2 tablespoons chopped kalamata or black olives

1. Preheat oven to 400 degrees. Line a baking sheet with parchment paper.

2. Pulse cauliflower in a food processor until reduced to the consistency of coarse breadcrumbs, working in batches as needed.

3. Place cauliflower crumbs in a large microwave-safe bowl; cover and microwave for 3½ minutes.

4. Uncover and stir. Re-cover and microwave for another 3½ minutes, or until hot and soft.

5. Transfer cauliflower crumbs to a fine-mesh strainer to drain. Let cool for 10 minutes, or until cool enough to handle.

6. Using a clean dish towel (or paper towels), firmly press out as much liquid as possible from the cauliflower crumbs in the strainer—there will be a lot of liquid!

7. Return cauliflower crumbs to the bowl, and add all remaining flatbread ingredients. Mix thoroughly.

8. To form the flatbreads, evenly divide cauliflower mixture into two squares on the parchment-lined baking sheet, each about 6 inches by 6 inches and ½ inch thick.

9. Bake until the tops have browned, about 35 minutes.

10. Meanwhile, bring a skillet sprayed with nonstick spray to medium-high heat. Add eggplant, garlic powder, and onion powder. Cook and stir until softened and lightly browned, about 3 minutes.

11. Sprinkle flatbreads with feta cheese, leaving ½-inch borders. Top with eggplant, chopped sun-dried tomatoes, and olives.

12. Bake until crispy, 5 to 7 minutes.

MAKES 2 SERVINGS

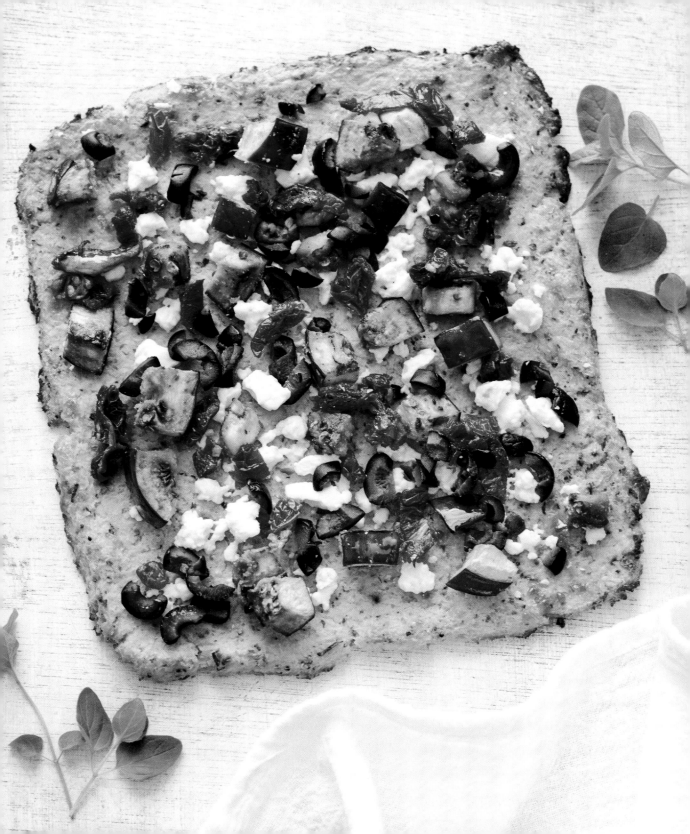

Cauliflower Rice 101

Turning cauliflower florets into rice is a piece of cake . . .

A standard blender is all you need. Just pulse the cauliflower until reduced to rice-sized pieces. For recipes with more than 2 cups of cauliflower to blend, work in batches.

When making the rice in the blender, you may need to stop and stir occasionally in order to finish the job. Rearrange the cauliflower in the blender, and then resume blending.

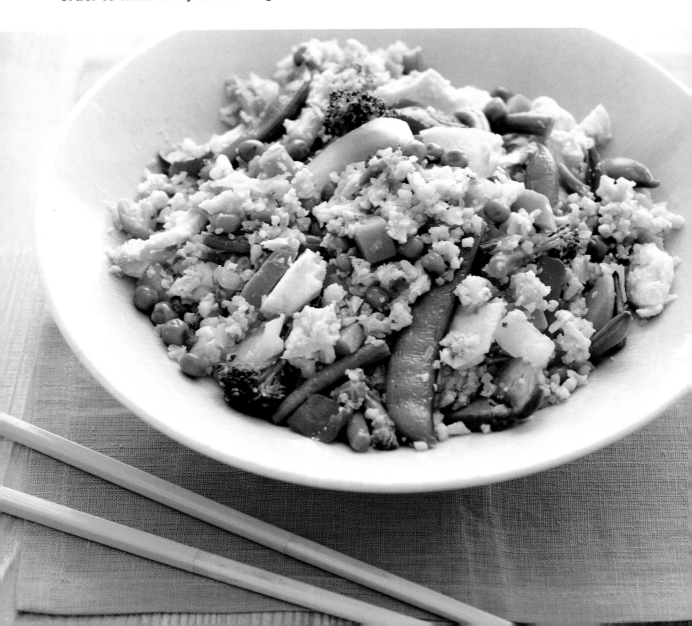

Cauliflower Power Fried Rice

⅛ᵗʰ of recipe (about 1⅓ cups): 131 calories, 3g total fat (0.5g sat fat), 285mg sodium, 17.5g carbs, 5.5g fiber, 7.5g sugars, 8.5g protein

Here's a healthy swap for a classic Chinese dish. Looking for more Chinese-food makeovers? Check out the Chicken Zucchini So Low Mein on page 195 . . .

You'll Need: blender, extra-large skillet, nonstick spray, large bowl

Prep: 15 minutes • **Cook:** 20 minutes

5 cups roughly chopped cauliflower

¾ cup (about 6) egg whites

3 cups frozen Asian-style stir-fry vegetables

1 cup frozen peas

1 cup chopped onion

1 tablespoon sesame oil

1 teaspoon chopped garlic

⅛ teaspoon salt

⅓ cup Clean & Hungry Teriyaki Sauce (recipe and store-bought alternatives on page 23)

1. Pulse cauliflower in a blender until reduced to rice-sized pieces, working in batches as needed.

2. Bring an extra-large skillet sprayed with nonstick spray to medium heat. Scramble egg whites until fully cooked, 3 to 4 minutes, breaking them up into bite-sized pieces. Transfer to a large bowl, and cover to keep warm.

3. Remove skillet from heat; clean, if needed. Re-spray, and bring to medium-high heat. Add stir-fry veggies, peas, and ¼ cup water. Cover and cook for 3 minutes, or until thawed. Add cauliflower rice, onion, sesame oil, garlic, and salt. Cook and stir until veggies have mostly softened, 6 to 8 minutes.

4. Add scrambled egg whites and teriyaki sauce. Cook and stir until hot and well mixed, about 2 minutes.

MAKES 5 SERVINGS

Hawaiian Shrimp Fried Rice with Pineapple

¼th of recipe (about 2 cups): 229 calories, 4.5g total fat (0.5g sat fat), 487mg sodium, 23.5g carbs, 7g fiber, 10.5g sugars, 23.5g protein

You'll Need: blender, extra-large skillet, nonstick spray, large bowl

Prep: 20 minutes • **Cook:** 20 minutes

5 cups roughly chopped cauliflower

¾ cup (about 6 large) egg whites

2 cups frozen Asian-style stir-fry vegetables

1 cup frozen peas

10 ounces (about 20) raw large shrimp, peeled, tails removed, deveined, chopped

1 cup chopped onion

1 tablespoon sesame oil

1 teaspoon chopped garlic

½ cup finely chopped pineapple

⅓ cup Clean & Hungry Teriyaki Sauce (recipe and store-bought alternatives on page 23)

Optional seasoning: salt

1. Pulse cauliflower in a blender until reduced to rice-sized pieces, working in batches as needed.

2. Bring an extra-large skillet sprayed with nonstick spray to medium heat. Scramble egg whites until fully cooked, 3 to 4 minutes, breaking them up into bite-sized pieces. Transfer to a large bowl, and cover to keep warm.

3. Remove skillet from heat; clean, if needed. Re-spray, and bring to medium-high heat. Add stir-fry veggies, peas, and ¼ cup water. Cover and cook for 3 minutes, or until thawed.

4. Add cauliflower rice, chopped shrimp, onion, sesame oil, and garlic. Cook and stir until veggies have mostly softened and shrimp are cooked through, 6 to 8 minutes.

5. Add scrambled egg whites, pineapple, and teriyaki sauce. Cook and stir until hot and well mixed, about 2 minutes.

MAKES 4 SERVINGS

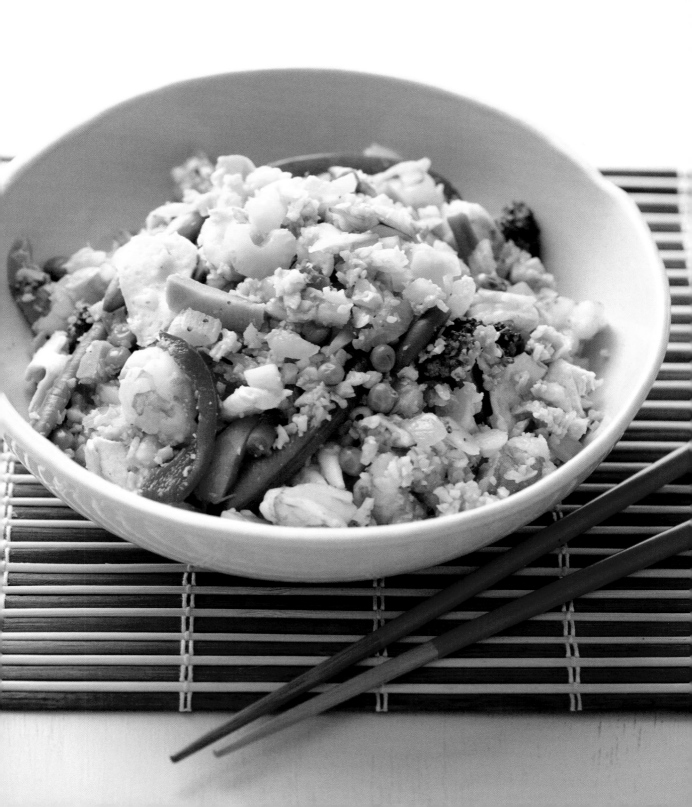

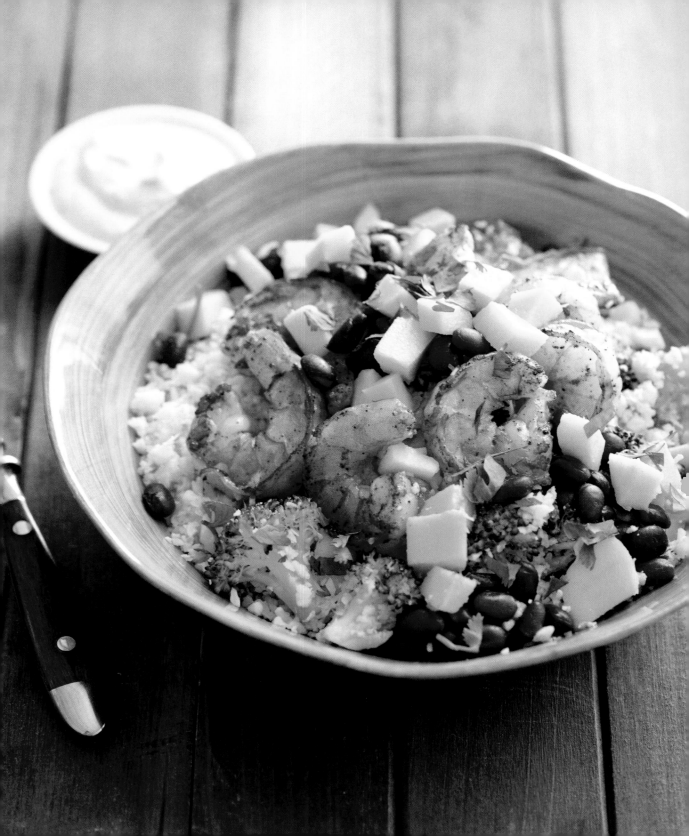

Island Shrimp Cauliflower Rice Bowl

Entire recipe: 327 calories, 4g total fat (0.5g sat fat), 896mg sodium, 38g carbs, 12.5g fiber, 15g sugars, 37.5g protein

You'll Need: small bowl, blender, large skillet, nonstick spray, medium-large bowl

Prep: 10 minutes   •   **Cook:** 10 minutes

Sauce

¼ cup fat-free plain Greek yogurt

½ ounce (about 1 tablespoon) mashed avocado

1 teaspoon lime juice

⅛ teaspoon ground cumin

Bowl

2 cups roughly chopped cauliflower

1 cup broccoli florets

⅛ teaspoon salt

4 ounces (about 8) raw large shrimp, peeled, tails removed, deveined

⅛ teaspoon ground cumin

⅛ teaspoon chili powder

¼ cup canned black beans, drained and rinsed

¼ cup chopped mango

2 tablespoons chopped fresh cilantro

1. Combine sauce ingredients in a small bowl. Mix until uniform.

2. Pulse cauliflower in a blender until reduced to rice-sized pieces.

3. Bring a large skillet sprayed with nonstick spray to medium-high heat. Add broccoli and ¼ cup water. Cover and cook for 3 minutes, or until broccoli is tender and water has evaporated.

4. Add cauliflower rice to the skillet. Cook and stir until hot and softened, 2 to 3 minutes. Transfer contents to a medium-large bowl. Stir in salt, and cover to keep warm.

5. Remove skillet from heat; clean, if needed. Re-spray, and bring to medium heat. Add shrimp, and season with cumin and chili powder. Cook and stir for about 4 minutes, until cooked through.

6. Top veggies with shrimp, beans, mango, cilantro, and sauce.

MAKES 1 SERVING

Southwest Chicken Cauliflower Rice Bowl

Entire recipe: 291 calories, 3.5g total fat (0.5g sat fat), 662mg sodium, 31.5g carbs, 10g fiber, 10g sugars, 34.5g protein

You'll Need: blender, small bowl, skillet, nonstick spray, medium bowl

Prep: 10 minutes • **Cook:** 20 minutes

2 cups roughly chopped cauliflower

¼ teaspoon chili powder

⅛ teaspoon ground cumin

⅛ teaspoon each salt and black pepper

Dash garlic powder

Dash paprika

One 4-ounce raw boneless skinless chicken breast cutlet, pounded to ½-inch thickness

2 tablespoons frozen sweet corn kernels

2 tablespoons chopped onion

¼ cup canned black beans, drained and rinsed

¼ cup chopped tomato

3 tablespoons Clean & Hungry Salsa (recipe and store-bought alternatives on page 18)

1. Pulse cauliflower in a blender until reduced to rice-sized pieces.

2. In a small bowl, mix all seasonings.

3. Bring a skillet sprayed with nonstick spray to medium heat. Season chicken with *half* the seasoning mixture. Cook for about 4 minutes per side, until cooked through. Transfer to a cutting board.

4. Remove skillet from heat; clean, if needed. Re-spray, and return to medium-high heat. Cook and stir corn until hot and slightly blackened, 1 to 2 minutes.

5. Add cauliflower rice, onion, and remaining seasoning mixture to the skillet. Cook and stir until veggies have mostly softened, 6 to 8 minutes.

6. Meanwhile, chop chicken.

7. Add chicken and beans to the skillet. Cook and stir until hot and well mixed, about 2 minutes.

8. Transfer to a medium bowl. Top with tomato and salsa.

MAKES 1 SERVING

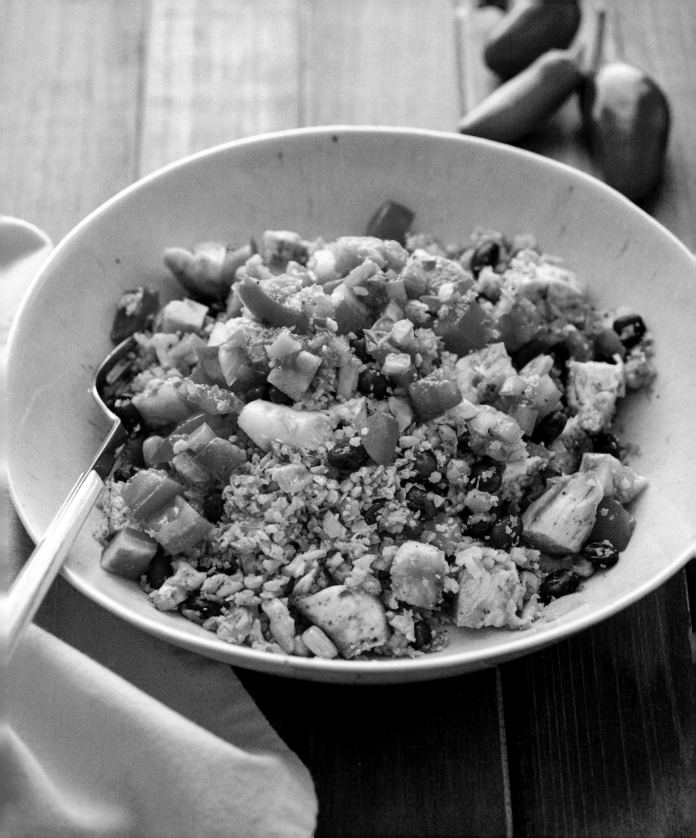

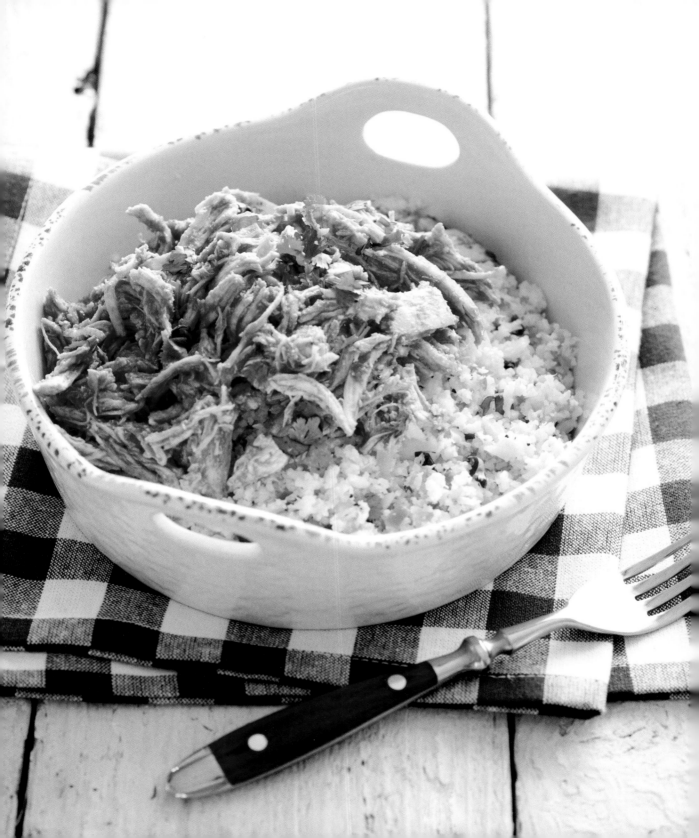

BBQ Chicken Cauliflower Rice Bowl

Entire recipe: 283 calories, 4g total fat (1g sat fat), 665mg sodium, 24.5g carbs, 7g fiber, 13.5g sugars, 37.5g protein

You'll Need: heavy-duty aluminum foil, baking sheet, nonstick spray, blender, 2 medium bowls (1 microwave-safe)

Prep: 10 minutes • **Cook:** 25 minutes

5 ounces raw boneless skinless chicken breast, pounded to ½-inch thickness

2 dashes each salt and black pepper

2 cups roughly chopped cauliflower

¼ cup finely chopped red onion

1 tablespoon finely chopped fresh cilantro

3 tablespoons Clean & Hungry BBQ Sauce (recipe and store-bought alternatives on page 19)

Optional seasonings: additional salt and black pepper

1. Preheat oven to 375 degrees. Lay a large piece of heavy-duty foil on a baking sheet, and spray with nonstick spray.

2. Place chicken on the center of the foil, and sprinkle with a dash each salt and pepper.

3. Cover with another large piece of foil. Fold together and seal all four edges of the foil pieces, forming a well-sealed packet.

4. Bake for 25 minutes, or until chicken is cooked through.

5. Meanwhile, pulse cauliflower in a blender until reduced to rice-sized pieces.

6. Transfer cauliflower rice to a medium microwave-safe bowl. Stir in onion. Cover and microwave for 3 minutes.

7. Uncover and stir. Re-cover and microwave for another 3 minutes, or until hot and soft. Stir in ½ tablespoon cilantro and remaining dash each salt and pepper. Re-cover to keep warm.

8. Cut packet to release hot steam before opening entirely. Transfer chicken to a medium bowl. Shred using two forks. Add BBQ sauce, and mix well.

9. Spoon saucy chicken over cauliflower rice. Top with remaining ½ tablespoon cilantro.

MAKES 1 SERVING

HG FYI

The chicken here is baked in a foil pack, making it very tender and easy to shred. For more foil-pack creations, flip to Chapter 6!

Cauliflower Rice Paella

¼th of recipe (about 1¾ cups): 251 calories, 2.5g total fat (0.5g sat fat), 771mg sodium, 22.5g carbs, 7g fiber, 9.5g sugars, 33.5g protein

You'll Need: blender, medium-large bowl, large pot with a lid, nonstick spray

Prep: 35 minutes • **Cook:** 40 minutes

4 cups roughly chopped cauliflower

1 teaspoon turmeric

1 teaspoon paprika

¼ teaspoon ground thyme

8 ounces raw boneless skinless chicken breast cutlets, pounded to ½-inch thickness

¼ teaspoon plus ⅛ teaspoon each salt and black pepper

1 cup sliced onion

1 cup chopped red bell pepper

1 tablespoon chopped garlic

2 cups chopped tomatoes

⅛ teaspoon cayenne pepper

1 cup frozen peas

¾ cup fat-free chicken broth

2 bay leaves

8 ounces (about 16) raw large shrimp, peeled, tails removed, deveined

6 ounces raw scallops, cut into bite-sized pieces

1 tablespoon lemon juice

Optional seasonings: additional salt and black pepper

1. Pulse cauliflower in a blender until reduced to rice-sized pieces, working in batches as needed.

2. Transfer cauliflower rice to a medium-large bowl. Sprinkle with ½ teaspoon turmeric, ½ teaspoon paprika, and ⅛ teaspoon thyme. Mix well.

3. Bring a large pot (with a lid) sprayed with nonstick spray to medium heat. Season chicken with ⅛ teaspoon each salt and black pepper. Cook for about 4 minutes per side, until cooked through. Transfer chicken to a cutting board.

4. Remove pot from heat; clean, if needed. Re-spray, and bring to medium-high heat. Add onion, bell pepper, and garlic. Cook and stir until veggies have softened, about 5 minutes.

5. Add tomatoes, cayenne pepper, and remaining ½ teaspoon turmeric, ½ teaspoon paprika, ⅛ teaspoon thyme, and ¼ teaspoon each salt and black pepper. Cook and stir until tomatoes have softened, about 3 minutes.

6. Add seasoned cauliflower rice, peas, broth, and bay leaves. Bring to a boil.

7. Reduce to a simmer. Cover and cook for 6 minutes.

8. Meanwhile, roughly chop chicken.

9. Add shrimp, scallops, and chopped chicken to the pot. Cook and stir until seafood is fully cooked, about 5 minutes.

10. Add lemon juice and stir. Cover and remove from heat. Let stand for 10 minutes.

11. Remove bay leaves.

MAKES 4 SERVINGS

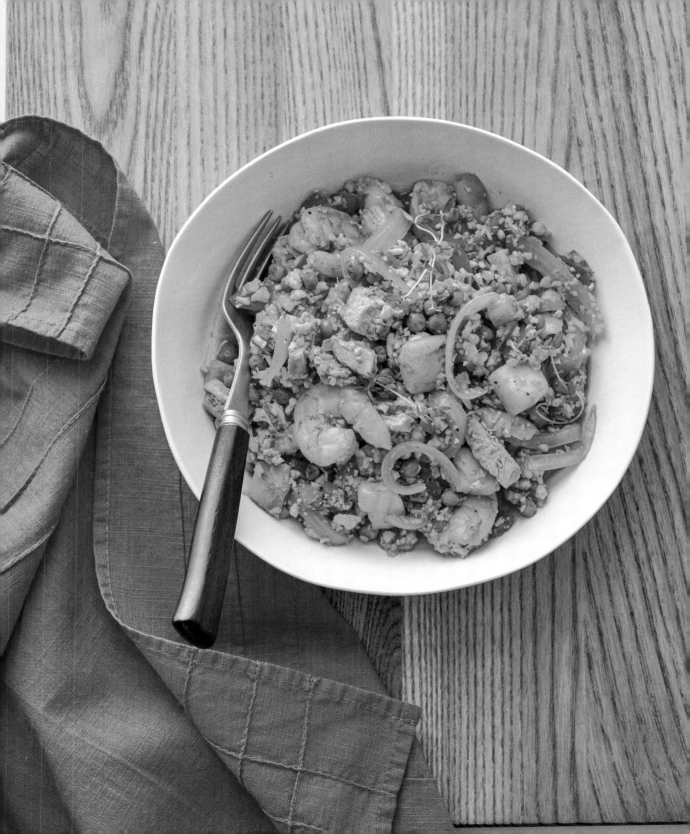

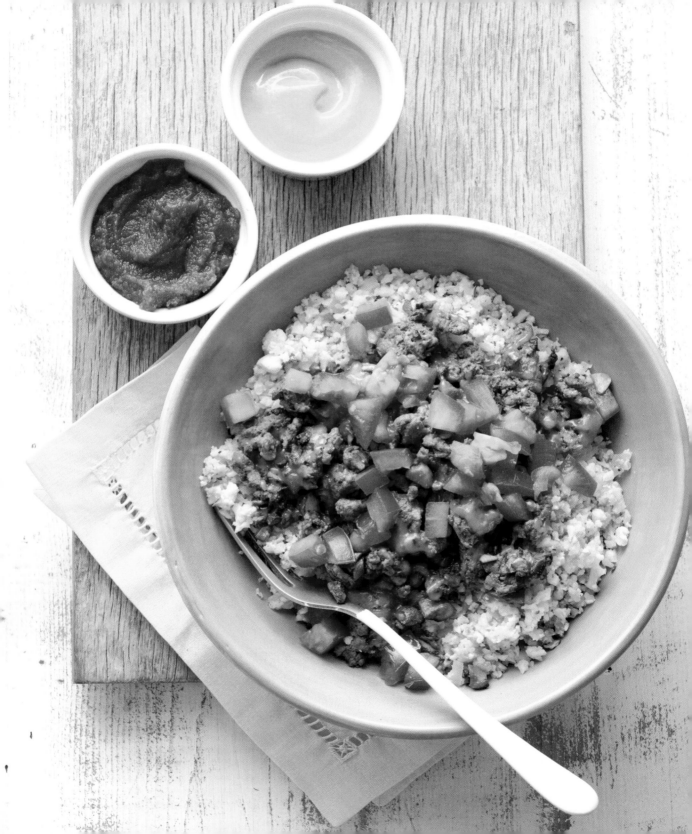

Cheeseburger Skillet

Entire recipe: 333 calories, 11g total fat (5.5g sat fat), 777mg sodium, 22.5g carbs, 7g fiber, 9.5g sugars, 38g protein

Who doesn't love the taste of a juicy cheeseburger? Get more good-burger goodness on page 279: Cheeseburger Crepes!

You'll Need: blender, large skillet, nonstick spray, medium-large bowl

Prep: 10 minutes • **Cook:** 10 minutes

2 cups roughly chopped cauliflower

¼ cup finely chopped onion

¼ teaspoon garlic powder

2 dashes each salt and black pepper

4 ounces raw extra-lean ground beef (4% fat or less)

1 cup finely chopped brown mushrooms

¼ cup shredded reduced-fat cheddar cheese

2 teaspoons yellow mustard

¼ cup chopped tomato

Optional topping: Clean & Hungry Ketchup (recipe and store-bought alternatives on page 24)

1. Pulse cauliflower in a blender until reduced to rice-sized pieces.

2. Bring a large skillet sprayed with nonstick spray to medium-high heat. Add cauliflower rice, onion, ⅛ teaspoon garlic powder, and a dash each salt and pepper. Cook and stir until hot and softened, 2 to 3 minutes. Transfer contents to a medium-large bowl. Cover to keep warm.

3. Remove skillet from heat; clean, if needed. Re-spray and return to medium-high heat. Add beef, and season with remaining ⅛ teaspoon garlic powder and dash each salt and pepper. Add mushrooms. Cook, stir, and crumble until beef is fully cooked and mushrooms have softened, about 5 minutes.

4. Add cheese and mustard. Cook and stir until melted and well mixed, about 1 minute.

5. Add beef mixture to the medium-large bowl, and top with tomato.

MAKES 1 SERVING

Chicken Fajita Stuffed Peppers

¼th of recipe (1 stuffed pepper): 179 calories, 4.5g total fat (2g sat fat), 348mg sodium, 15.5g carbs, 5g fiber, 7.5g sugars, 21g protein

You'll Need: deep 8-inch by 8-inch baking pan, blender, large skillet, nonstick spray

Prep: 10 minutes • **Cook:** 25 minutes

4 large green bell peppers (look for peppers that sit flat when stem ends are up)

2½ cups roughly chopped cauliflower

8 ounces raw boneless skinless chicken breast cutlets, pounded to ½-inch thickness

¼ teaspoon ground cumin

¼ teaspoon chili powder

¼ teaspoon garlic powder

¼ teaspoon salt

½ cup chopped onion

½ cup shredded reduced-fat Mexican-blend cheese

¼ cup fat-free plain Greek yogurt

¼ cup Clean & Hungry Salsa (recipe and store-bought alternatives on page 18)

1. Preheat oven to 350 degrees.

2. Carefully slice off and discard the stem ends of the bell peppers, about half an inch from the top. Remove and discard seeds. Place peppers cut-side up in a deep 8-inch by 8-inch baking pan. If peppers do not sit flat, gently lean them against the pan sides for support.

3. Bake until peppers are soft, 20 to 25 minutes.

4. Meanwhile, pulse cauliflower in a blender until reduced to rice-sized pieces, working in batches as needed.

5. Bring a large skillet sprayed with nonstick spray to medium heat. Season chicken with ⅛ teaspoon of each seasoning, and place in the skillet. Cook for about 4 minutes per side, until cooked through. Transfer to a cutting board.

6. Remove skillet from heat; clean, if needed. Re-spray, and bring to medium-high heat. Add cauliflower rice, onion, and remaining ⅛ teaspoon of each seasoning. Cook and stir until veggies have mostly softened, about 4 minutes.

7. Chop chicken, and add to the skillet. Cook and stir until veggies are soft, about 2 minutes.

8. Blot away excess moisture from bell peppers. Evenly distribute filling among the peppers. Sprinkle with cheese.

9. Top each pepper with 1 tablespoon each yogurt and salsa.

MAKES 4 SERVINGS

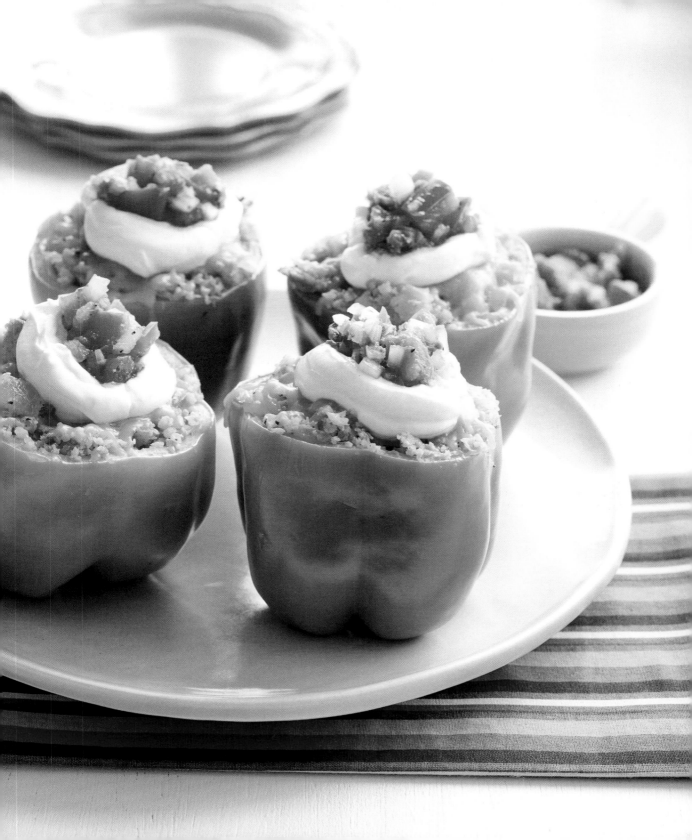

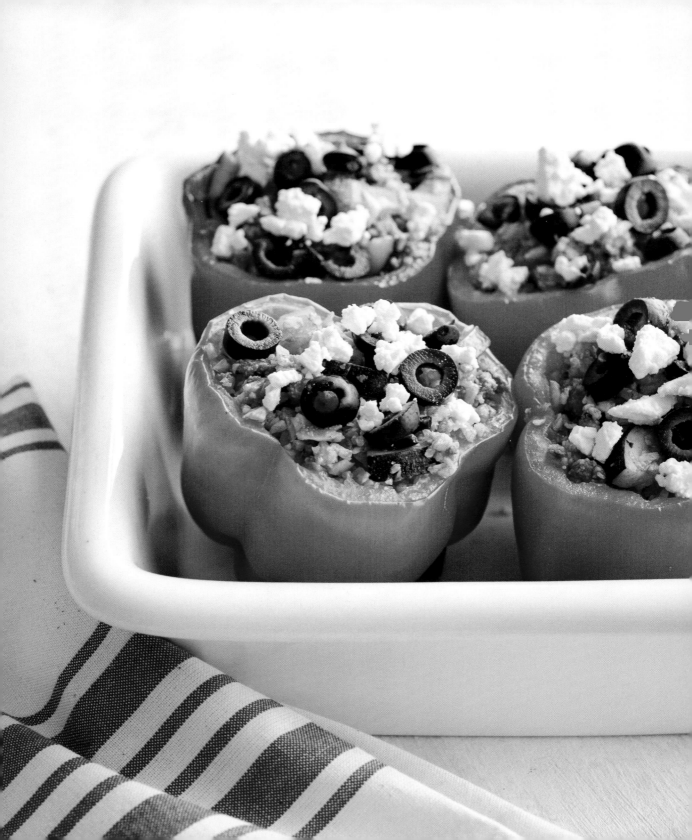

Greek Stuffed Peppers

¼th of recipe (1 stuffed pepper): 190 calories, 5.5g total fat (3g sat fat), 440mg sodium, 20.5g carbs, 6.5g fiber, 11g sugars, 17g protein

You'll Need: deep 8-inch by 8-inch baking pan, blender, large skillet, nonstick spray

Prep: 15 minutes • **Cook:** 25 minutes

4 large red bell peppers (look for peppers that sit flat when stem ends are up)

2½ cups roughly chopped cauliflower

8 ounces raw extra-lean ground beef (4% fat or less)

¼ teaspoon oregano

¼ teaspoon each salt and black pepper

½ cup chopped onion

½ cup chopped zucchini

½ teaspoon chopped garlic

¾ cup canned crushed tomatoes

¼ cup crumbled feta cheese

¼ cup sliced black olives

1. Preheat oven to 350 degrees.

2. Carefully slice off and discard the stem ends of the bell peppers, about half an inch from the top. Remove and discard seeds. Place peppers cut-side up in a deep 8-inch by 8-inch baking pan. If peppers do not sit flat, gently lean them against the pan sides for support.

3. Bake until peppers are soft, 20 to 25 minutes.

4. Meanwhile, pulse cauliflower in a blender until reduced to rice-sized pieces, working in batches as needed.

5. Bring a large skillet sprayed with nonstick spray to medium-high heat. Add beef, and sprinkle with ⅛ teaspoon each oregano, salt, and black pepper. Cook and crumble for 4 minutes.

6. Add cauliflower rice, onion, zucchini, and garlic to the skillet. Cook and stir until beef is fully cooked and veggies have softened, about 3 minutes.

7. Add crushed tomatoes to the skillet, along with remaining ⅛ teaspoon each oregano, salt, and black pepper. Cook and stir until hot and well mixed, about 2 minutes.

8. Blot away excess moisture from bell peppers. Evenly distribute filling among the peppers.

9. Top with feta cheese and olives.

MAKES 4 SERVINGS

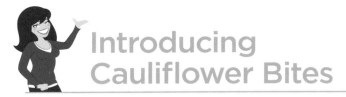

Introducing
Cauliflower Bites

These breaded 'n baked cauliflower florets are the ultimate appetizer or 4-serving snack. They taste best when eaten immediately . . . That's when they're nice and crispy!

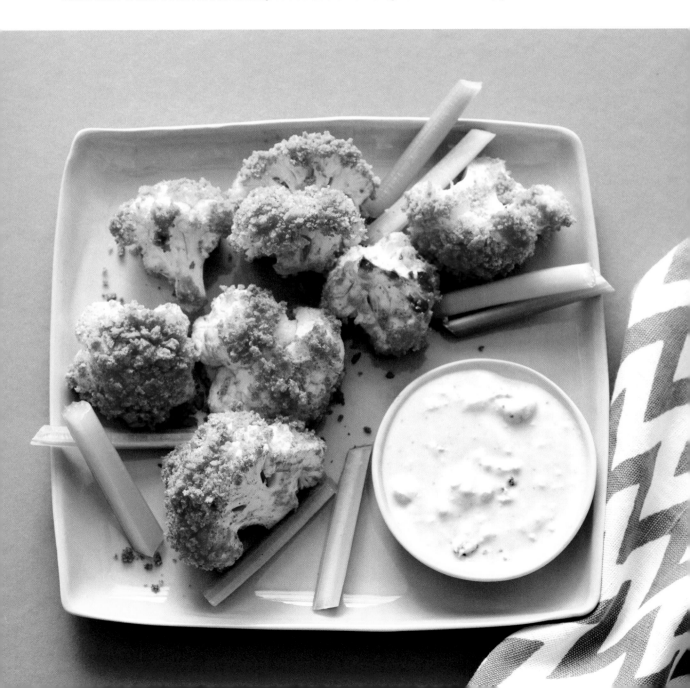

Big Buffalo Cauliflower Bites

¼th of recipe (about 7 pieces): 82 calories, 0.5g total fat (0g sat fat), 373mg sodium, 15.5g carbs, 5g fiber, 4.5g sugars, 6g protein

You'll Need: large baking sheet, nonstick spray, 3 large bowls, whisk

Prep: 15 minutes   •   **Cook:** 30 minutes

¼ cup (about 2 large) egg whites

¼ teaspoon cayenne pepper

6 cups large cauliflower florets (about 2 inches wide)

½ cup whole-wheat panko breadcrumbs

¼ teaspoon garlic powder

¼ teaspoon onion powder

2 tablespoons Frank's RedHot Original Cayenne Pepper Sauce

Optional dip: Clean & Hungry Chunky Blue Cheese Dressing (recipe and store-bought alternatives on page 22)

1. Preheat oven to 375 degrees. Spray a large baking sheet with nonstick spray.

2. In a large bowl, combine cayenne pepper with egg whites. Whisk well. Add cauliflower, and toss to coat.

3. In another large bowl, mix breadcrumbs with garlic powder and onion powder.

4. One at a time, shake cauliflower florets to remove excess egg whites, and coat with seasoned breadcrumbs. Place on the baking sheet, evenly spaced.

5. Bake until cauliflower is slightly crispy on the outside and tender on the inside, about 30 minutes.

6. Transfer cauliflower to a large bowl, and toss with hot sauce.

MAKES 4 SERVINGS

Mega Mexican Cauliflower Bites

¼th of recipe (about 7 pieces): 126 calories, 3.5g total fat (2g sat fat), 192mg sodium, 16g carbs, 5g fiber, 4.5g sugars, 9.5g protein

You'll Need: large baking sheet, nonstick spray, 2 large bowls, whisk

Prep: 15 minutes • **Cook:** 35 minutes

½ cup whole-wheat panko breadcrumbs

1 teaspoon ground cumin

¼ teaspoon cayenne pepper

¼ teaspoon garlic powder

¼ teaspoon onion powder

¼ cup (about 2 large) egg whites

6 cups large cauliflower florets (about 2 inches wide)

½ cup shredded reduced-fat cheddar cheese

Optional topping: chopped fresh cilantro

Optional dip: Clean & Hungry Salsa (recipe and store-bought alternatives on page 18)

1. Preheat oven to 375 degrees. Spray a large baking sheet with nonstick spray.

2. In a large bowl, combine breadcrumbs, ½ teaspoon cumin, and ⅛ teaspoon each cayenne pepper, garlic powder, and onion powder. Mix well.

3. In another large bowl, combine egg whites with remaining ½ teaspoon cumin and remaining ⅛ teaspoon each cayenne pepper, garlic powder, and onion powder. Whisk well. Add cauliflower, and toss to coat.

4. One at a time, shake cauliflower florets to remove excess egg whites, and coat with seasoned breadcrumbs. Place on the baking sheet, evenly spaced.

5. Bake until cauliflower is slightly crispy on the outside and tender on the inside, about 30 minutes.

6. Remove baking sheet from oven, and increase temperature to broil.

7. Arrange cauliflower florets on the center of the sheet so that they are touching. Sprinkle with cheese.

8. Broil until cheese has melted, about 2 minutes.

MAKES 4 SERVINGS

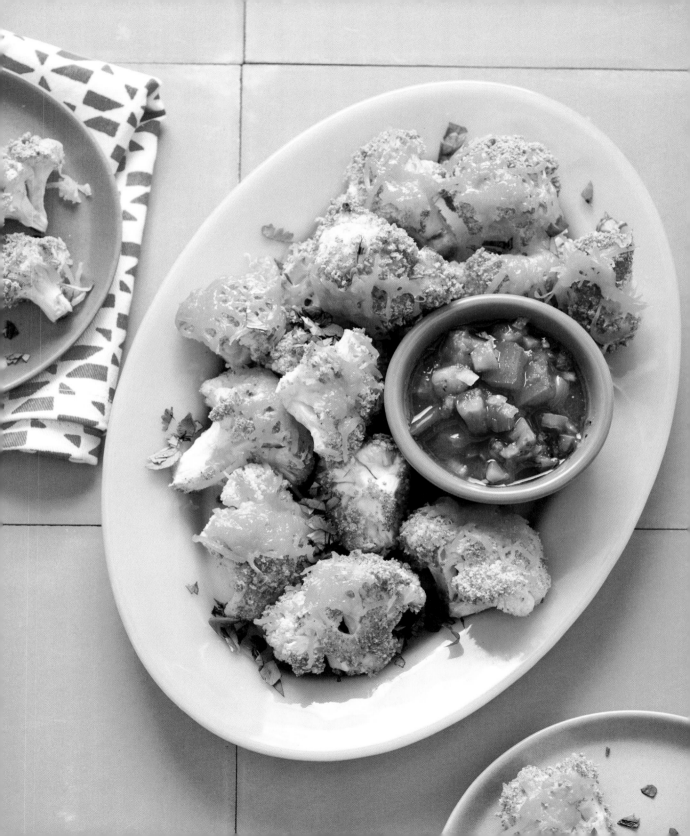

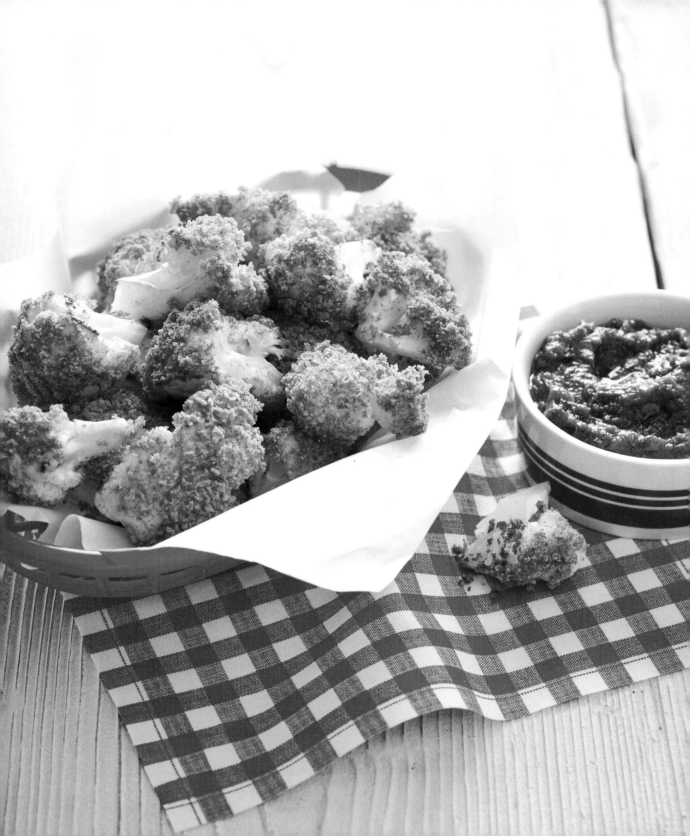

Big BBQ Cauliflower Bites

¼th of recipe (about 7 pieces with 2 tablespoons dip):
112 calories, 0.5g total fat (0g sat fat), 313mg sodium, 22g carbs,
6g fiber, 9g sugars, 7g protein

You'll Need: large baking sheet, nonstick spray, 2 large bowls, whisk, small bowl

Prep: 15 minutes • **Cook:** 30 minutes

½ cup whole-wheat panko breadcrumbs

⅛ teaspoon salt

1 teaspoon paprika

½ teaspoon garlic powder

½ teaspoon onion powder

¼ teaspoon cayenne pepper

¼ cup (about 2 large) egg whites

6 cups large cauliflower florets (about 2 inches wide)

½ cup Clean & Hungry BBQ Sauce (recipe and store-bought alternatives on page 19)

¼ cup finely chopped fresh cilantro

1. Preheat oven to 375 degrees. Spray a large baking sheet with nonstick spray.

2. In a large bowl, combine breadcrumbs with salt. Add ½ teaspoon paprika, ¼ teaspoon garlic powder, ¼ teaspoon onion powder, and ⅛ teaspoon cayenne pepper. Mix well.

3. In another large bowl, combine egg whites with remaining ½ teaspoon paprika, ¼ teaspoon garlic powder, ¼ teaspoon onion powder, and ⅛ teaspoon cayenne pepper. Whisk well. Add cauliflower, and toss to coat.

4. One at a time, shake cauliflower florets to remove excess egg whites, and coat with seasoned breadcrumbs. Place on the baking sheet, evenly spaced.

5. Bake until cauliflower is slightly crispy on the outside and tender on the inside, about 30 minutes.

6. Meanwhile, in a small bowl, stir cilantro into BBQ sauce.

7. Serve cauliflower with BBQ sauce for dipping.

MAKES 4 SERVINGS

Hungry for More Cauliflower Creations?

Check these out . . .

10

Carb-Slashed Sandwiches, Burgers & More

The best part of a sandwich is *not* the doughy mess of a bun . . . it's all the tasty stuff inside! From gigantic burger patties to delicious chicken wraps, this chapter is exploding with savory goodness.

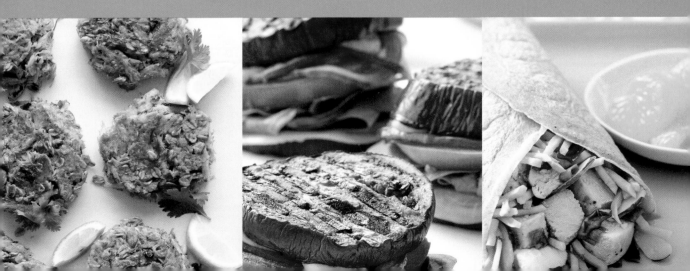

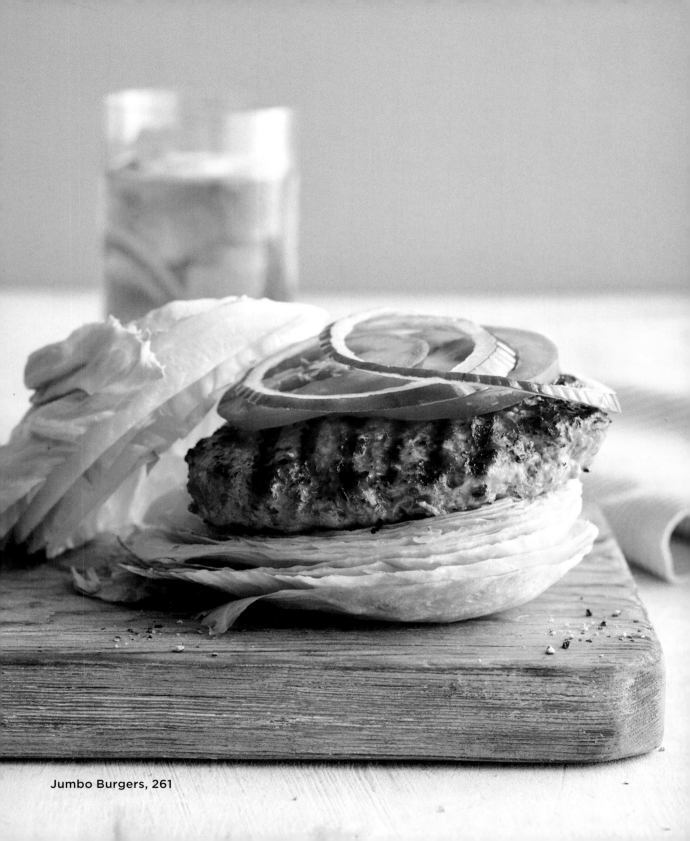

Jumbo Burgers, 261

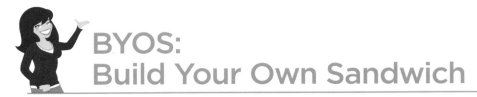

BYOS:
Build Your Own Sandwich

For this chapter, we kept the burger and patty recipes bun-free. Why? Because guilt-free clean bread options aren't easy to find, and not everyone wants to spend their calories on carby buns . . . especially when there are great alternatives like lettuce buns and cabbage wraps! Keep reading for the 411 . . .

Step 1   CHOOSE YOUR BASE:

Lettuce buns: These are a Hungry Girl favorite: cool and crisp! You'll need 4 large leaves of iceberg or butter lettuce: 2 leaves for the bottom half of the bun and 2 leaves for the top. Each lettuce bun has only around 15 calories, plus a gram of fiber.

Cabbage wraps: Here's another fantastic option. You'll need 2 extra-large leaves of green cabbage that have been steamed or boiled. (Want cabbage-cooking assistance? See the next page!) Just stack the cooked leaves, place your sandwich fillings on one half, and wrap the other half of the leaves around it. Each 2-leaf cabbage wrap has about 20 calories and 1.5 grams of fiber. Nice!

Whole-grain buns/bread: Look for minimally processed, all-natural, whole-grain buns or bread slices—the fewer calories, the better. Watch out for oversized buns and added sugar. Food for Life's Ezekiel line of sprouted bread products is great. The brand even makes gluten-free options.

Step 2   PICK YOUR PATTY:

Black Bean Burger (page 257)

Falafel Burger (page 258)

Jumbo Burger (page 261)

Step 3   ADD YOUR EXTRAS:

Fresh veggies: Sliced tomato and red onion are classic. Diced sweet onion is great too. And for the Falafel Burgers, try thinly sliced cucumber!

Condiments: Those Falafel Burgers have their very own sauce, but as for the other burgers? Try the Clean & Hungry BBQ Sauce or Clean & Hungry Ketchup (recipes and store-bought alternatives on pages 19 and 24). Mustard is another great low-calorie condiment.

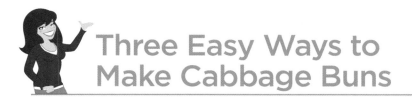

Three Easy Ways to Make Cabbage Buns

fastest **IN THE MICROWAVE:**

Carefully halve a head of green cabbage. In a large microwave-safe bowl, microwave for about 4 minutes, until the outer leaves begin to loosen. Once cool enough to handle, gently remove outer leaves, and place them back in the bowl. (Reserve the rest of the cabbage for another time.) Add 2 tablespoons water to the bowl. Cover and microwave for about 2 minutes, until very soft.

easiest **IN A SLOW COOKER:**

Carefully halve a head of green cabbage, and place in a slow cooker. Add 1 cup of water. Cover and cook on high for 1½ hours, or until soft. Gently remove leaves from the head once cool.

classic **ON THE STOVE:**

Carefully halve a head of green cabbage. Place in an extra-large pot, and cover with water. Bring to a boil. Cover and cook, rotating cabbage occasionally, until leaves soften, loosen, and begin to fall off the head, 8 to 10 minutes. Drain cabbage. Once cool, gently remove leaves.

Leftovers Alert: How to Freeze and Reheat Burger Patties

The burger recipes in this chapter each make four patties . . . Store extras in the freezer, and you'll have delicious, healthy options on hand the next time your fridge is empty! (P.S. These methods work for the Tuna Patties and Crab Cakes too.)

To freeze: Tightly wrap each cooled patty in plastic wrap. Place individually wrapped patties in a sealable container or bag, seal, and store in the freezer.

To reheat on the stove: Bring a grill pan (or skillet) with a lid sprayed with nonstick spray to medium heat. Cook (unwrapped) patties until hot and slightly softened, 4 to 6 minutes per side. (Jumbo Burgers will take longer: 6 to 8 minutes per side.)

To reheat in the microwave: Place a single (unwrapped) patty on a microwave-safe plate. Microwave on high for about 45 seconds per side.

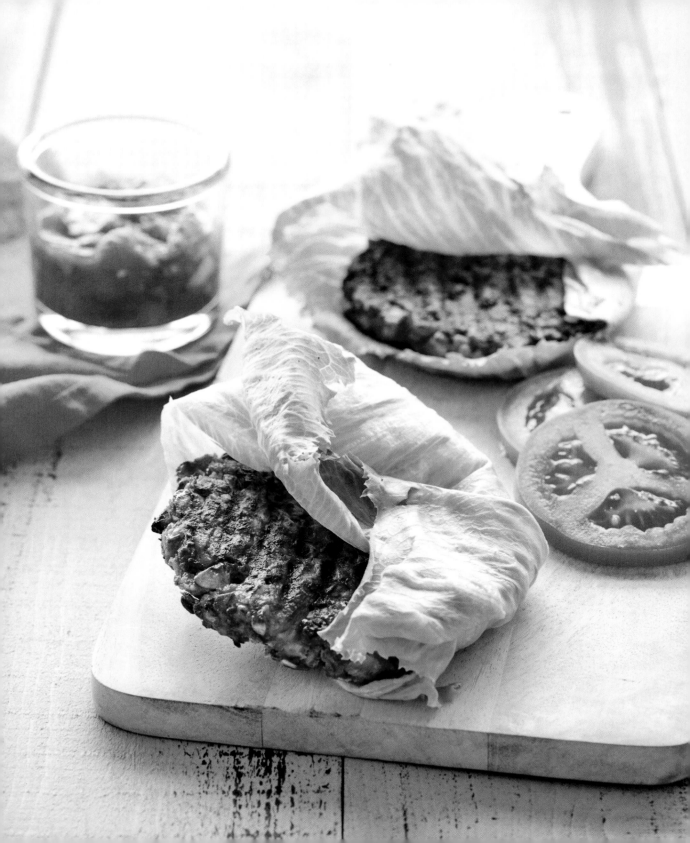

Black Bean Burgers

¼ᵗʰ of recipe (1 patty): 121 calories, 1g total fat (0g sat fat), 345mg sodium, 19.5g carbs, 4.5g fiber, 2.5g sugars, 9g protein

These meat-free, no-gluten veggie burgers are better than any meatless patties you'll find in the freezer aisle ... PROMISE.

You'll Need: medium bowl, large bowl, potato masher, grill pan (or large skillet), nonstick spray

Prep: 20 minutes • **Cook:** 10 minutes

½ cup old-fashioned oats

1 cup canned black beans, drained and rinsed

1½ cups finely chopped brown mushrooms

½ cup (about 4 large) egg whites

¼ cup finely chopped onion

1 teaspoon ground cumin

½ teaspoon garlic powder

½ teaspoon onion powder

¼ teaspoon each salt and black pepper

1. In a medium bowl, combine oats with ⅓ cup hot water. Mix well, and let sit for 5 minutes.

2. Meanwhile, in a large bowl, thoroughly mash black beans with a potato masher.

3. Add soaked oats and remaining ingredients to the large bowl. Mix thoroughly.

4. Bring a grill pan (or large skillet) sprayed with nonstick spray to medium-high heat. Evenly distribute mixture into 4 mounds. Flatten into patties, each about ½ inch thick.

5. Cook patties until golden brown and cooked through, about 5 minutes per side.

MAKES 4 SERVINGS

Falafel Burgers

¼th of recipe (1 patty with about 2 tablespoons sauce):
171 calories, 2g total fat (0g sat fat), 587mg sodium, 29g carbs,
6.5g fiber, 4g sugars, 11.5g protein

You'll Need: small blender or food processor, large bowl, potato masher, grill pan (or large skillet), nonstick spray

Prep: 20 minutes • **Cook:** 10 minutes

Sauce

½ cup fat-free plain Greek yogurt

¼ cup peeled, seeded, and chopped cucumber

1 teaspoon dried dill

¼ teaspoon garlic powder

⅛ teaspoon salt

Dash black pepper

Burgers

One 15-ounce can chickpeas (garbanzo beans), drained and rinsed

1 cup very finely chopped onion

¼ cup whole-wheat flour

¼ cup (about 2 large) egg whites

3 tablespoons finely chopped fresh parsley

1½ tablespoons chopped garlic

1 tablespoon chopped fresh cilantro

1 tablespoon ground cumin

½ teaspoon salt

¼ teaspoon lemon juice

⅛ teaspoon paprika

⅛ teaspoon black pepper

1. Place sauce ingredients in a small blender or food processor. Pulse until just blended. Cover and refrigerate.

2. Place chickpeas in a large bowl, and thoroughly mash with a potato masher. Add remaining burger ingredients, and mix thoroughly.

3. Firmly form into 4 patties, each about ½ inch thick.

4. Bring a grill pan (or large skillet) sprayed with nonstick spray to medium-high heat. Cook patties until golden brown and cooked through, about 5 minutes per side.

5. Top patties with sauce, or serve sauce on the side.

MAKES 4 SERVINGS

HG FYI

In order to thoroughly blend the sauce, you'll need a small blender or food processor—the Magic Bullet is our top pick.

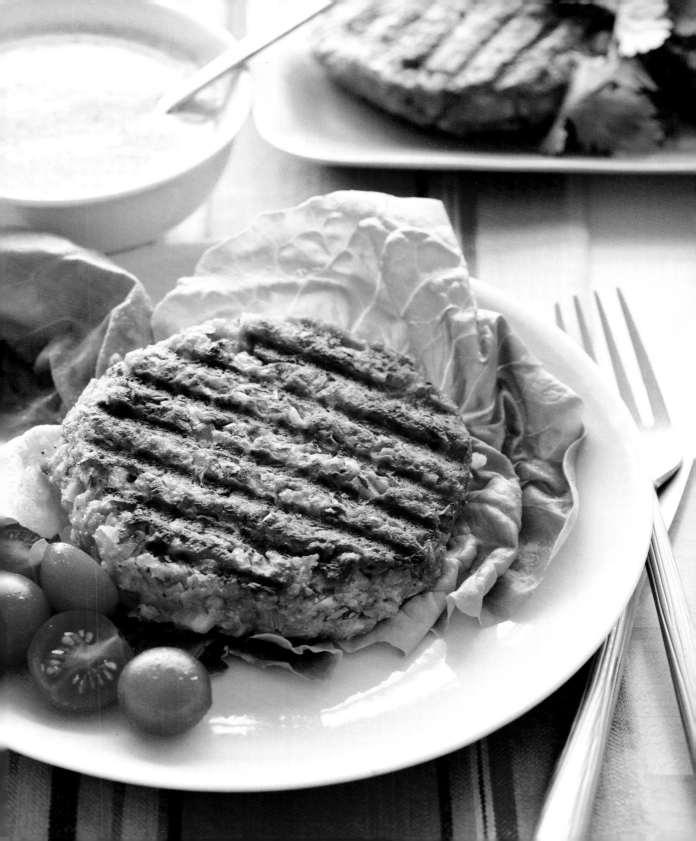

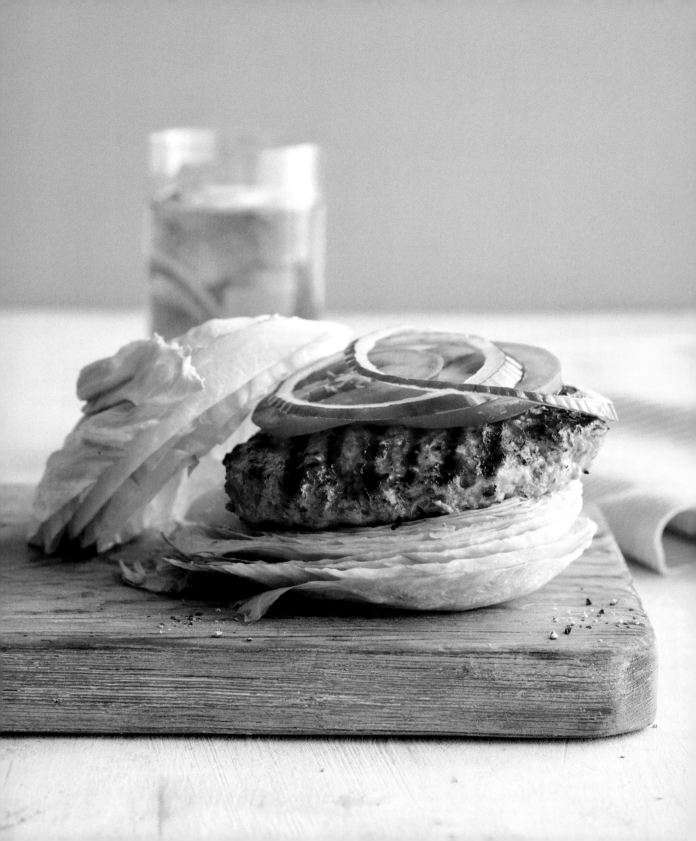

Jumbo Burgers

¼th of recipe (1 patty): 188 calories, 5g total fat (2g sat fat), 403mg sodium, 7g carbs, 2g fiber, 2g sugars, 27g protein

Riced cauliflower helps super-size these yummy patties. For more fun with cauliflower, check out Chapter 9: Cauliflower Rice & More Cauliflower Creations.

You'll Need: blender, large bowl, grill pan (or large skillet), nonstick spray

Prep: 20 minutes • **Cook:** 25 minutes

2 cups roughly chopped cauliflower

1 pound raw extra-lean ground beef (4% fat or less)

¼ cup (about 2 large) egg whites

¼ cup old-fashioned oats

½ teaspoon garlic powder

½ teaspoon onion powder

½ teaspoon each salt and black pepper

1. Pulse cauliflower in a blender until reduced to rice-sized pieces. Transfer to a large bowl.

2. Add all remaining ingredients, and mix thoroughly. Evenly form into 4 patties, each about ¾ inch thick.

3. Bring a grill pan (or large skillet) sprayed with nonstick spray to medium-high heat. Cook 2 patties for about 6 minutes per side, until cooked to your preference. (Reduce cook time for rare; increase for well done.)

4. Remove skillet from heat; clean if needed. Re-spray, and repeat cooking process with remaining 2 patties.

MAKES 4 SERVINGS

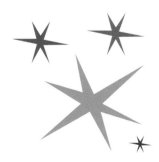

Tuna Patties

¼ᵗʰ of recipe (1 patty): 172 calories, 2.5g total fat (1g sat fat), 507mg sodium, 6g carbs, 1g fiber, 0.5g sugars, 29g protein

These things are OUTSTANDING. So much flavor! Try 'em and see . . .

You'll Need: large bowl, extra-large skillet, nonstick spray

Prep: 15 minutes • **Cook:** 10 minutes

15 ounces thoroughly drained albacore tuna (previously packed in water), flaked

½ cup (about 4 large) egg whites

⅓ cup old-fashioned oats

2 tablespoons chopped chives

1 tablespoon Dijon mustard

2 teaspoons lemon juice

1 teaspoon garlic powder

⅛ teaspoon each salt and black pepper

Dash cayenne pepper

1. Combine all ingredients in a large bowl, and mix until uniform.

2. Bring an extra-large skillet sprayed with nonstick spray to medium-high heat. Evenly distribute mixture into 4 mounds. Flatten into patties, each about ½ inch thick.

3. Cook patties until golden brown and cooked through, about 4 minutes per side.

MAKES 4 SERVINGS

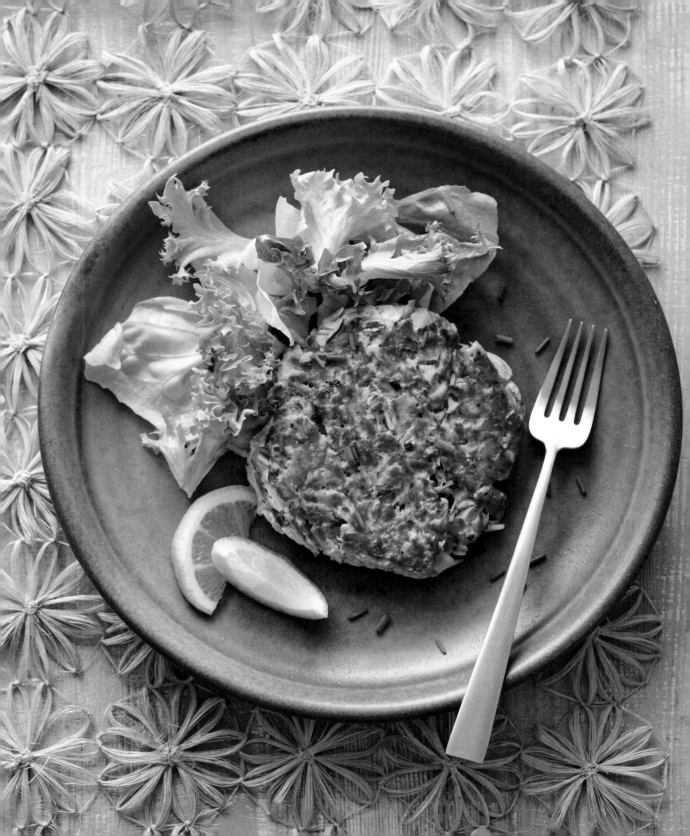

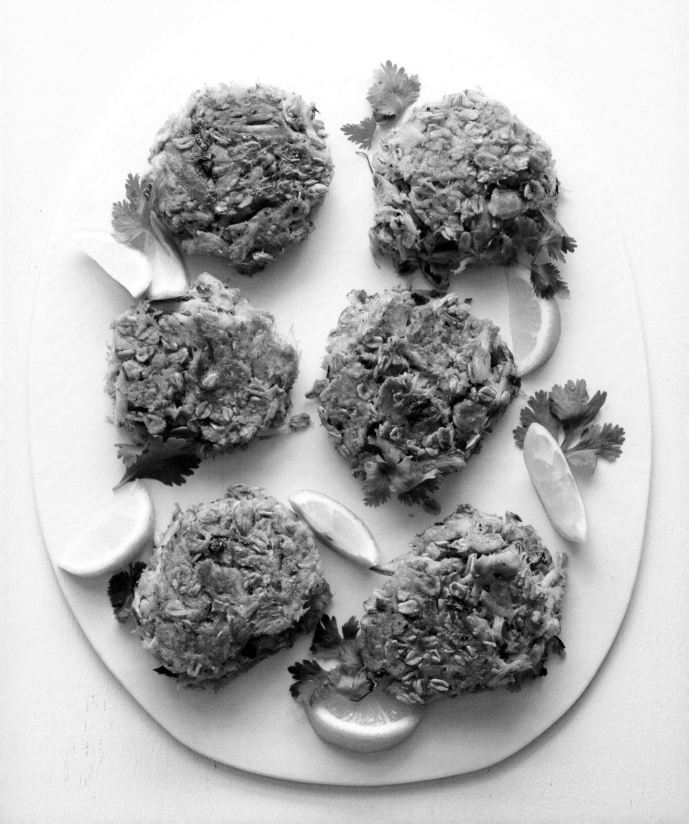

Crab Cakes

⅙ᵗʰ of recipe (1 crab cake): 107 calories, 1g total fat (<0.5g sat fat), 395mg sodium, 5.5g carbs, 0.5g fiber, 0.5g sugars, 18g protein

You'll Need: large bowl, large skillet, nonstick spray

Prep: 10 minutes • **Cook:** 20 minutes

16 ounces thoroughly drained ready-to-eat crabmeat

½ cup old-fashioned oats

½ cup (about 4 large) egg whites

¼ cup chopped fresh cilantro

1½ tablespoons lime juice

¼ teaspoon garlic powder

¼ teaspoon each salt and black pepper

⅛ teaspoon cayenne pepper

1. Combine ingredients in large bowl, and mix until uniform.

2. Firmly form into 6 patties, each about ½ inch thick.

3. Bring a large skillet sprayed with nonstick spray to medium-high heat. Working in batches as needed, cook patties until golden brown and cooked through, about 4 minutes per side, flipping carefully.

MAKES 6 SERVINGS

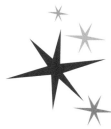

For more healthy recipes, plus the latest food news, tips & tricks, and more, sign up for free daily emails at Hungry-Girl.com!

Chinese Chicken Salad Wrap

Entire recipe: 262 calories, 8g total fat (1g sat fat), 642mg sodium, 17g carbs, 4g fiber, 2.5g sugars, 31.5g protein

You'll Need: medium bowl

Prep: 10 minutes

3 ounces cooked and chopped skinless chicken breast

⅓ cup bagged broccoli cole slaw, roughly chopped

2 tablespoons Clean & Hungry Sesame Ginger Dressing (recipe and store-bought alternatives on page 21)

1 tablespoon chopped scallions

¼ ounce (about 1 tablespoon) sliced almonds

1 Clean & Hungry Whole-Wheat Tortilla (recipe and store-bought alternatives on page 25)

1. In a medium bowl, combine all ingredients *except* tortilla. Mix well.

2. Place mixture across the middle of the tortilla.

3. Gently wrap tortilla up by first folding in one side (to keep filling from escaping) and then tightly rolling it up from the bottom.

MAKES 1 SERVING

HG Tip

We recommend warming your tortilla in the microwave for about 10 seconds to make it more pliable.

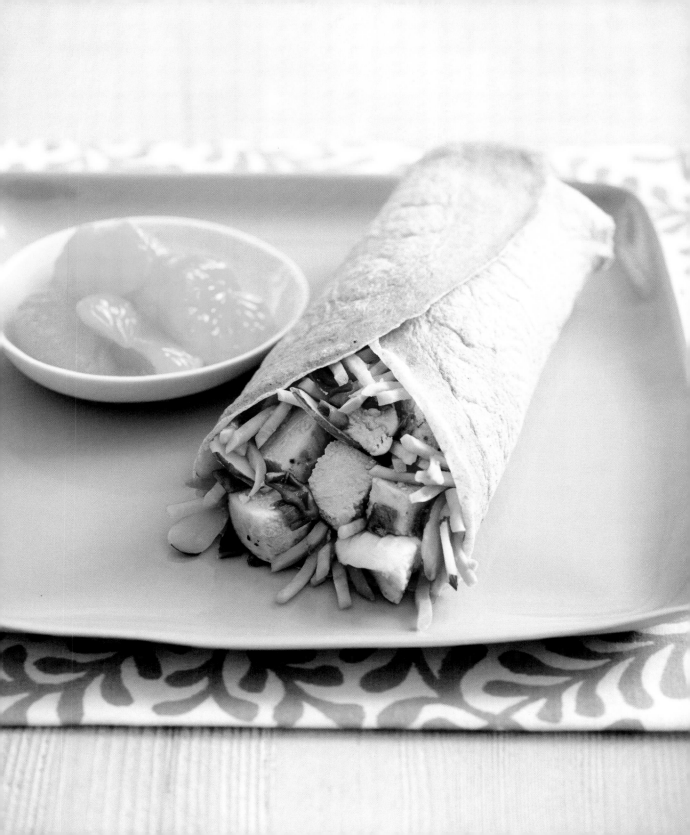

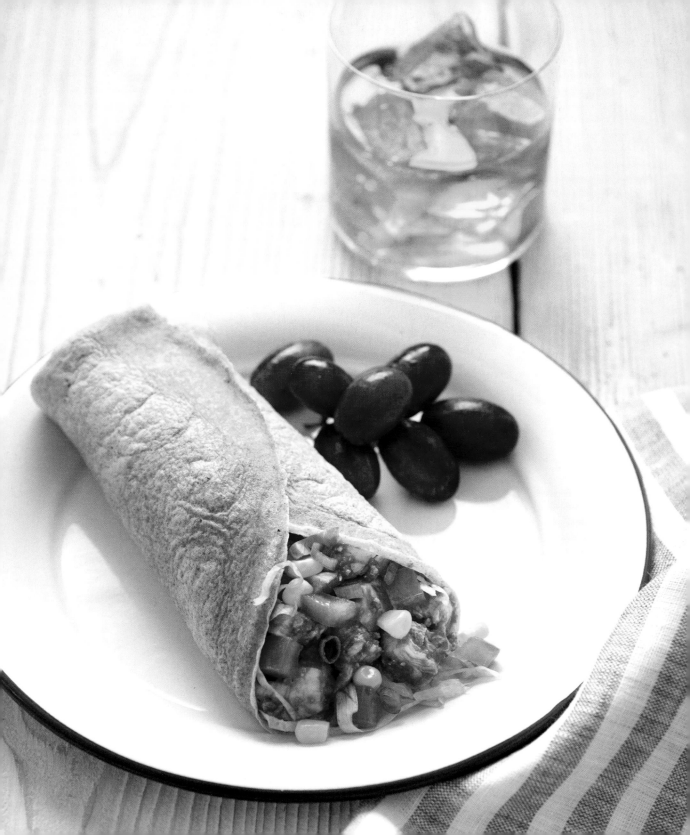

BBQ Chicken Wrap

Entire recipe: 248 calories, 2g total fat (0.5g sat fat), 661mg sodium, 26.5g carbs, 4g fiber, 9g sugars, 31g protein

You'll Need: medium bowl

Prep: 10 minutes

3 ounces cooked and chopped skinless chicken breast

3 tablespoons Clean & Hungry BBQ Sauce (recipe and store-bought alternatives on page 19)

1 Clean & Hungry Whole-Wheat Tortilla (recipe and store-bought alternatives on page 25)

⅓ cup shredded lettuce

2 tablespoons frozen sweet corn kernels, thawed

2 tablespoons chopped tomato

1 tablespoon chopped scallions

1. In a medium bowl, coat chicken with BBQ sauce.

2. Lay lettuce across the middle of the tortilla. Top with saucy chicken, corn, tomato, and scallions.

3. Gently wrap tortilla up by first folding in one side (to keep filling from escaping) and then tightly rolling it up from the bottom.

MAKES 1 SERVING

HG Tip

We recommend warming your tortilla in the microwave for about 10 seconds to make it more pliable.

Fork 'n Knife Eggplant "Sandwiches"

¼th of recipe (1 sandwich): 124 calories, 4.5g total fat (2.5g sat fat), 405mg sodium, 14.5g carbs, 7g fiber, 6g sugars, 8.5g protein

Maybe it's a stretch to call these eggplant stacks "sandwiches" ... But this recipe is so good, you won't care!

You'll Need: small bowl, grill pan (or large skillet), nonstick spray, plate

Prep: 10 minutes • **Cook:** 30 minutes

1 tablespoon reduced-sodium/lite soy sauce

1½ tablespoons Dijon mustard

Eight ¾-inch-thick eggplant slices (cut widthwise from the center of a wide eggplant), patted dry

⅛ teaspoon black pepper

4 thin slices red onion, rings intact

4 slices reduced-fat provolone cheese

1 cup baby spinach leaves

4 large slices tomato

1. In a small bowl, mix soy sauce with 1 teaspoon mustard. Spread mixture over eggplant slices, and sprinkle with pepper.

2. Bring a grill pan (or large skillet) sprayed with nonstick spray to medium heat. Cook onion until soft, about 2 minutes per side.

3. Remove onion, and set aside.

4. Remove grill pan from heat; clean, if needed. Re-spray and return to medium heat. Cook 4 eggplant slices until soft, about 5 minutes per side.

5. Set cooked eggplant aside; these are the top halves of your sandwiches.

6. Cook remaining 4 eggplant slices until soft, about 5 minutes per side. Still in the pan, top each eggplant slice with a slice of cheese, and cook until melted, about 1 minute.

7. Transfer cheese-topped eggplant slices to a plate; these are the bottom halves of your sandwiches. Top with spinach, tomato, and onion.

8. Spread remaining cooked eggplant slices with remaining 3½ teaspoons mustard, and place each one over a sandwich.

MAKES 4 SERVINGS

Gluten FYI

Certain brands add gluten to their soy sauce. If you avoid gluten, read labels carefully. Or grab a specially marked product like Kikkoman Gluten-Free Soy Sauce.

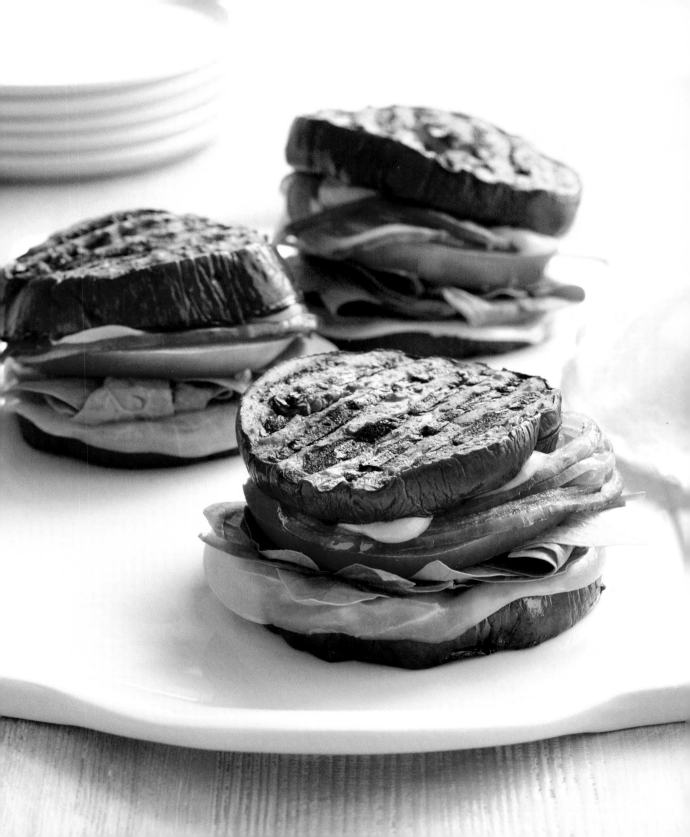

11

Stir-Frys, Savory Crepes & Skillet Meals

Everyone needs some go-to recipes that can easily be whipped up in a skillet. This chapter serves up TEN of 'em! All healthy and delicious, of course . . .

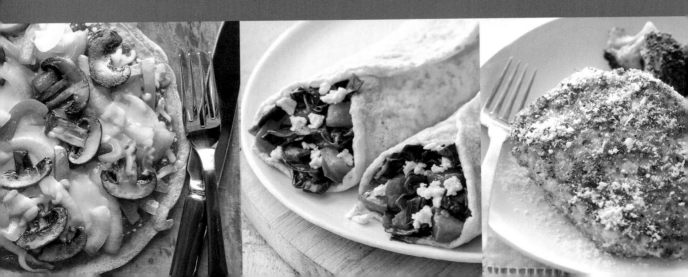

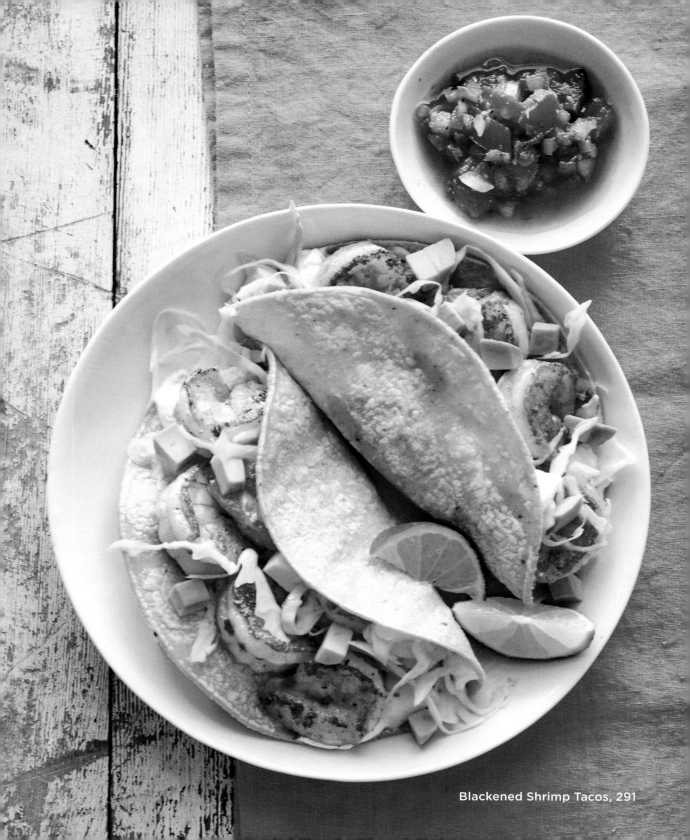

Blackened Shrimp Tacos, 291

Sweet Tomato Shrimp Stir-Fry

Entire recipe: 273 calories, 2g total fat (0.5g sat fat), 854mg sodium, 37.5g carbs, 8g fiber, 19g sugars, 28g protein

You'll Need: large skillet, nonstick spray

Prep: 10 minutes • **Cook:** 10 minutes

1 cup sliced red bell pepper

1 cup sliced onion

1 teaspoon chopped garlic

¾ cup canned stewed tomatoes, drained

4 ounces (about 8) raw large shrimp, peeled, tails removed, deveined

1 tablespoon balsamic vinegar

4 cups roughly chopped spinach

Optional seasonings: salt and black pepper

1. Bring a large skillet sprayed with nonstick spray to medium-high heat. Add bell pepper and onion. Cook and stir until slightly browned and softened, about 4 minutes.

2. Add garlic, and cook and stir until fragrant, about 1 minute.

3. Add tomatoes, shrimp, and balsamic vinegar. Cook and stir for about 3 minutes, until veggies have softened and shrimp are cooked through.

4. Add spinach, and cook and stir until wilted, about 1 minute.

MAKES 1 SERVING

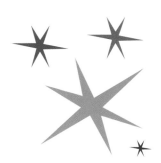

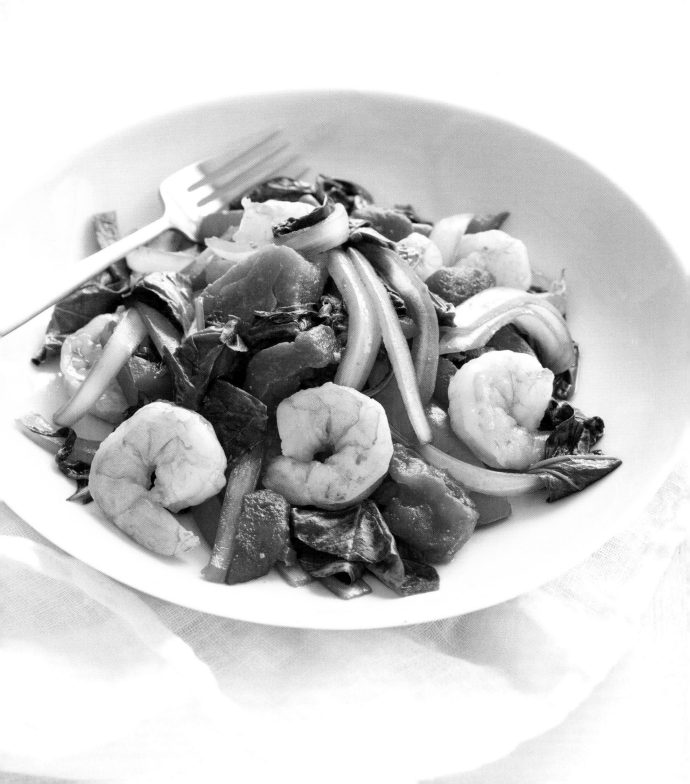

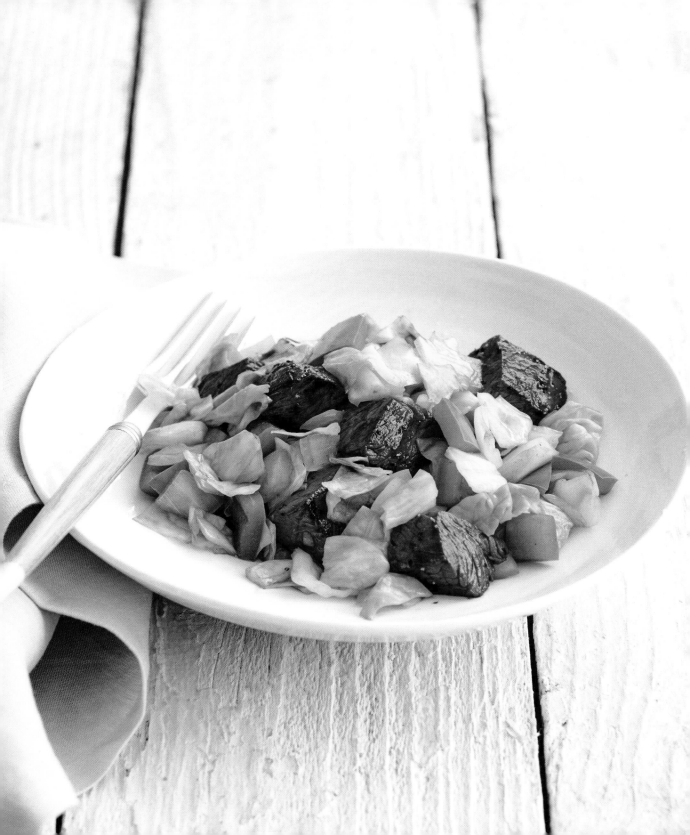

Spicy Steak 'n Cabbage Stir-Fry

Entire recipe: 284 calories, 7.5g total fat (2.5g sat fat),
790mg sodium, 24g carbs, 5g fiber, 12.5g sugars, 29.5g protein

This is comfort food with a kick! If you're not a fan of spicy food, just leave out the hot sauce and cayenne pepper.

You'll Need: small wide bowl, skillet, nonstick spray

Prep: 10 minutes • **Marinate:** 15 minutes • **Cook:** 10 minutes

1 tablespoon balsamic vinegar

1 tablespoon reduced-sodium/lite soy sauce

1 teaspoon yellow mustard

½ teaspoon chopped garlic

½ teaspoon Frank's RedHot Original Cayenne Pepper Sauce

4 ounces raw lean beefsteak filet, cut into bite-sized pieces

⅛ teaspoon black pepper

Dash garlic powder

Dash cayenne pepper

1½ cups chopped cabbage

½ cup chopped green bell pepper

½ cup chopped onion

1. In a small wide bowl, combine balsamic vinegar, soy sauce, mustard, garlic, and hot sauce. Mix until uniform.

2. Sprinkle beef with seasonings, and add to the vinegar mixture. Toss to coat. Cover and let marinate in the fridge for 15 minutes.

3. Bring a skillet sprayed with nonstick spray to medium-high heat. Add veggies and ¼ cup water. Cover and cook for 4 minutes, or until veggies have partially softened and water has evaporated.

4. Add beef and marinade. Cook and stir until veggies are soft and beef is cooked through, about 3 minutes.

MAKES 1 SERVING

Gluten FYI

Certain brands add gluten to their soy sauce. If you avoid gluten, read labels carefully. Or grab a specially marked product like Kikkoman Gluten-Free Soy Sauce.

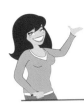

Get to Know
Hungry Girl Crepes

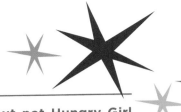

Traditional crepes are flour based and tricky to prepare . . . but not Hungry Girl crepes. These crepes are made from egg whites and protein powder, which means they're protein PACKED and *very* satisfying. And they couldn't be easier to whip up!

Not all protein powder is created equal. For shopping tips and brand picks, flip to page 5.

A 10-inch skillet is a must. Any smaller, and your crepe will be too thick; any larger, and your crepe will be too thin.

Also essential: An offset spatula or flexible rubber spatula. An offset spatula is just a flipping utensil with a handy bend in the blade, which lets you flip the crepe without breaking it. A flexible rubber spatula works too.

When you're mixing up the batter, don't worry if it isn't completely uniform. Any bits of protein powder will break up while the batter cooks.

Pssst . . . Don't miss the dessert crepes on pages 326, 329, and 330!

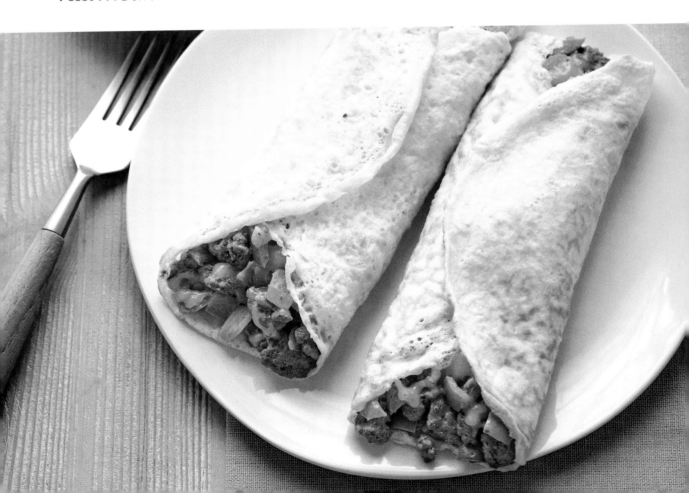

Cheeseburger Crepes

Entire recipe: 298 calories, 9g total fat (4.5g sat fat), 756mg sodium, 10g carbs, 1.5g fiber, 5g sugars, 42.5g protein

That's right: Cheeseburger Crepes! For another skillet-made cheeseburger creation, flip to page 241 for a Cheeseburger Skillet recipe.

You'll Need: medium bowl, whisk, 10-inch skillet, nonstick spray, offset spatula or flexible rubber spatula, plate

Prep: 10 minutes   •   **Cook:** 15 minutes

½ cup (about 4 large) egg whites

1½ tablespoons plain protein powder with about 100 calories per serving

¼ teaspoon garlic powder

¼ teaspoon onion powder

3 ounces raw extra-lean ground beef (4% fat or less)

Dash each salt and black pepper

¼ cup chopped bell pepper

¼ cup chopped onion

3 tablespoons shredded reduced-fat cheddar cheese

1 tablespoon yellow mustard

Optional topping: Clean & Hungry Ketchup (recipe and store-bought alternatives on page 24)

1. To make the crepe batter, in a medium bowl, combine egg whites, protein powder, and ⅛ teaspoon each garlic powder and onion powder. Whisk until uniform.

2. Bring a 10-inch skillet sprayed with nonstick spray to medium heat. Pour half of the batter into the pan, quickly tilting the skillet in all directions to evenly coat the bottom. Cook until lightly browned on the bottom, about 2 minutes.

3. Carefully flip with an offset spatula or flexible rubber spatula. Cook until lightly browned on the other side, about 1 minute.

4. Transfer the crepe to a plate, and repeat with remaining egg mixture to make another crepe. Cover to keep warm.

5. Remove skillet from heat; clean, if needed. Re-spray, and bring to medium-high heat. Add beef, and season with salt, black pepper, and remaining ⅛ teaspoon each garlic powder and onion powder. Add bell pepper and onion. Cook, stir, and crumble until beef is fully cooked and veggies have softened, about 5 minutes.

6. Remove skillet from heat. Immediately add cheese and mustard to the skillet. Stir until melted and well mixed, about 1 minute.

7. Evenly divide mixture between the centers of the crepes. Fold both sides of each crepe over the filling.

MAKES 1 SERVING

Cheesy Chicken & Broccoli Crepes

Entire recipe: 271 calories, 7.5g total fat (3.5g sat fat), 569mg sodium, 5.5g carbs, 1g fiber, 2g sugars, 44g protein

You'll Need: medium bowl, whisk, 10-inch skillet, nonstick spray, offset spatula or flexible rubber spatula, plate

Prep: 10 minutes • **Cook:** 15 minutes

½ cup (about 4 large) egg whites

1½ tablespoons plain protein powder with about 100 calories per serving

⅛ teaspoon garlic powder

⅛ teaspoon onion powder

½ cup chopped broccoli

3 ounces raw boneless skinless chicken breast, cut into bite-sized pieces

Dash each salt and black pepper

3 tablespoons shredded reduced-fat cheddar cheese

1. To make the crepe batter, in a medium bowl, combine egg whites, protein powder, garlic powder, and onion powder. Whisk until uniform.

2. Bring a 10-inch skillet sprayed with nonstick spray to medium heat. Pour half of the batter into the pan, quickly tilting the skillet in all directions to evenly coat the bottom. Cook until lightly browned on the bottom, about 2 minutes.

3. Carefully flip with an offset spatula or flexible rubber spatula. Cook until lightly browned on the other side, about 1 minute.

4. Transfer the crepe to a plate, and repeat with remaining egg mixture to make another crepe. Cover to keep warm.

5. Remove skillet from heat; clean, if needed. Re-spray, and return to medium heat. Add broccoli and 2 tablespoons water. Cover and cook for 3 minutes, or until broccoli has slightly softened and water has evaporated.

6. Add chicken, and season with salt and pepper. Cook and stir until broccoli is soft and chicken is fully cooked, about 4 minutes.

7. Sprinkle cheese over the broccoli and chicken in the skillet. Cook until melted, about 1 minute.

8. Evenly divide mixture between the centers of the crepes. Fold both sides of each crepe over the filling.

MAKES 1 SERVING

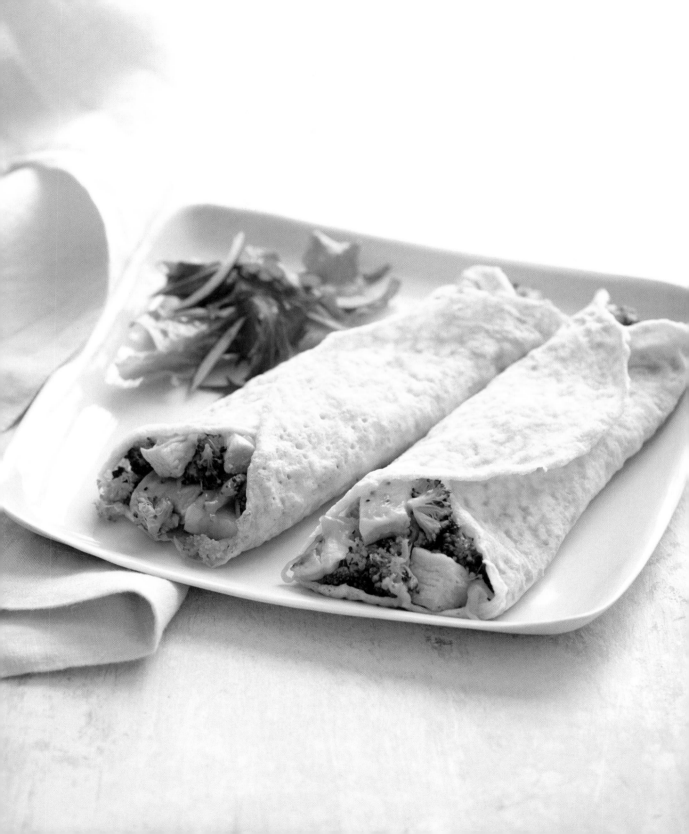

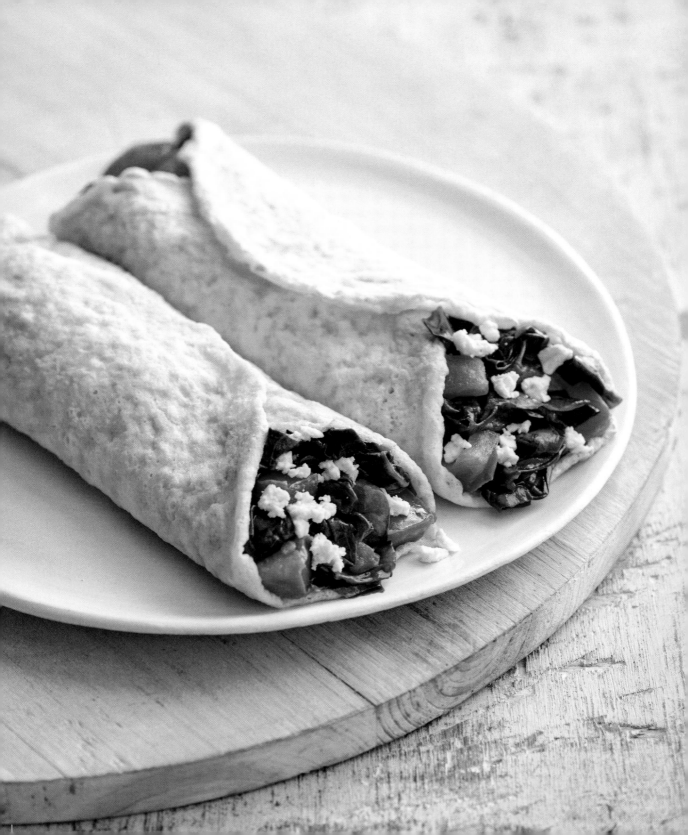

Spinach & Feta Crepes

Entire recipe: 219 calories, 7g total fat (4.5g sat fat), 811mg sodium, 12.5g carbs, 4g fiber, 5.5g sugars, 27.5g protein

You'll Need: medium bowl, whisk, 10-inch skillet, nonstick spray, offset spatula or flexible rubber spatula, plate

Prep: 15 minutes • **Cook:** 15 minutes

½ cup (about 4 large) egg whites

1½ tablespoons plain protein powder with about 100 calories per serving

¼ teaspoon garlic powder

¼ teaspoon onion powder

4 cups spinach leaves

¾ cup seeded and chopped tomato

Dash each salt and black pepper

¼ cup crumbled feta cheese

1. To make the crepe batter, in a medium bowl, combine egg whites, protein powder, garlic powder, and onion powder. Whisk until uniform.

2. Bring a 10-inch skillet sprayed with nonstick spray to medium heat. Pour half of the batter into the pan, quickly tilting the skillet in all directions to evenly coat the bottom. Cook until lightly browned on the bottom, about 2 minutes.

3. Carefully flip with an offset spatula or flexible rubber spatula. Cook until lightly browned on the other side, about 1 minute.

4. Transfer the crepe to a plate, and repeat with remaining egg mixture to make another crepe. Cover to keep warm.

5. Remove skillet from heat; clean, if needed. Re-spray, and return to medium heat. Cook and stir spinach until partially wilted, about 2 minutes. Add tomato, and sprinkle with salt and pepper. Cook and stir until spinach has wilted and tomato is hot, about 1 minute.

6. Evenly divide veggie mixture between the centers of the crepes. Sprinkle with feta cheese, and fold both sides of each crepe over the filling.

MAKES 1 SERVING

Crispy Bruschetta Chicken

Entire recipe: 344 calories, 9g total fat (1.5g sat fat), 491mg sodium, 21.5g carbs, 3g fiber, 7g sugars, 41.5g protein

This recipe is a personal favorite. Juicy chicken, crunchy coating, and flavorful toppings all add up to one fantastic dish!

You'll Need: medium bowl, 2 wide bowls, skillet, nonstick spray

Prep: 10 minutes • **Cook:** 10 minutes

½ **cup seeded and chopped tomatoes**

2 tablespoons chopped fresh basil

1½ **tablespoons balsamic vinegar**

1 teaspoon olive oil

½ **teaspoon chopped garlic**

½ **teaspoon Italian seasoning**

¼ **teaspoon black pepper**

One 5-ounce raw boneless skinless chicken breast cutlet, pounded to ¼-inch thickness

¼ **cup (about 2 large) egg whites**

¼ **cup whole-wheat panko breadcrumbs**

⅛ **teaspoon salt**

1. In a medium bowl, combine tomatoes, basil, balsamic vinegar, olive oil, garlic, ¼ teaspoon Italian seasoning, and ⅛ teaspoon black pepper. Stir to mix.

2. Place chicken in a wide bowl, and top with egg whites. Flip to coat.

3. In another wide bowl, combine breadcrumbs, salt, remaining ¼ teaspoon Italian seasoning, and remaining ⅛ teaspoon black pepper.

4. Shake chicken to remove excess egg whites, and coat with seasoned breadcrumbs.

5. Bring a skillet sprayed with nonstick spray to medium heat. Cook chicken for about 4 minutes per side, until cooked through.

6. Top chicken with tomato mixture. Cover and cook until hot, about 2 minutes.

MAKES 1 SERVING

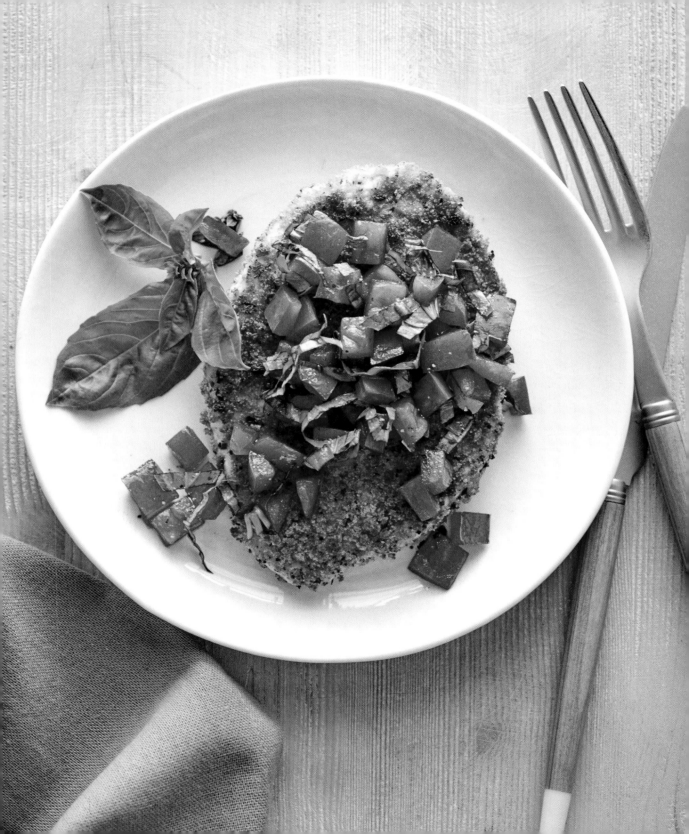

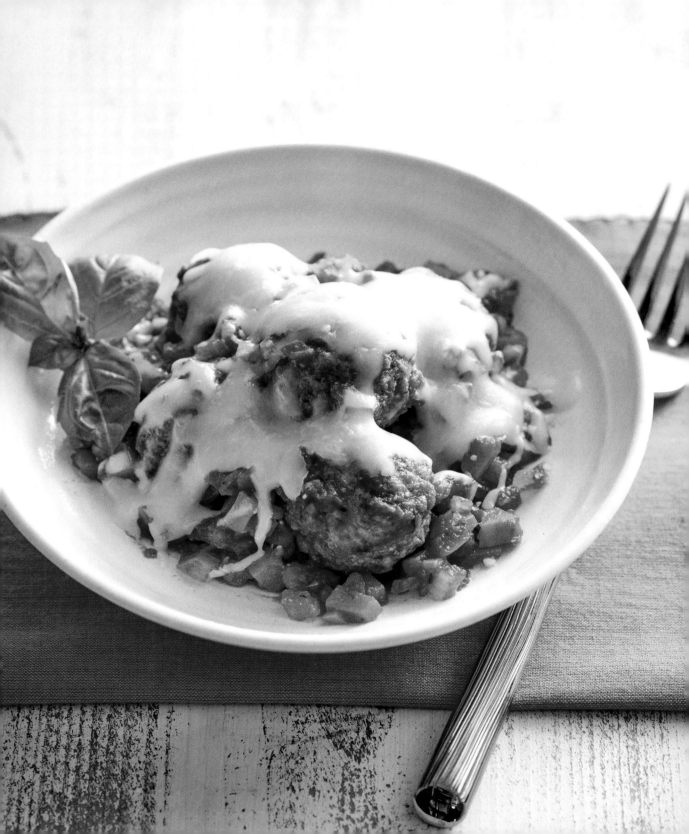

Cheesy 'n Saucy Skillet Meatballs

¼th of recipe (5 meatballs with sauce): 276 calories, 8.5g total fat (4g sat fat), 579mg sodium, 16.5g carbs, 3.5g fiber, 6g sugars, 32.5g protein

You'll Need: 2 large bowls, extra-large skillet, nonstick spray

Prep: 20 minutes • **Cook:** 25 minutes

1 pound raw extra-lean ground beef (4% fat or less)

¼ cup whole-wheat panko breadcrumbs

¼ cup (about 2 large) egg whites

¼ teaspoon each salt and black pepper

1 cup finely chopped onion

1 cup finely chopped carrot

1 teaspoon chopped garlic

1 cup Clean & Hungry Marinara Sauce (recipe and store-bought alternatives on page 20)

½ cup shredded part-skim mozzarella cheese

1 tablespoon grated Parmesan cheese

1. In a large bowl, combine beef, breadcrumbs, egg whites, salt, and pepper. Thoroughly mix. Firmly and evenly form into 20 meatballs.

2. Bring an extra-large skillet sprayed with nonstick spray to medium-high heat. Cook and stir onion and carrot until slightly softened, about 4 minutes. Add garlic, and cook and stir until fragrant, about 2 minutes. Transfer to another large bowl. Add marinara sauce, and mix well.

3. Remove skillet from heat; clean, if needed. Re-spray, and return to medium-high heat. Place meatballs in the skillet. Cook and rotate until browned on all sides, about 5 minutes.

4. Reduce heat to medium low. Carefully add sauce mixture, covering the meatballs. Cover and cook for 10 minutes, or until meatballs are cooked through.

5. Rearrange meatballs so they are close together in the center of the skillet. Sprinkle with mozzarella and Parm. Re-cover and cook for 2 minutes, or until mozzarella has melted.

MAKES 4 SERVINGS

Fork 'n Knife Skillet Pizza

Entire recipe: 357 calories, 12.5g total fat (7g sat fat), 969mg sodium, 35g carbs, 8.5g fiber, 10g sugars, 27.5g protein

This pizza is unique and completely amazing. And if you love pizza, don't miss the Cauliflower Crust Pizza on page 225.

You'll Need: 2 medium bowls, whisk, small bowl, 10-inch skillet, nonstick spray, offset spatula or flexible rubber spatula

Prep: 15 minutes • **Cook:** 10 minutes

¼ cup chickpea flour

2 tablespoons (about 1 large) egg white

⅛ teaspoon salt

½ cup canned crushed tomatoes

½ teaspoon garlic powder

½ teaspoon onion powder

½ teaspoon Italian seasoning

¼ cup sliced mushrooms

¼ cup sliced onion

¼ cup sliced green bell pepper

½ cup shredded part-skim mozzarella cheese

1. To make the batter for the crust, in a medium bowl, combine chickpea flour, egg white, and salt. Add ¼ cup water, and whisk until smooth and uniform. Let thicken for 10 minutes.

2. Meanwhile, in a small bowl, combine tomatoes with seasonings. Mix well.

3. Bring a 10-inch skillet sprayed with nonstick spray to medium heat. Add mushrooms, onion, and pepper. Cook and stir until mostly softened, about 3 minutes. Transfer to a medium bowl, and cover to keep warm.

4. Remove skillet from heat; clean, if needed. Re-spray, and return to medium heat. Pour batter into the skillet, quickly tilting the skillet in all directions to evenly coat the bottom. Cook until lightly browned and cooked through, about 2 minutes per side, flipping carefully with an offset spatula or flexible rubber spatula.

5. Still in the skillet, top with seasoned tomatoes, leaving a ¼-inch border. Sprinkle with cheese, and top with cooked veggies.

6. Cover and cook until cheese has melted, about 2 minutes.

MAKES 1 SERVING

Ingredient FYI

Chickpea flour is a must for this recipe, and it's worth seeking out. Sometimes called garbanzo bean, besan, or gram flour, this gluten-free ingredient has fewer carbs and more fiber than wheat. Look for it in the ethnic-foods aisle (it's a staple in Indian cooking), or order it online. Bob's Red Mill is our go-to brand.

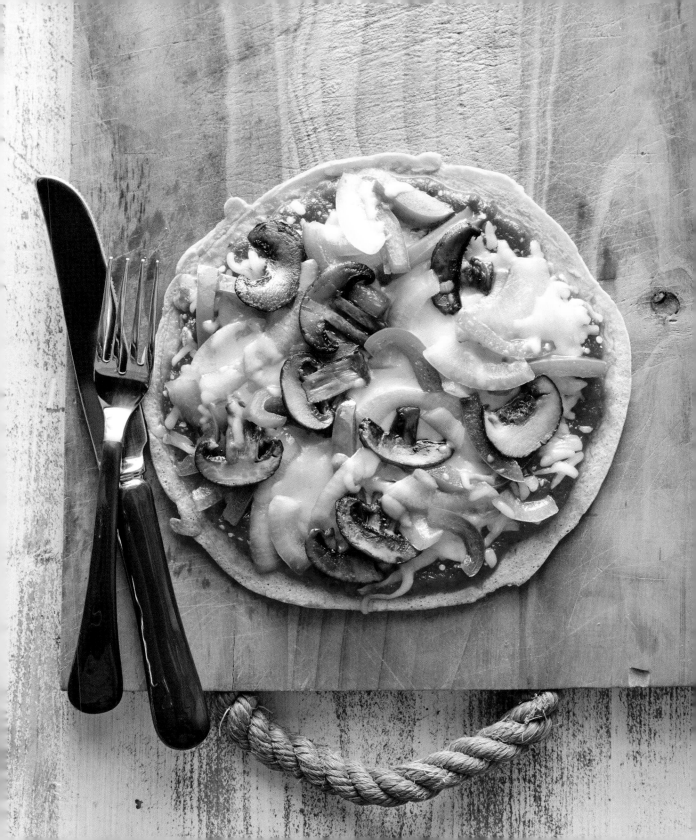

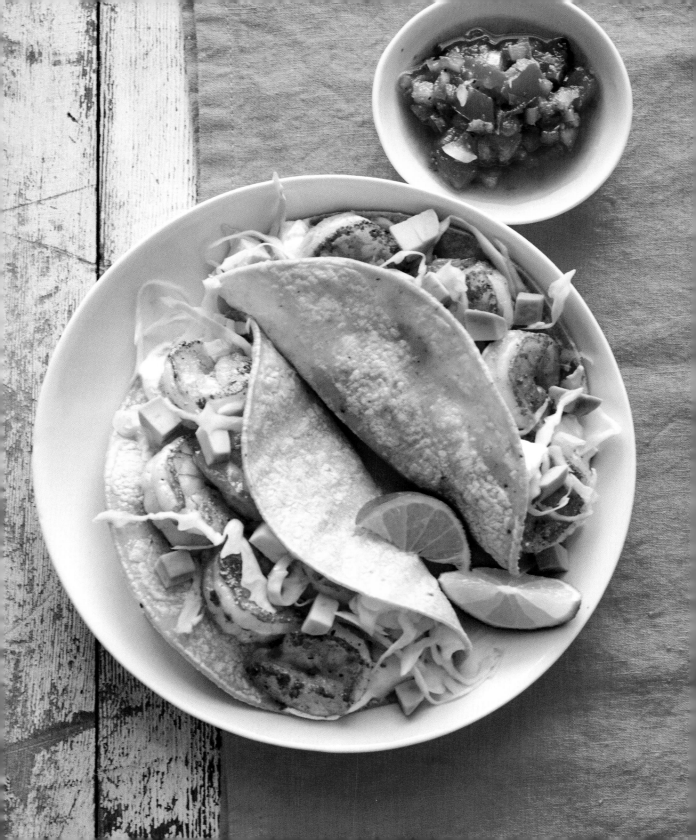

Blackened Shrimp Tacos

Entire recipe: 306 calories, 7g total fat (1g sat fat), 607mg sodium, 27.5g carbs, 4.5g fiber, 3.5g sugars, 32g protein

You'll Need: medium bowl, grill pan (or large skillet), nonstick spray, plate

Prep: 10 minutes • **Cook:** 10 minutes

5 ounces (about 10) raw large shrimp, peeled, tails removed, deveined

¼ teaspoon garlic powder

¼ teaspoon onion powder

⅛ teaspoon paprika

Dash cayenne pepper

Dash cumin

Dash each salt and black pepper

Two 6-inch natural corn tortillas

2 tablespoons fat-free plain Greek yogurt

⅓ cup shredded cabbage

1 lime wedge

1 ounce (about 2 tablespoons) chopped avocado

Optional topping: Clean & Hungry Salsa (recipe and store-bought alternatives on page 18)

1. In a medium bowl, coat shrimp with seasonings.

2. Bring a grill pan (or large skillet) sprayed with nonstick spray to medium-high heat. Cook and stir shrimp for about 4 minutes, until cooked through and blackened.

3. Remove pan from heat; clean, if needed. Re-spray, and return to medium-high heat. Cook each tortilla until hot and lightly browned, about 1 minute per side.

4. Plate tortillas, and spread Greek yogurt down the centers. Top with cabbage, and squirt with juice from the lime wedge.

5. Top with blackened shrimp and avocado, and fold 'em up.

MAKES 1 SERVING

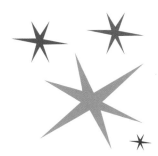

Parm-Crusted Chicken

½ of recipe (1 cutlet): 261 calories, 7.5g total fat (3g sat fat), 435mg sodium, 7g carbs, 1g fiber, 1g sugars, 39g protein

You'll Need: 2 wide bowls, large skillet, nonstick spray

Prep: 10 minutes • **Cook:** 10 minutes

¼ **cup whole-wheat panko breadcrumbs**

½ **teaspoon Italian seasoning**

¼ **teaspoon garlic powder**

⅛ **teaspoon each salt and black pepper**

2 tablespoons plus 2 teaspoons grated Parmesan cheese

Two 5-ounce raw boneless skinless chicken breast cutlets, pounded to ¼-inch thickness

¼ **cup (about 2 large) egg whites**

1. In a wide bowl, combine breadcrumbs, all seasonings, and 2 tablespoons Parm. Mix well.

2. Place chicken in another wide bowl. Top with egg whites, and flip to coat.

3. One at a time, shake chicken cutlets to remove excess egg, and coat with breadcrumb mixture.

4. Bring a large skillet sprayed with nonstick spray to medium heat. Cook chicken for about 4 minutes per side, until cooked through.

5. Serve topped with remaining 2 teaspoons Parm.

MAKES 2 SERVINGS

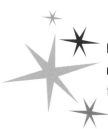

For more healthy recipes, plus the latest food news, tips & tricks, and more, sign up for free daily emails at Hungry-Girl.com!

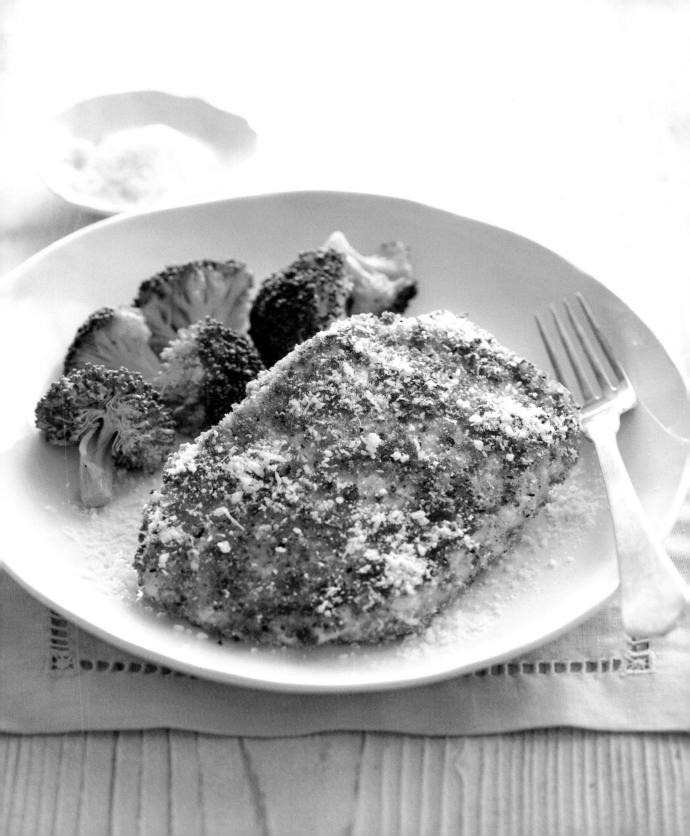

Baked Goodies, Frozen Treats & Other Sweets

All I can say is WOW. Not only are these desserts completely clean and low in calories, they're also some of the BEST sweet treats to ever come out of the Hungry Girl kitchen. Enjoy!

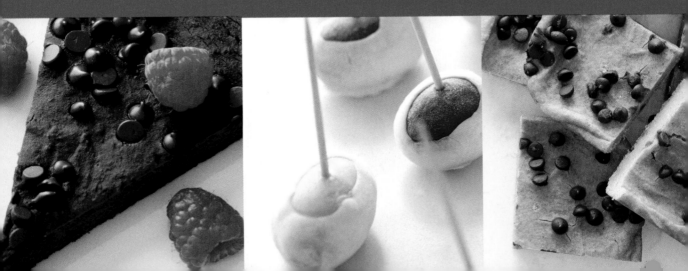

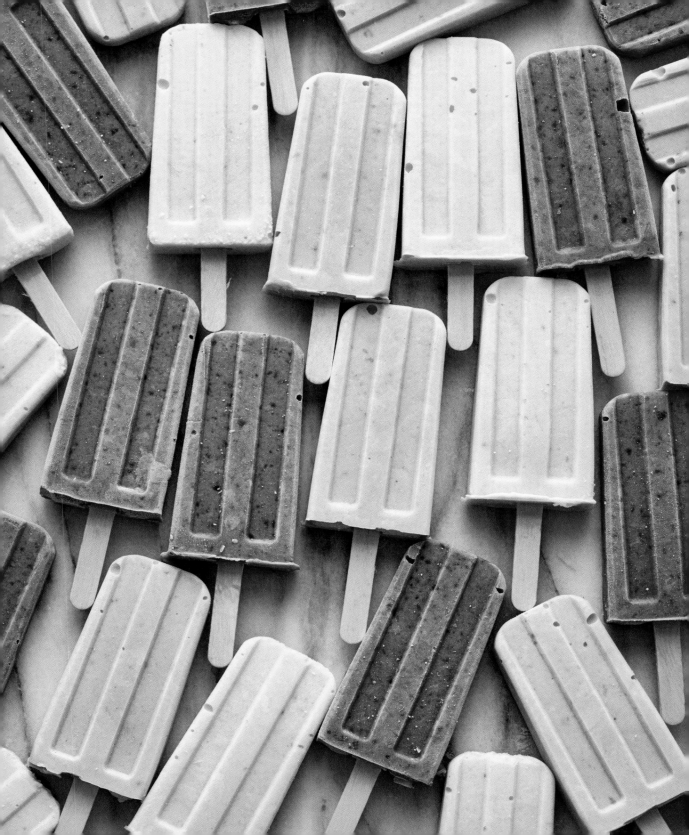

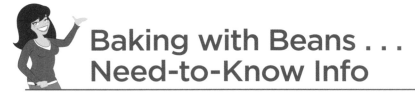

Baking with Beans . . . Need-to-Know Info

I nearly lost it the first time I made brownies with black beans . . . They're unbelievably delicious. Since then, a slew of desserts using either black beans or chickpeas (garbanzo beans) have been created in the Hungry Girl kitchen. And they're ALL amazing! Here's the 411 . . .

- **These treats taste NOTHING like beans.** All you'll taste is a rich, decadent dessert! Don't believe me? Try 'em and see.

- **Keep cool!** There's a reason these recipes say to let your treats cool completely. Doing so perfects the texture and makes them tastier and easier to slice.

- **Cover up.** Whether you store these in the fridge (our recommendation!) or on the counter, you'll want to cover 'em to keep them fresh.

- **Chill out!** These treats taste FANTASTIC chilled. They'll also stay fresh longer when stored in the fridge.

- **They freeze and thaw perfectly.** Yup. Bake up a batch, toss them in the freezer, and portion-controlled treats will be just a minute away. Here's how . . .

To Freeze: Tightly wrap each cooled serving in plastic wrap. Place individually wrapped treats in a sealable container or bag, seal, and store in the freezer.

To Thaw: Unwrap a treat, and place on a microwave-safe plate. Microwave at 50 percent power for 45 seconds, or until it reaches your desired temperature. Alternatively, refrigerate overnight to thaw.

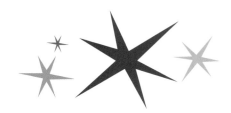

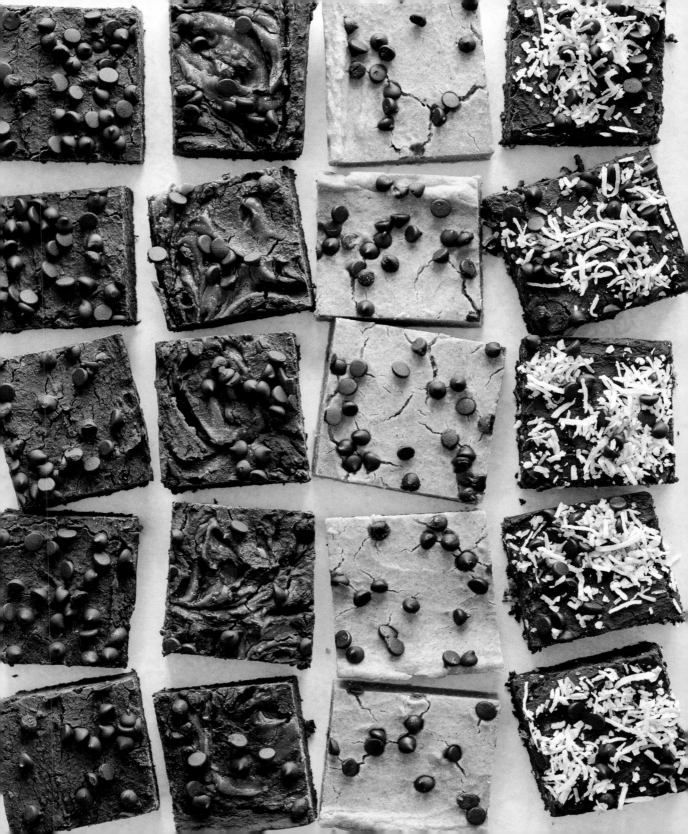

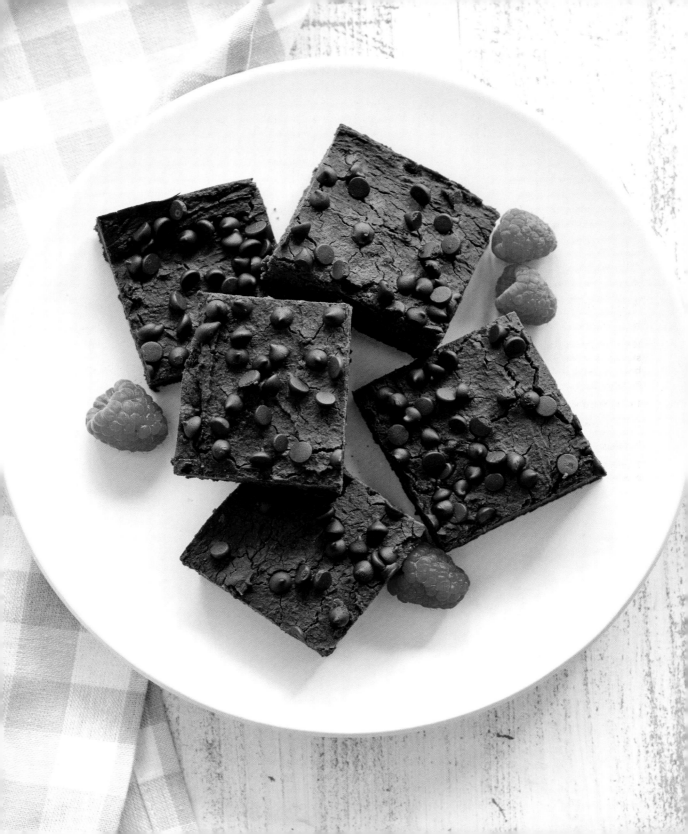

Clean & Hungry Brownies

⅑ᵗʰ of pan (about 2½ inches by 2½ inches): 98 calories, 2.5g total fat (1.5g sat fat), 225mg sodium, 22g carbs, 4.5g fiber, 4g sugars, 4.5g protein

You'll Need: 8-inch by 8-inch baking pan, nonstick spray, food processor

Prep: 15 minutes • **Cook:** 30 minutes • **Cool:** 1 hour

One 15-ounce can black beans, drained and rinsed

½ cup unsweetened cocoa powder

⅓ cup unsweetened applesauce

¼ cup canned pure pumpkin

¼ cup (about 2 large) egg whites

¼ cup whole-wheat flour

¼ cup Truvia spoonable no-calorie sweetener (or another natural brand that's about twice as sweet as sugar)

1 teaspoon vanilla extract

¾ teaspoon baking powder

¼ teaspoon salt

3 tablespoons mini (or chopped) semi-sweet chocolate chips

1. Preheat oven to 350 degrees. Spray an 8-inch by 8-inch baking pan with nonstick spray.

2. Place all ingredients *except* chocolate chips in a food processor. Puree until completely smooth and uniform.

3. Fold in 1 tablespoon chocolate chips.

4. Spread mixture into the baking pan, and smooth out the top.

5. Evenly top with remaining 2 tablespoons chocolate chips, and lightly press into the batter.

6. Bake until a toothpick (or knife) inserted into the center comes out mostly clean, 25 to 30 minutes.

7. Let cool completely, about 1 hour.

MAKES 9 SERVINGS

Sweetener Alternative

If using Stevia In The Raw bakers bag (or another no-calorie sweetener that's approximately as sweet as sugar), use ½ cup in this recipe.

Peanut Butter Brownies

⅑th of pan (about 2½ inches by 2½ inches): 116 calories, 3.5g total fat (1g sat fat), 255mg sodium, 23.5g carbs, 5g fiber, 4g sugars, 6.5g protein

You'll Need: 8-inch by 8-inch baking pan, nonstick spray, food processor, medium bowl

Prep: 15 minutes • **Cook:** 30 minutes • **Cool:** 1 hour

Brownies

One 15-ounce can black beans, drained and rinsed

½ cup unsweetened cocoa powder

⅓ cup unsweetened applesauce

¼ cup canned pure pumpkin

¼ cup (about 2 large) egg whites

¼ cup whole-wheat flour

¼ cup Truvia spoonable no-calorie sweetener (or another natural brand that's about twice as sweet as sugar)

1 teaspoon vanilla extract

¾ teaspoon baking powder

¼ teaspoon salt

2 tablespoons mini (or chopped) semi-sweet chocolate chips

Topping

⅓ cup powdered peanut butter or defatted peanut flour

1 tablespoon Truvia spoonable no-calorie sweetener (or another natural brand that's about twice as sweet as sugar)

Dash salt

1 tablespoon creamy peanut butter (no sugar added)

1. Preheat oven to 350 degrees. Spray an 8-inch by 8-inch baking pan with nonstick spray.

2. Place all brownie ingredients *except* chocolate chips in a food processor. Puree until completely smooth and uniform.

3. Fold in 1 tablespoon chocolate chips.

4. Spread mixture into the baking pan, and smooth out the top.

5. In a medium bowl, combine all topping ingredients *except* creamy peanut butter. Add ¼ cup water, and mix until smooth and uniform. Add peanut butter, and stir until uniform.

6. Spoon topping onto the brownie batter, and swirl it in with a knife. Sprinkle with remaining 1 tablespoon chocolate chips, and lightly press into the batter.

7. Bake until a toothpick (or knife) inserted into the center comes out mostly clean, 25 to 30 minutes.

8. Let cool completely, about 1 hour.

MAKES 9 SERVINGS

Sweetener Alternative

If using Stevia In The Raw bakers bag (or another no-calorie sweetener that's approximately as sweet as sugar), use ½ cup in the brownies and 2 tablespoons in the topping.

Ingredient FYI

Unfamiliar with powdered peanut butter, a.k.a. defatted peanut flour? Get the scoop on page 4.

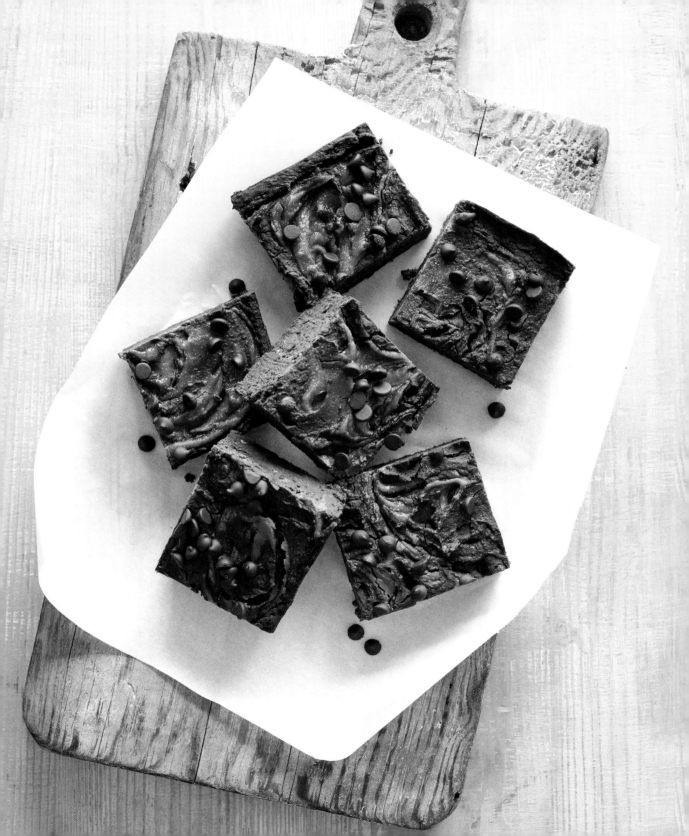

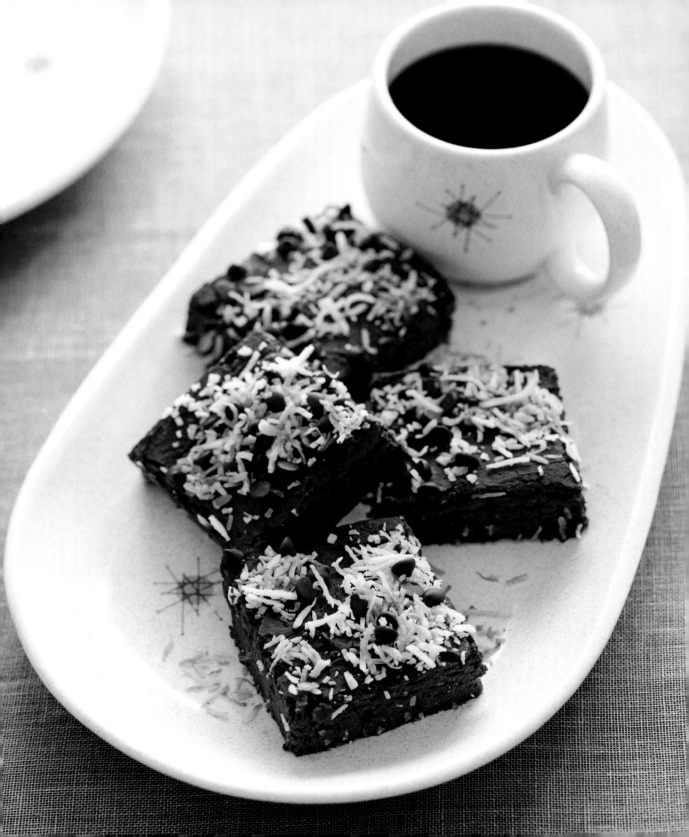

Island Coconut Brownies

⅑th of pan (about 2½ inches by 2½ inches): 108 calories, 3.5g total fat (2.5g sat fat), 225mg sodium, 22g carbs, 4.5g fiber, 4.5g sugars, 4.5g protein

You'll Need: 8-inch by 8-inch baking pan, nonstick spray, food processor

Prep: 15 minutes • **Cook:** 30 minutes • **Cool:** 1 hour

One 15-ounce can black beans, drained and rinsed

½ cup unsweetened cocoa powder

⅓ cup unsweetened applesauce

¼ cup canned pure pumpkin

¼ cup (about 2 large) egg whites

¼ cup whole-wheat flour

¼ cup Truvia spoonable no-calorie sweetener (or another natural brand that's about twice as sweet as sugar)

¾ teaspoon coconut extract

¾ teaspoon baking powder

¼ teaspoon vanilla extract

¼ teaspoon salt

3 tablespoons mini (or chopped) semi-sweet chocolate chips

3 tablespoons unsweetened shredded coconut

1. Preheat oven to 350 degrees. Spray an 8-inch by 8-inch baking pan with nonstick spray.

2. Place all ingredients *except* chocolate chips and shredded coconut in a food processor. Puree until completely smooth and uniform.

3. Fold in 1 tablespoon chocolate chips and 1 tablespoon coconut.

4. Spread mixture into the baking pan, and smooth out the top.

5. Evenly top with remaining 2 tablespoons chocolate chips and 2 tablespoons shredded coconut, and lightly press into the batter.

6. Bake until a toothpick (or knife) inserted into the center comes out mostly clean, 25 to 30 minutes.

7. Let cool completely, about 1 hour.

MAKES 9 SERVINGS

Sweetener Alternative

If using Stevia In The Raw bakers bag (or another no-calorie sweetener that's approximately as sweet as sugar), use ½ cup in this recipe.

Fudgy Flourless Chocolate Cake

⅛ᵗʰ of cake: 100 calories, 2.5g total fat (1.5g sat fat), 310mg sodium, 22g carbs, 4.5g fiber, 5g sugars, 5.5g protein

You'll Need: 9-inch round cake pan, aluminum foil, nonstick spray, food processor

Prep: 15 minutes • **Cook:** 40 minutes • **Cool:** 1 hour

One 15-ounce can black beans, drained and rinsed

½ cup unsweetened cocoa powder

½ cup (about 4 large) egg whites

⅓ cup unsweetened applesauce

⅓ cup canned pure pumpkin

¼ cup Truvia spoonable no-calorie sweetener (or another natural brand that's about twice as sweet as sugar)

1½ teaspoons baking powder

1 teaspoon vanilla extract

¼ teaspoon salt

3 tablespoons mini (or chopped) semi-sweet chocolate chips

1. Preheat oven to 350 degrees. Line a 9-inch round cake pan with foil, and generously spray with nonstick spray.

2. Place all ingredients *except* chocolate chips in a food processor. Puree until completely smooth and uniform.

3. Fold in 1 tablespoon chocolate chips.

4. Spread mixture into the baking pan, and smooth out the top.

5. Evenly top with remaining 2 tablespoons chocolate chips, and lightly press into the batter.

6. Bake until a toothpick (or knife) inserted into the center comes out mostly clean, 35 to 40 minutes.

7. Let cool completely, about 1 hour.

MAKES 8 SERVINGS

Sweetener Alternative

If using Stevia In The Raw bakers bag (or another no-calorie sweetener that's approximately as sweet as sugar), use ½ cup in this recipe.

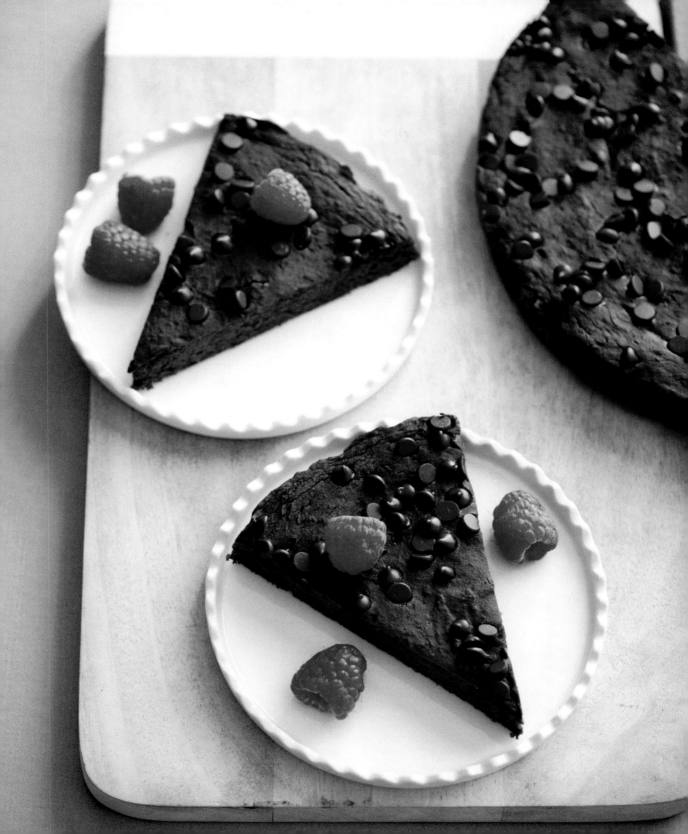

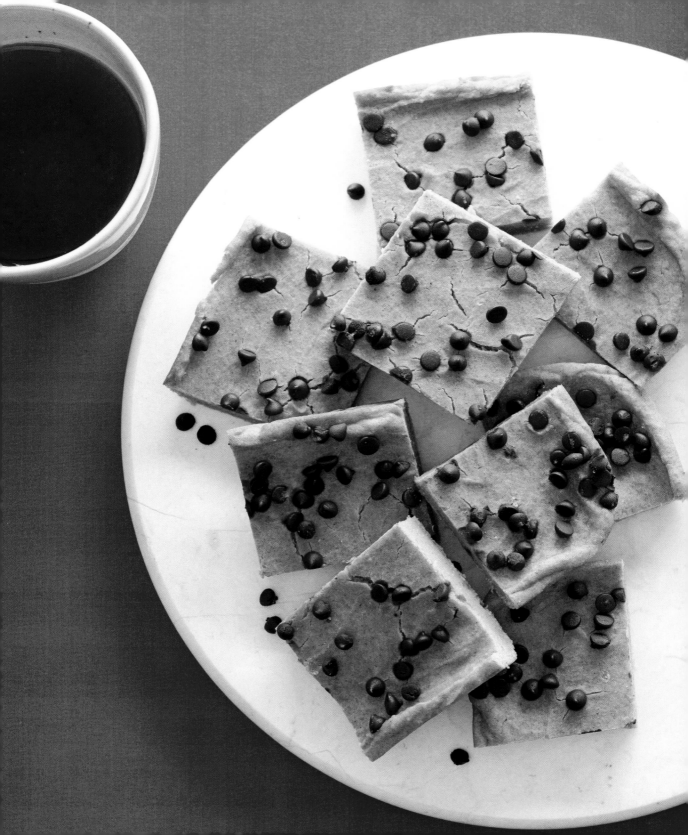

Clean & Hungry Blondies

⅑th of pan (about 2½ inches by 2½ inches): 111 calories, 3.5g total fat (1g sat fat), 197mg sodium, 19g carbs, 3.5g fiber, 3.5g sugars, 4.5g protein

You'll Need: 8-inch by 8-inch baking pan, nonstick spray, food processor

Prep: 15 minutes • **Cook:** 30 minutes • **Cool:** 1 hour

One 15-ounce can chickpeas (garbanzo beans), drained and rinsed

¼ cup plus 2 tablespoons whole-wheat flour

⅓ cup unsweetened applesauce

¼ cup (about 2 large) egg whites

3 tablespoons Truvia spoonable no-calorie sweetener (or another natural brand that's about twice as sweet as sugar)

2 tablespoons creamy peanut butter (no sugar added)

2 tablespoons canned pure pumpkin

1½ tablespoons vanilla extract

¾ teaspoon baking powder

¼ teaspoon salt

2 tablespoons mini (or chopped) semi-sweet chocolate chips

1. Preheat oven to 350 degrees. Spray an 8-inch by 8-inch baking pan with nonstick spray.

2. Place all ingredients *except* chocolate chips in a food processor. Puree until completely smooth and uniform.

3. Gently fold in ½ tablespoon chocolate chips.

4. Spread mixture into the baking pan, and smooth out the top. Evenly top with remaining 1½ tablespoons chocolate chips, and lightly press into the batter.

5. Bake until a toothpick (or knife) inserted into the center comes out mostly clean, 25 to 30 minutes.

6. Let cool completely, about 1 hour.

MAKES 9 SERVINGS

Sweetener Alternative

If using Stevia In The Raw bakers bag (or another no-calorie sweetener that's approximately as sweet as sugar), use 6 tablespoons in this recipe.

Apple Walnut Bars

⅑ᵗʰ of pan (about 2½ inches by 2½ inches): 119 calories, 4g total fat (0.5g sat fat), 197mg sodium, 21g carbs, 4g fiber, 3g sugars, 5g protein

You'll Need: 8-inch by 8-inch baking pan, nonstick spray, food processor

Prep: 20 minutes • **Cook:** 30 minutes • **Cool:** 1 hour

One 15-ounce can chickpeas (garbanzo beans), drained and rinsed

¼ cup plus 2 tablespoons whole-wheat flour

¼ cup (about 2 large) egg whites

¼ cup Truvia spoonable no-calorie sweetener (or another natural brand that's about twice as sweet as sugar)

2 tablespoons creamy peanut butter (no sugar added)

2 tablespoons canned pure pumpkin

1½ tablespoons vanilla extract

1 tablespoon cinnamon

¾ teaspoon baking powder

½ teaspoon nutmeg

¼ teaspoon salt

1¼ cups finely chopped Fuji or Gala apple

¾ ounce (about 3 tablespoons) chopped walnuts

1. Preheat oven to 350 degrees. Spray an 8-inch by 8-inch baking pan with nonstick spray.

2. Place all ingredients *except* apple and walnuts in a food processor. Puree until completely smooth and uniform.

3. Gently fold in 1 cup apple.

4. Spread mixture into the baking pan, and smooth out the top. Evenly top with remaining ¼ cup apple. Sprinkle with walnuts, and lightly press apple and walnuts into the batter.

5. Bake until a toothpick (or knife) inserted into the center comes out mostly clean, 25 to 30 minutes.

6. Let cool completely, about 1 hour.

MAKES 9 SERVINGS

Sweetener Alternative

If using Stevia In The Raw bakers bag (or another no-calorie sweetener that's approximately as sweet as sugar), use ½ cup in this recipe.

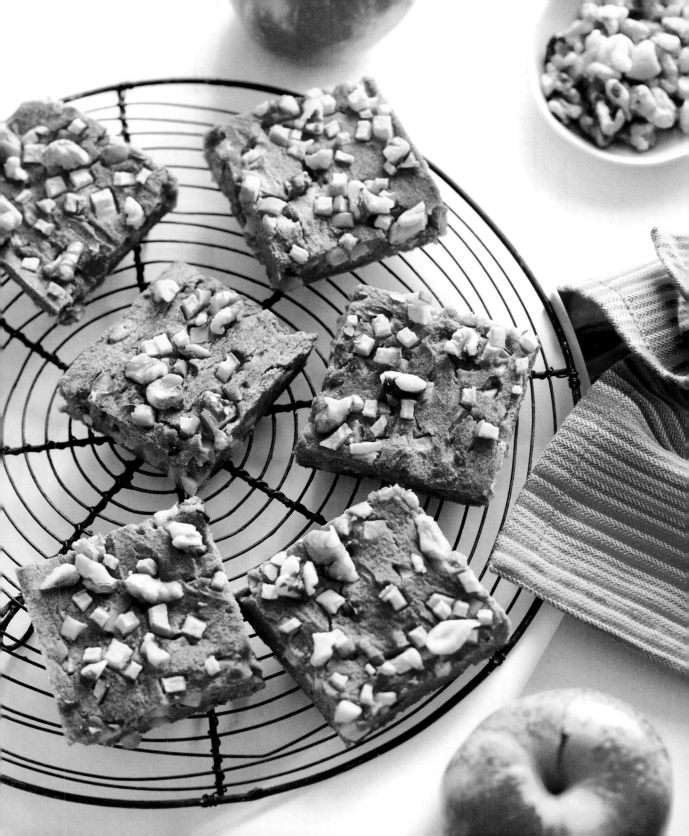

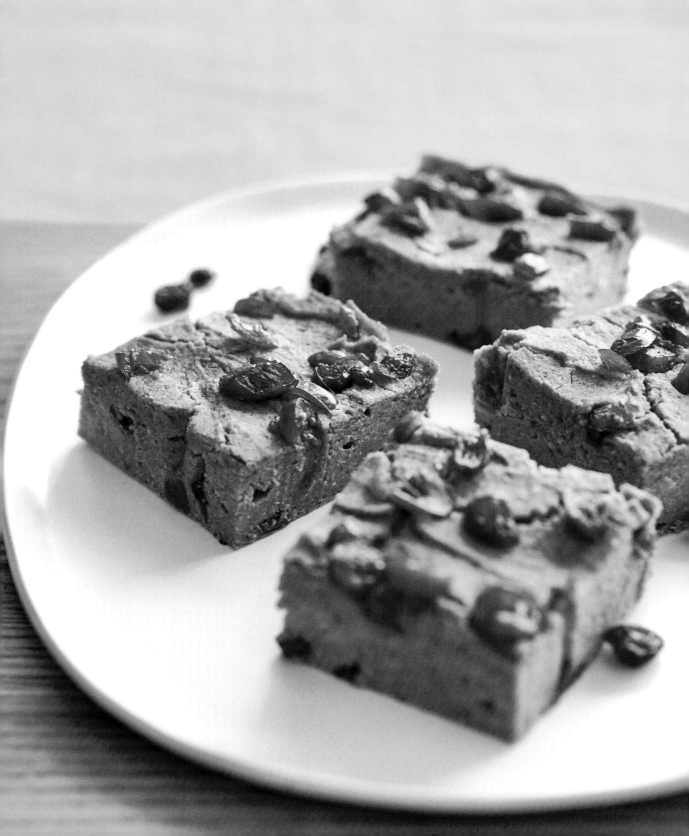

Pumpkin Cranberry Bars

⅑th of pan (about 2½ inches by 2½ inches): 117 calories, 2.5g total fat (<0.5g sat fat), 198mg sodium, 23g carbs, 4g fiber, 5.5g sugars, 4.5g protein

You'll Need: 8-inch by 8-inch baking pan, nonstick spray, food processor

Prep: 15 minutes • **Cook:** 30 minutes • **Cool:** 1 hour

One 15-ounce can chickpeas (garbanzo beans), drained and rinsed

⅓ cup unsweetened applesauce

¼ cup plus 2 tablespoons whole-wheat flour

¼ cup (about 2 large) egg whites

¼ cup canned pure pumpkin

3½ tablespoons Truvia spoonable no-calorie sweetener (or another natural brand that's about twice as sweet as sugar)

2 tablespoons creamy peanut butter (no sugar added)

1½ tablespoons vanilla extract

1 tablespoon pumpkin pie spice

1 teaspoon cinnamon

¾ teaspoon baking powder

¼ teaspoon salt

¼ cup plus 2 tablespoons naturally sweetened dried cranberries, chopped

1. Preheat oven to 350 degrees. Spray an 8-inch by 8-inch baking pan with nonstick spray.

2. Place all ingredients *except* cranberries in a food processor. Puree until completely smooth and uniform.

3. Gently fold in half of the chopped cranberries.

4. Spread mixture into the baking pan, and smooth out the top. Evenly top with remaining chopped cranberries, and lightly press into the batter.

5. Bake until a toothpick (or knife) inserted into the center comes out mostly clean, 25 to 30 minutes.

6. Let cool completely, about 1 hour.

MAKES 9 SERVINGS

Sweetener Alternative

If using Stevia In The Raw bakers bag (or another no-calorie sweetener that's approximately as sweet as sugar), use 7 tablespoons in this recipe.

Banana Walnut Bars

⅑ᵗʰ of pan (about 2½ inches by 2½ inches): 130 calories, 4g total fat (0.5g sat fat), 197mg sodium, 22g carbs, 4g fiber, 4g sugars, 5g protein

You'll Need: 8-inch by 8-inch baking pan, nonstick spray, food processor

Prep: 15 minutes • **Cook:** 30 minutes • **Cool:** 1 hour

One 15-ounce can chickpeas (garbanzo beans), drained and rinsed

1 cup (about 2 medium) mashed extra-ripe bananas

¼ cup plus 2 tablespoons whole-wheat flour

¼ cup (about 2 large) egg whites

3 tablespoons Truvia spoonable no-calorie sweetener (or another natural brand that's about twice as sweet as sugar)

2 tablespoons creamy peanut butter (no sugar added)

1½ tablespoons vanilla extract

2 teaspoons cinnamon

¾ teaspoon baking powder

¼ teaspoon salt

¾ ounce (about 3 tablespoons) chopped walnuts

1. Preheat oven to 350 degrees. Spray an 8-inch by 8-inch baking pan with nonstick spray.

2. Place all ingredients *except* walnuts in a food processor. Puree until completely smooth and uniform.

3. Spread mixture into the baking pan, and smooth out the top. Sprinkle with walnuts, and lightly press into the batter.

4. Bake until a toothpick (or knife) inserted into the center comes out mostly clean, 25 to 30 minutes.

5. Let cool completely, about 1 hour.

MAKES 9 SERVINGS

Sweetener Alternative

If using Stevia In The Raw bakers bag (or another no-calorie sweetener that's approximately as sweet as sugar), use 6 tablespoons in this recipe.

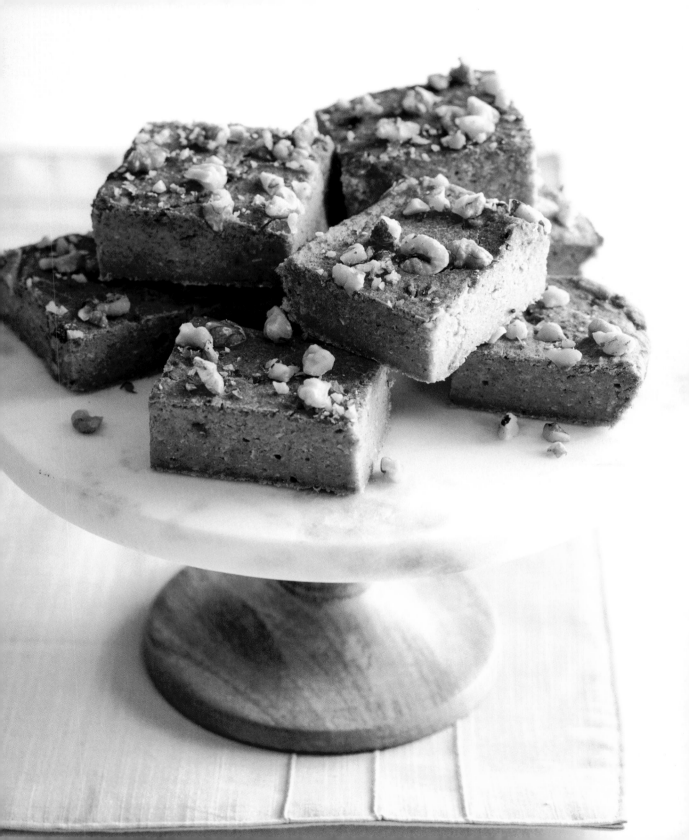

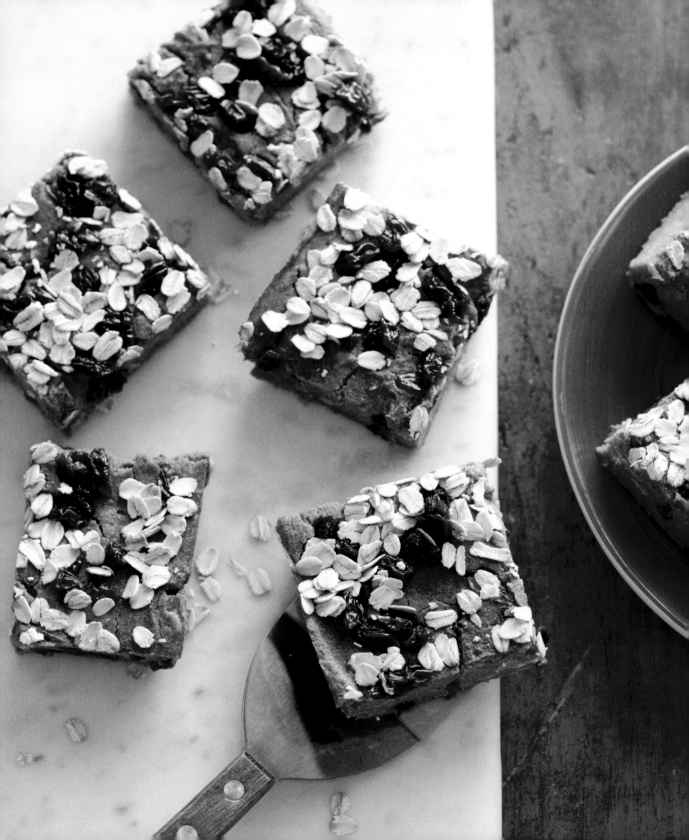

Oatmeal Raisin Bars

⅑th of pan (about 2½ inches by 2½ inches): 129 calories, 2.5g total fat (0.5g sat fat), 199mg sodium, 24.5g carbs, 4.5g fiber, 6.5g sugars, 5g protein

You'll Need: 8-inch by 8-inch baking pan, nonstick spray, food processor

Prep: 15 minutes • **Cook:** 30 minutes • **Cool:** 1 hour

One 15-ounce can chickpeas (garbanzo beans), drained and rinsed

⅓ cup unsweetened applesauce

¼ cup plus 2 tablespoons whole-wheat flour

¼ cup canned pure pumpkin

¼ cup (about 2 large) egg whites

3 tablespoons Truvia spoonable no-calorie sweetener (or another natural brand that's about twice as sweet as sugar)

2 tablespoons creamy peanut butter (no sugar added)

1½ tablespoons vanilla extract

1 tablespoon cinnamon

¾ teaspoon baking powder

½ teaspoon nutmeg

¼ teaspoon salt

¼ cup plus 2 tablespoons raisins, chopped

¼ cup old-fashioned oats

1. Preheat oven to 350 degrees. Spray an 8-inch by 8-inch baking pan with nonstick spray.

2. Place all ingredients *except* raisins and oats in a food processor. Puree until completely smooth and uniform.

3. Gently fold in half of the chopped raisins and 2 tablespoons oats.

4. Spread mixture into the baking pan, and smooth out the top. Evenly top with remaining chopped raisins and 2 tablespoons oats, and lightly press into the batter.

5. Bake until a toothpick (or knife) inserted into the center comes out mostly clean, 25 to 30 minutes.

6. Let cool completely, about 1 hour.

MAKES 9 SERVINGS

Sweetener Alternative

If using Stevia In The Raw bakers bag (or another no-calorie sweetener that's approximately as sweet as sugar), use 6 tablespoons in this recipe.

Blueberry Lemon Bars

¹⁄₁₂ᵗʰ of pan (about 3 inches by 3 inches): 127 calories, 4g total fat (1.5g sat fat), 116mg sodium, 25.5g carbs, 3.5g fiber, 6g sugars, 2.5g protein

You'll Need: 9-inch by 13-inch baking pan, nonstick spray, 2 large bowls

Prep: 25 minutes • **Cook:** 30 minutes • **Cool:** 1 hour

Dough

1½ cups old-fashioned oats

¾ cup whole-wheat flour

⅓ cup whipped butter

¼ cup unsweetened applesauce

2 tablespoons Truvia spoonable no-calorie sweetener (or another natural brand that's about twice as sweet as sugar)

1 teaspoon cinnamon

½ teaspoon baking powder

¼ teaspoon salt

Filling

2 tablespoons Truvia spoonable calorie-free sweetener (or another natural brand that's about twice as sweet as sugar)

1½ tablespoons arrowroot powder/starch

4 cups blueberries (fresh or thawed from frozen)

2 tablespoons lemon juice

1 tablespoon lemon zest

⅛ teaspoon salt

1. Preheat oven to 375 degrees. Spray a 9-inch by 13-inch baking pan with nonstick spray.

2. Combine dough ingredients in a large bowl. Mash and stir until uniform and crumbly.

3. Spread three-quarters of the dough (about 2½ cups) into the baking pan, pressing firmly into an even layer.

4. To make the filling, in another large bowl, mix sweetener with arrowroot powder. Add remaining filling ingredients, and stir to coat.

5. Evenly pour filling over the dough in the pan. Break remaining dough mixture into pieces, and sprinkle over the filling.

6. Bake until topping is golden brown and filling is bubbly, 25 to 30 minutes.

7. Let cool completely, about 1 hour.

8. Refrigerate leftovers.

MAKES 12 SERVINGS

Ingredients FYIs

➤ Arrowroot powder is a clean cornstarch alternative. Cornstarch can be substituted. More info on page 5!

➤ If using frozen blueberries, check the ingredient list to make sure sugar hasn't been added.

Sweetener Alternative

If using Stevia In The Raw bakers bag (or another no-calorie sweetener that's approximately as sweet as sugar), use 4 tablespoons in the dough and 4 tablespoons in the filling.

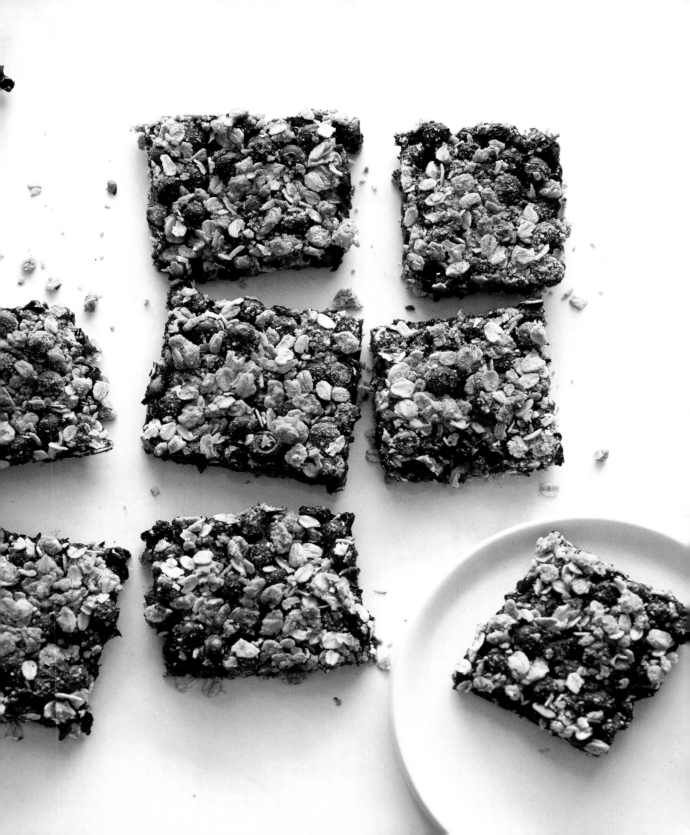

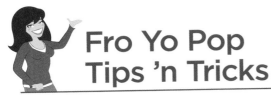

Fro Yo Pop
Tips 'n Tricks

Look for a 6-piece popsicle mold set made from BPA-free plastic. Each mold should hold about 3 ounces of liquid.

If using molds that don't come with handles and require popsicle sticks to be added, freeze the pops until partially frozen, about 2 hours. Then gently slide a stick into the center of each pop (it should stand on its own), and return to the freezer until solid, about 1 hour.

To make the popsicle easier to remove from the mold, try this trick just before eating: Run the mold under warm water for about 30 seconds, and then gently pull out by the handle or stick.

Each of these pop recipes calls for sliced and frozen banana. Once blended, the banana brings incredible creamy texture to the treats. Keep some banana slices in the freezer at all times for recipes like these. They'll also come in handy for the Creamy Peanut Butter Smoothie (page 111) and Purple Power Smoothie (page 119).

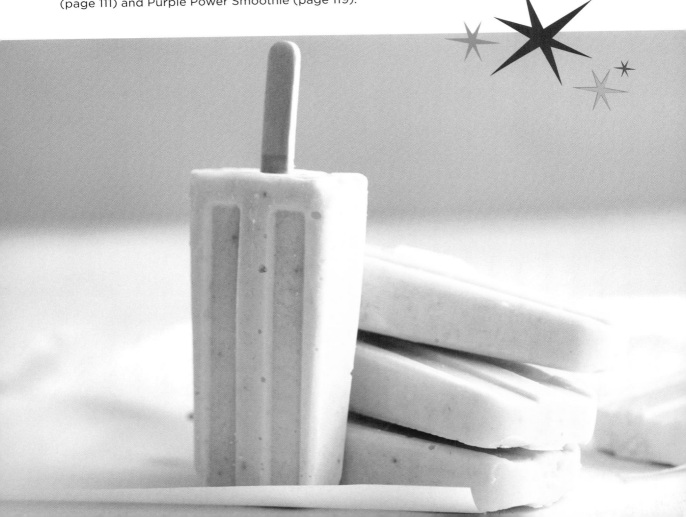

Tropical Mango Fro Yo Pops

⅙th of recipe (1 pop): 67 calories, 0g total fat (0g sat fat), 16mg sodium, 13g carbs, 1.5g fiber, 9.5g sugars, 4g protein

You'll Need: food processor or blender, 6-piece popsicle mold set

Prep: 10 minutes • **Freeze:** 3 hours

1 cup frozen mango chunks (no sugar added), slightly thawed

1 cup sliced and frozen banana, slightly thawed

1 cup fat-free plain Greek yogurt

2 packets natural no-calorie sweetener

1 teaspoon coconut extract

1. Combine all ingredients in a food processor or blender. Blend until completely smooth and uniform, stopping and stirring if needed.

2. Evenly distribute mixture into a 6-piece popsicle mold set, leaving about ½ inch of space at the top. (Pops will expand as they freeze.)

3. Insert popsicle handles. Freeze until solid, at least 3 hours.

MAKES 6 SERVINGS

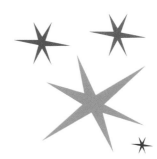

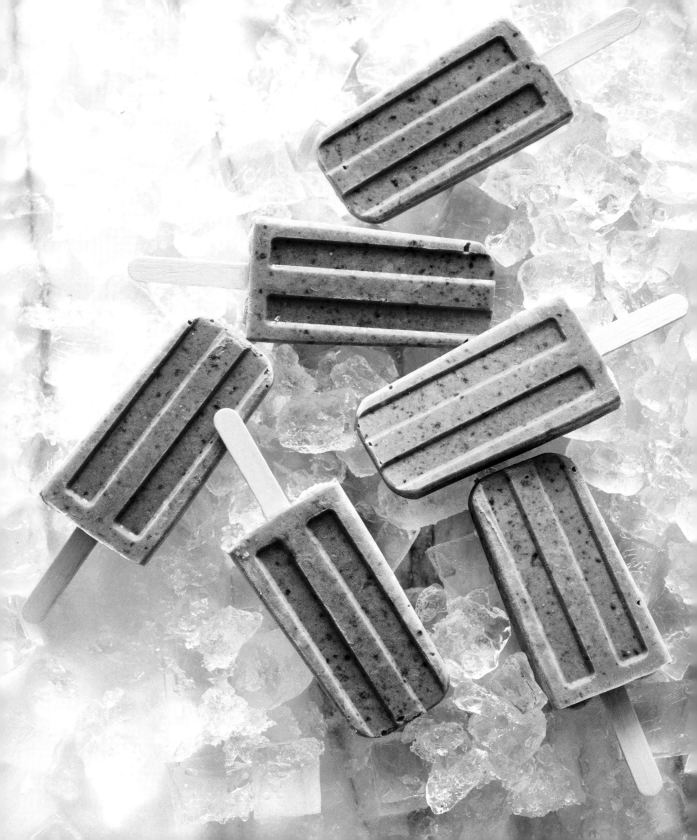

Black Cherry Chip Fro Yo Pops

⅙ᵗʰ of recipe (1 pop): 75 calories, 0.5g total fat (0.5g sat fat), 16mg sodium, 13g carbs, 1.5g fiber, 9g sugars, 4.5g protein

You'll Need: food processor or blender, 6-piece popsicle mold set

Prep: 10 minutes • **Freeze:** 3 hours

1 cup frozen pitted dark sweet cherries (no sugar added), slightly thawed

1 cup frozen banana slices, slightly thawed

1 cup fat-free plain Greek yogurt

3 packets natural no-calorie sweetener

1 teaspoon vanilla extract

1 tablespoon mini (or chopped) semi-sweet chocolate chips

1. In a food processor or blender, combine all ingredients *except* chocolate chips. Blend until completely smooth and uniform, stopping and stirring if needed.

2. Stir in chocolate chips.

3. Evenly distribute mixture into a 6-piece popsicle mold set, leaving about ½ inch of space at the top. (Pops will expand as they freeze.)

4. Insert popsicle handles. Freeze until solid, at least 3 hours.

MAKES 6 SERVINGS

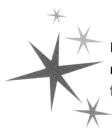

For more healthy recipes, plus the latest food news, tips & tricks, and more, **sign up for free daily emails at Hungry-Girl.com!**

Peanut Butter Banana Fro Yo Pops

⅙ᵗʰ of recipe (1 pop): 103 calories, 1.5g total fat (0g sat fat), 38.5mg sodium, 16g carbs, 2.5g fiber, 8.5g sugars, 8.5g protein

You'll Need: food processor or blender, 6-piece popsicle mold set

Prep: 10 minutes • **Freeze:** 3 hours

2 cups sliced and frozen bananas, slightly thawed

1 cup fat-free plain Greek yogurt

½ cup powdered peanut butter or defatted peanut flour

2 packets natural no-calorie sweetener

1 teaspoon vanilla extract

1. Combine all ingredients in a food processor or blender. Blend until completely smooth and uniform, stopping and stirring if needed.

2. Evenly distribute mixture into a 6-piece popsicle mold set, leaving about ½ inch of space at the top. (Pops will expand as they freeze.)

3. Insert popsicle handles. Freeze until solid, at least 3 hours.

MAKES 6 SERVINGS

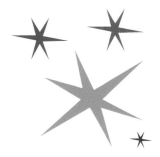

Ingredient FYI

Unfamiliar with powdered peanut butter, a.k.a. defatted peanut flour? Get the scoop on page 4.

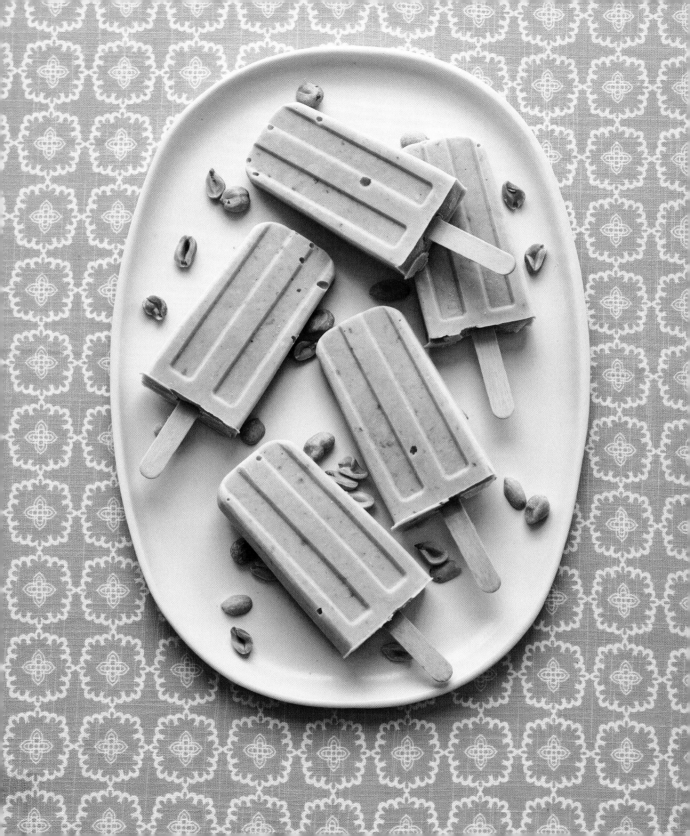

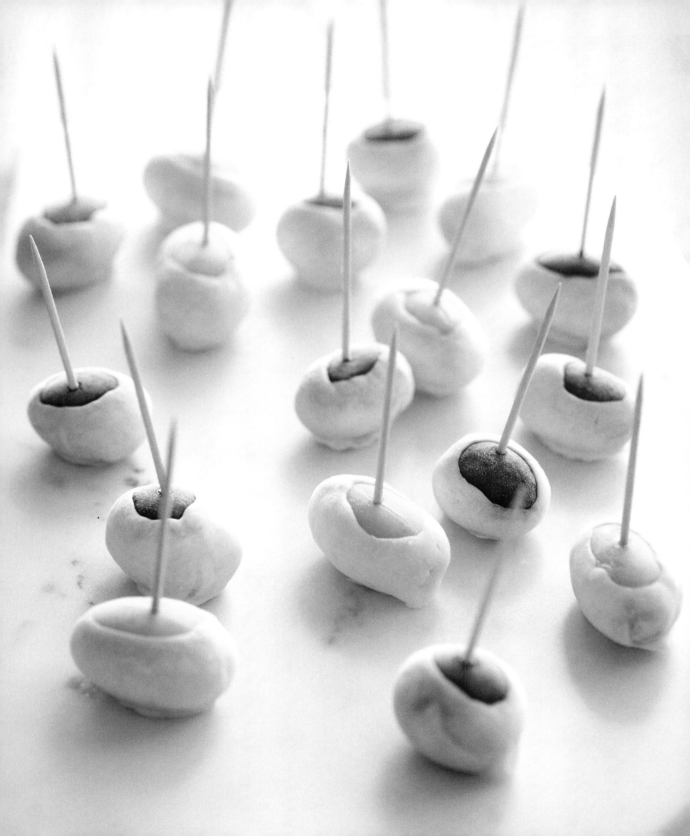

Fro Yo Grapesicles

¼ᵗʰ of recipe (about 10 grapes): 70 calories, <0.5g total fat (0g sat fat), 13mg sodium, 15.5g carbs, 1g fiber, 13g sugars, 3.5g protein

You'll Need: baking sheet, parchment paper, medium bowl, toothpicks

Prep: 20 minutes • **Freeze:** 1 hour

½ cup fat-free plain Greek yogurt

2 packets natural no-calorie sweetener

⅛ teaspoon vanilla extract

2 cups red or green seedless grapes

1. Line a baking sheet with parchment paper.

2. In medium bowl, combine yogurt, sweetener, and vanilla extract. Mix well.

3. Pierce one grape with a toothpick, dunk into the yogurt mixture, and rotate to lightly coat. Transfer to the baking sheet, toothpick end up.

4. Repeat with remaining grapes, evenly spacing them on the baking sheet.

5. Freeze until solid, at least 1 hour.

MAKES 4 SERVINGS

Cannoli Crepes

½ of recipe (1 crepe): 148 calories, 4.5g total fat (2.5g sat fat), 192mg sodium, 11.5g carbs, 1.5g fiber, 8.5g sugars, 16g protein

You'll Need: 2 medium bowls, whisk, 10-inch skillet, nonstick spray, offset spatula or flexible rubber spatula, plate

Prep: 10 minutes • **Cook:** 10 minutes

Filling

½ cup light/low-fat ricotta cheese

2 teaspoons mini (or chopped) semi-sweet chocolate chips

1 packet natural no-calorie sweetener

¼ teaspoon vanilla extract

Crepes

½ cup (about 4 large) egg whites

2 tablespoons plain protein powder with about 100 calories per serving

1 packet natural no-calorie sweetener

¼ teaspoon vanilla extract

⅛ teaspoon cinnamon

Topping

½ cup sliced strawberries

1. In a medium bowl, combine all filling ingredients. Mix well.

2. In another medium bowl, combine all crepe ingredients. Whisk until uniform.

3. Bring a 10-inch skillet sprayed with nonstick spray to medium heat. Pour half of the crepe batter into the pan, quickly tilting the skillet in all directions to evenly coat the bottom. Cook until lightly browned on the bottom, about 2 minutes.

4. Carefully flip with an offset spatula or flexible rubber spatula. Cook until lightly browned on the other side, about 1 minute.

5. Transfer the crepe to a plate, and repeat with remaining batter to make another crepe.

6. Divide filling between the crepes. Fold both sides of each crepe over the filling.

7. Top with strawberries.

MAKES 2 SERVINGS

HG FYI

For more about Hungry Girl crepes, flip to page 278.

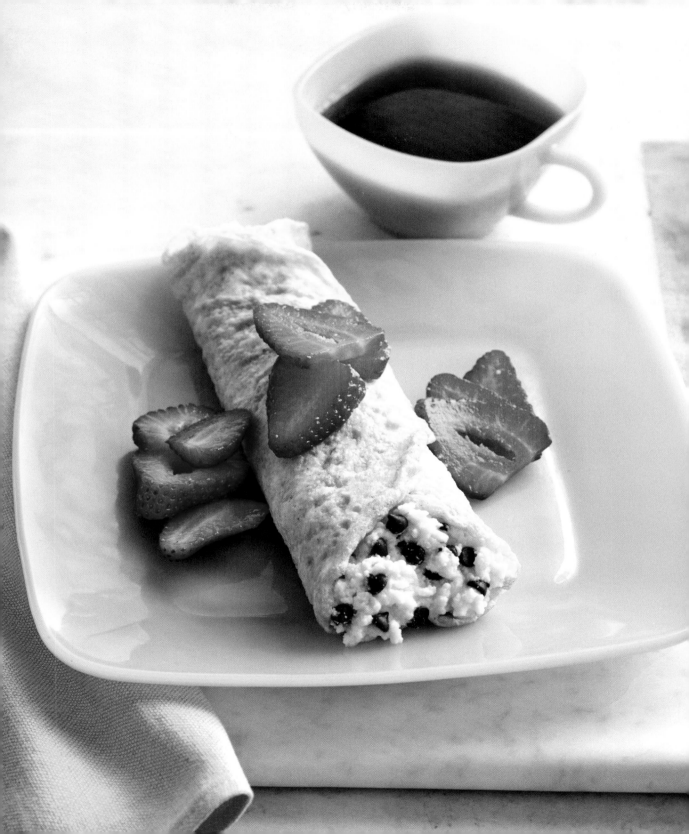

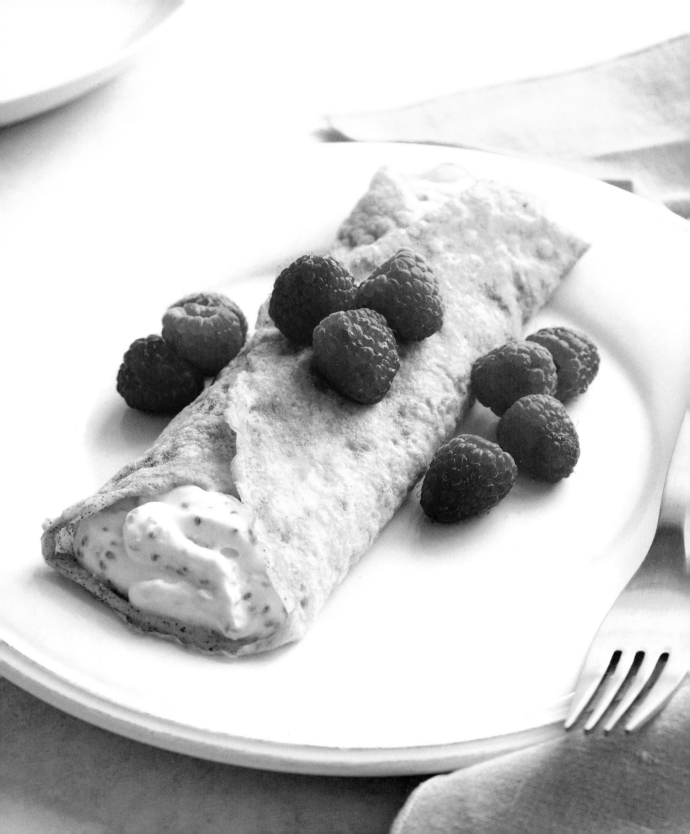

Raspberry Key Lime Crepes

½ of recipe (1 crepe): 117 calories, 1.5g total fat (<0.5g sat fat), 133mg sodium, 9.5g carbs, 3.5g fiber, 4.5g sugars, 17g protein

You'll Need: 2 medium bowls, whisk, 10-inch skillet, nonstick spray, offset spatula or flexible rubber spatula, plate

Prep: 10 minutes • **Cook:** 10 minutes

Filling

½ cup fat-free plain Greek yogurt

2 teaspoons lime juice (key lime, if available)

1½ teaspoons chia seeds

1 packet natural no-calorie sweetener

⅛ teaspoon vanilla extract

Crepes

½ cup (about 4 large) egg whites

2 tablespoons plain protein powder with about 100 calories per serving

1 packet natural no-calorie sweetener

¼ teaspoon vanilla extract

⅛ teaspoon cinnamon

Topping

½ cup raspberries

1. In a medium bowl, combine all filling ingredients. Mix well.

2. In another medium bowl, combine all crepe ingredients. Whisk until uniform.

3. Bring a 10-inch skillet sprayed with nonstick spray to medium heat. Pour half of the crepe batter into the pan, quickly tilting the skillet in all directions to evenly coat the bottom. Cook until lightly browned on the bottom, about 2 minutes.

4. Carefully flip with an offset spatula or flexible rubber spatula. Cook until lightly browned on the other side, about 1 minute.

5. Transfer the crepe to a plate, and repeat with remaining batter to make another crepe.

6. Divide filling between crepes. Fold both sides of each crepe over the filling.

7. Top with raspberries.

MAKES 2 SERVINGS

Blueberry Lemon Crepes

½ of recipe (1 crepe): 123 calories, 1.5g total fat (<0.5g sat fat), 133mg sodium, 11g carbs, 2.5g fiber, 7g sugars, 16.5g protein

You'll Need: 2 medium bowls, whisk, 10-inch skillet, nonstick spray, offset spatula or flexible rubber spatula, plate

Prep: 10 minutes • **Cook:** 10 minutes

Filling

½ cup fat-free plain Greek yogurt

1 tablespoon lemon juice

1½ teaspoons chia seeds

1 packet natural no-calorie sweetener

Crepes

½ cup (about 4 large) egg whites

2 tablespoons plain protein powder with about 100 calories per serving

1 packet natural no-calorie sweetener

¼ teaspoon vanilla extract

⅛ teaspoon cinnamon

Topping

½ cup blueberries

1. In a medium bowl, combine all filling ingredients. Mix well.

2. In another medium bowl, combine all crepe ingredients. Whisk until uniform.

3. Bring a 10-inch skillet sprayed with nonstick spray to medium heat. Pour half of the crepe batter into the pan, quickly tilting the skillet in all directions to evenly coat the bottom. Cook until lightly browned on the bottom, about 2 minutes.

4. Carefully flip with an offset spatula or flexible rubber spatula. Cook until lightly browned on the other side, about 1 minute.

5. Transfer the crepe to a plate, and repeat with remaining batter to make another crepe.

6. Divide filling between crepes. Fold both sides of each crepe over the filling.

7. Top with blueberries.

MAKES 2 SERVINGS

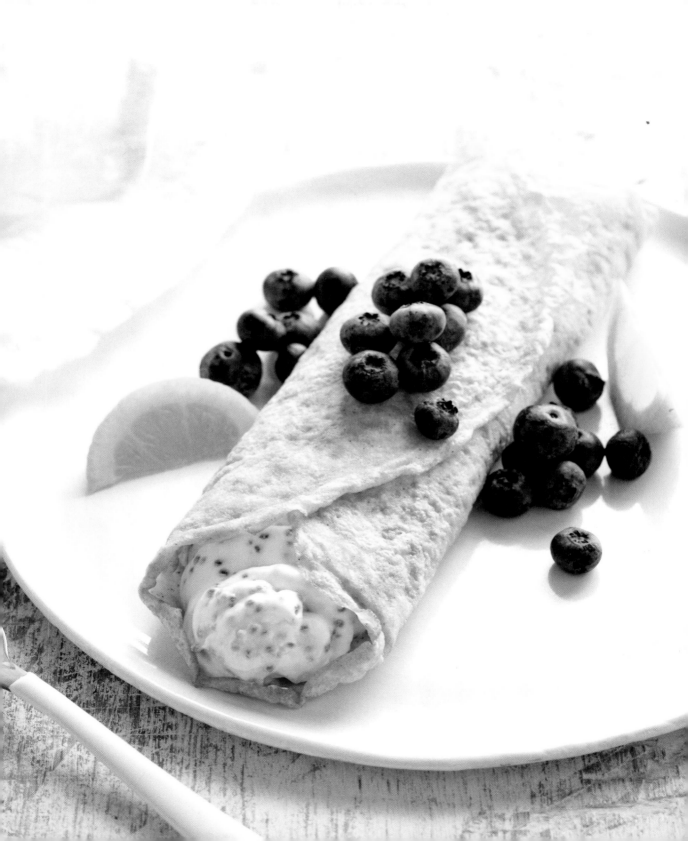

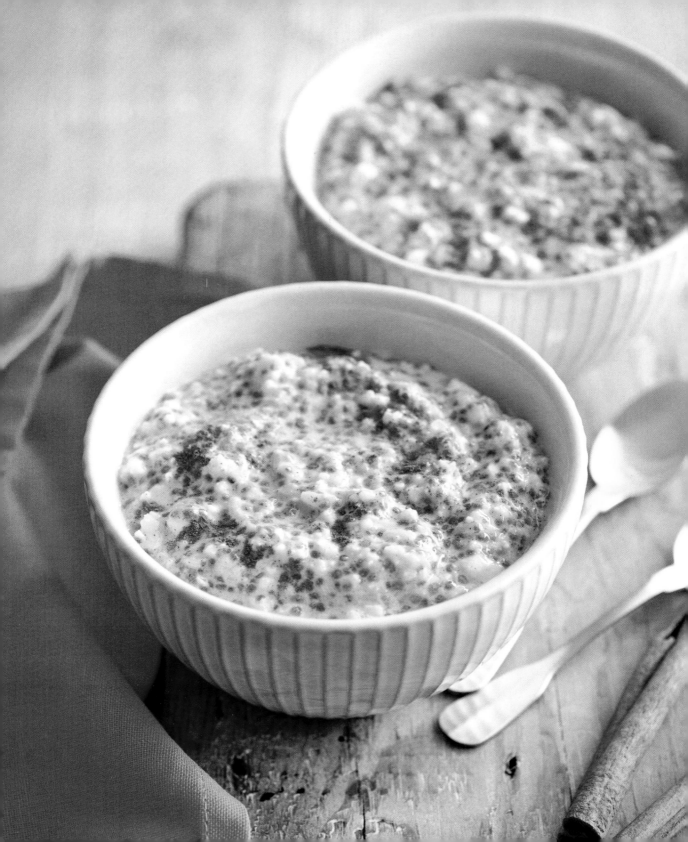

Clean & Hungry Rice Pudding

¼th of recipe (about ¾ cup): 139 calories, 5.5g total fat (0.5g sat fat), 177mg sodium, 18.5g carbs, 7g fiber, 1.5g sugars, 5g protein

You'll Need: small nonstick pot, medium bowl, blender, medium microwave-safe bowl

Prep: 10 minutes • **Cook:** 40 minutes • **Chill:** 3 hours

¼ cup uncooked brown rice

2 cups roughly chopped cauliflower

2 cups unsweetened vanilla almond milk

¼ cup chia seeds

4 packets natural no-calorie sweetener

1 teaspoon vanilla extract

½ teaspoon cinnamon, or more to taste

⅛ teaspoon salt

1. Add ½ cup water to a small nonstick pot. Set temperature to high, and bring to a boil.

2. Reduce heat to low. Carefully add rice. Cover and cook for 35 minutes, or until rice is cooked and water has been absorbed. Transfer to a medium bowl.

3. Meanwhile, pulse cauliflower in a blender until reduced to rice-sized pieces.

4. Place cauliflower rice in a medium microwave-safe bowl; cover and microwave for 2 minutes.

5. Uncover and stir. Re-cover and microwave for another 2 minutes, or until hot and soft.

6. Add cauliflower rice to the medium bowl, along with remaining ingredients. Mix until uniform.

7. Cover and refrigerate for at least 3 hours, until mixture has reached a pudding-like consistency.

MAKES 4 SERVINGS

HG Time-Saving Tip

Use quick-cooking or instant brown rice instead of standard grains.

There you have it!
141 amazingly delicious Clean & Hungry recipes.
I hope you try 'em all! Have questions, comments, or
just want to say hi? Email me at ask@hungry-girl.com.
And for all the latest food news, product finds,
and brand-new recipes, sign up for FREE daily
emails at hungry-girl.com.

'Til next time . . . Chew the right thing!

Lisa :)

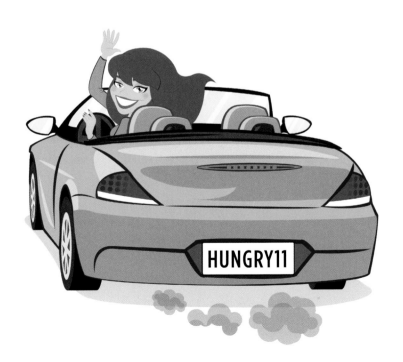

Index